PSYCHOLOGICAL PROBLEMS OF THE CHILD AND HIS FAMILY

Psychological Problems of

EDITED BY

AND

A TEXTBOOK OF BASIC CHILD AND ADOLESCENT PSYCHIATRY FOR STUDENTS AND PRACTITIONERS OF MEDICINE AND THE MENTAL HEALTH PROFESSIONS.

the Child and His Family

Paul D. Steinhauer
Quentin Rae-Grant

MACMILLAN OF CANADA

First published in Canada in 1977 by
The Macmillan Company of Canada Ltd

First published in the U.K. in 1978 by
THE MACMILLAN PRESS LTD
London and Basingstoke
Associated companies in Delhi Dublin
Hong Kong Johannesburg Lagos Melbourne
New York Singapore and Tokyo

British Library Cataloguing in Publication Data

Psychological problems of the child and his family
1. Child psychiatry
I. Steinhauer, Paul D II. Rae-Grant, Quentin
618.9'28'9 RJ499

ISBN 0-333-24020-0

This book is sold subject to the standard conditions of the Net Book Agreement

Printed in the United States for
The Macmillan Company of Canada Limited
70 Bond Street, Toronto, Ontario
M5B 1X3

The editors would like to dedicate this book to
DRS. E. JAMES ANTHONY, LEON EISENBERG, and the late **HYMAN S. LIPPMAN**
whose example and friendship have had such an influence
on their careers in academic child psychiatry,
and to their colleagues on the
Committee on Child and Adolescent Psychiatry,
Department of Psychiatry,
University of Toronto

Contents

Contributing Authors

Dr. Harvey R. Alderton
Associate Professor, Department of Psychiatry, University of Toronto.
Formerly, Director of Training and Research, Thistletown Regional Centre.

Dr. Graham Berman
Assistant Professor, Department of Psychiatry, University of Toronto.
Staff Psychiatrist, Hospital for Sick Children.

Dr. Elsa Broder
Assistant Professor, Department of Psychiatry, University of Toronto.
Staff Psychiatrist, C. M. Hincks Treatment Centre.

Dr. David Dickman
Assistant Professor, Department of Psychiatry, University of Toronto.
Staff Psychiatrist, Hospital for Sick Children.

Dr. Arthur P. Froese
Assistant Professor, Department of Psychiatry, University of Toronto.
Staff Psychiatrist, Hospital for Sick Children.

Dr. Barry Garfinkel
Lecturer, Department of Psychiatry, University of Toronto.
Staff Psychiatrist, C. M. Hincks Treatment Centre.

Dr. Sol Goldstein
Assistant Professor, Department of Psychiatry, University of Toronto.
Staff Psychiatrist, Hospital for Sick Children.

Dr. Harvey Golombek
Assistant Professor, Department of Psychiatry, University of Toronto.
Staff Psychiatrist, C.M. Hincks Treatment Centre.

Dr. Milada Havelkova
Assistant Professor, Department of Psychiatry, University of Toronto.
Staff Psychiatrist, Hospital for Sick Children.

Dr. William A. Hawke
Special Lecturer, Department of Psychiatry, University of Toronto.
Emeritus of Pediatrics, University of Toronto,
Honorary Consultant, Hospital for Sick Children.

Dr. Simon Kreindler
Lecturer, Department of Psychiatry, University of Toronto.
Staff Psychiatrist, Hospital for Sick Children.

Dr. Stanley R. Lesser
Associate Professor, Department of Psychiatry, University of Toronto.
Associate Psychoanalyst, Columbia University.
Senior Staff Psychiatrist, Hospital for Sick Children.

Dr. Saul Levine
Associate Professor, Departments of Psychiatry and Psychology, University of Toronto.
Senior Staff Psychiatrist, Hospital for Sick Children.

Dr. Klaus Minde
Associate Professor and Director of Research in Child Psychiatry, Department of Psychiatry, University of Toronto.
Senior Staff Psychiatrist, Hospital for Sick Children.

Dr. David N. Mushin
Honorary Assistant Child Psychiatrist, Prince Henry's Hospital, Melbourne, Australia.

Dr. Ed Pakes
Assistant Professor, Department of Psychiatry, University of Toronto.
Senior Staff Psychiatrist, Hospital for Sick Children.

Dr. Quentin Rae-Grant
Professor of Child Psychiatry, Department of Psychiatry, University of Toronto.
Psychiatrist-in-Chief, Hospital for Sick Children.

Dr. Bonnie Robson
Assistant Professor, Department of Psychiatry, University of Toronto.
Staff Psychiatrist, C. M. Hincks Treatment Centre.

Dr. Robert Simmons

Assistant Professor, Department of Psychiatry, University of Toronto.
Staff Psychiatrist, Hospital for Sick Children.

Dr. Paul D. Steinhauer

Associate Professor and Director of Training in Child Psychiatry, Department of Psychiatry, University of Toronto.
Senior Staff Psychiatrist, Hospital for Sick Children.

Dr. James VanLeeuwen

Assistant Professor, Department of Psychiatry, University of Toronto.
Senior Staff Psychiatrist, Hospital for Sick Children.

Dr. Gordon Warme

Associate Professor, Department of Psychiatry, University of Toronto.
Chief, Child and Adolescent Service, Clarke Institute of Psychiatry.
Staff Psychiatrist, Hospital for Sick Children.

Dr. James Wilkes

Honorary Lecturer, Department of Psychiatry, University of Toronto.
Director, Child and Adolescent Psychiatry, Scarborough Centenary Hospital.

Preface

Preparing an introductory text presents an intriguing series of challenges to the editors. The text must be basic enough to be readily comprehensible, while approaching its subject matter in an authoritative and comprehensive way. It must order and present a large number of facts and key concepts in a language and in a manner that are clear, organized, and sequential. Highly technical terms and concepts must be so presented that even the reader new to the area can relate them to his own experience or to concrete illustrations supplied by the text. If it is to succeed in its task, it is not enough that it be read and memorized; it must be understood and even enjoyed.

Psychological Problems of the Child and His Family is intended to present the basic principles of child and adolescent psychiatry while meeting the above criteria. It attempts to cover the broad subject area of child and adolescent psychiatry from biological, developmental, psychoanalytic, and systems perspectives. Even more important, it attempts to integrate these conceptual approaches so that readers from a variety of disciplines are guided towards a practical approach in understanding and dealing with patients and their families.

Throughout the text, the child is viewed as both an individual, with his own internal network of drives and defences, and as a member of a family and social system. An integration between these inner (intrapsychic) and outer (interpersonal and social) aspects of the child's reality is continually kept in focus. Consistent emphasis is placed on the process of development and on the effects of blocks and deviations in the development of the child's personality and functioning.

It is hoped that the concepts and topic areas of psychological disturbance in the child and his family are conveyed in a clear and well-organized manner. Determined efforts have been made to minimize the use of jargon. Students and practitioners of medicine and allied professions do not require familiarity with psychiatric terminology to understand and follow the text. Where technical terms are used, they are clearly defined. Key concepts are illustrated by schematic diagrams and brief clinical vignettes. A glossary of medical and technical terms is included, and key references are annotated to help the interested reader pursue in greater depth areas of his own inclination.

The editors would like to express their appreciation to their colleagues on the Committee on Child and Adolescent Psychiatry, Department of Psychiatry, University of Toronto, who have made available at all times their knowledge, their experience, and their friendship. In addition, we would like to thank the following, without whose assistance the text could not have been prepared: Mr. Allan Kaplan, for his help in the preparation of the bibliography and in indexing; Mr. John Fanning, for his assistance in the preparation of the glossary; Mr. David Steinhauer, for proofreading and editorial assistance; the secretarial staff of the Department of Psychiatry, Hospital for Sick Children, with special thanks to Miss Barbara Wood for the typing and preparation of the manuscript.

The guidance and encouragement of Mr. Rolf Lockwood and Mr. Virgil Duff of Macmillan of Canada with regard to technical aspects of preparing the manuscript has been much appreciated.

P.D.S. and Q.R.-G.

UNIT ONE: The Child and His Family

BONNIE ROBSON
KLAUS MINDE

1. Normal Child Development

Child psychiatry was recognized as a specialty within psychiatry only twenty years ago. Its basic aims—to provide knowledge about children's emotional needs and to attempt to help both children and those who assist them in their growth and development—reflect the roots that child psychiatry as a distinct profession has in both psychology and the social sciences. The following chapters describe a great number of psychiatric syndromes and clinical manifestations in children of various ages. Diagnostic categories are related to different genetic and environmental forces that influence the behaviour of the child and his family. Yet common to all chapters is the awareness that disturbed children have failed, for whatever reason, in some part of their social, cognitive, or emotional development.

To understand disturbed children and their families and to adequately assess their developmental deviations, the student must first have an intimate knowledge of normal developmental processes. How do children change as they grow up? What are the determinants of these changes? In the present chapter we investigate these issues in two ways. First, some general developmental principles are discussed; this discussion allows us to see the features common to various theories of human development. It also gives us an opportunity to describe some of the constitutional and environmental forces that produce developmental changes in children. In the second part of the chapter, the effects of particular general developmental principles in specific aspects of a child's development at a variety of ages are illustrated.

Historical Review

In the history of Western culture, childhood was not considered important until relatively recently. Until the seventeenth century, children were seen as "little adults". Parents and teachers did not regard the child, once past infancy, as having specific educational or emotional needs. Towards the end of the seventeenth century, through the more systematic observation of individual children by educators and parents, the particular nature of childhood began to be recognized. Children came to be seen as "innocent" yet "primitive" and "irrational", in need of safeguarding from pollution by life and sex. In many respects these concepts proved beneficial for younger children, for example, by reducing the amount of heavy work they were permitted to do. But the child was considered in need of protection not only from the corrupting influences of the outer world but also from his own primitive psychic forces. These forces, including many basic biological drives, were seen as a potential source of damnation, very much in need of containment. Society took upon itself the mandate of "civilizing" children by taming the essentially "savage" and "bestial" aspect of their natures. This led to the creation of an educational system that saw as its prime responsibility the task of suppressing such potentially dangerous impulses.

Confirmation for this "predeterminist" concept of development seemed to come from biology. Here scientists claimed that "ontogeny recapitulates phylogeny" (i.e. the development of the individual repeats that of the species), which meant that each human embryo, in the course of its intrauterine development, passes through each stage of the evolutionary process. Starting as a single cell, the embryo proceeds up the evolutionary ladder, its structure resembling at one point that of a reptile and finally that of a mammal. This theory was seen as further proof of the close association between humans and animals. It contributed to the philosophical rationale for seeing humans as always having a bit of the beast lurking beneath the surface needing to be tamed, and for viewing all children as endowed with the sins and failures of their phylogenetic ancestors.

Various scientific advances during the past fifty years have called the predeterminist position into question. There was, for example, the recognition that the physical or psychological characteristics that an individual *inherits* (i.e. the genotype) may not be identical with the psychological and physical characteristics that the individual *shows* (i.e. the phenotype). The phenotype was seen to reflect the genetic base after its modification by the environment. Thus scientists came to accept that the genetic constitution contributed the potential for development, but that throughout the process of growth and maturation environmental forces continually influenced the outcome. Furthermore, some environmental influences appeared to be more significant at specific, "critical" times in the child's development than at other times. For example, it was felt that the absence of the biological mother during the first years of life would necessarily produce a psychologically deviant older child and adult. This notion has since been replaced by the recognition that while children need stable predictable relationships, these can be provided by other than the biological parents. The notion of important or "critical" times in the over-all process of development led naturally to the "epigenetic" or "stage" concept of development.

This concept notes that certain groups, or "segments", of behaviour routinely occur together; for example, the child begins to show stranger-anxiety just about the time he realizes the difference between strange and familiar faces. The epigenetic theory implies that these behavioural segments are routinely followed by other specific behaviours or functions. Development, therefore, is seen as proceeding in an orderly, step-like manner through a series of stages, each representing a higher level of function than its predecessor. While still acknowledging that individual development is biologically influenced, this theory suggests that a group of behaviours would occur only if its more elementary precursors had first been mastered.

The importance of the "stage", or "epigenetic", concept of development cannot be overstated, as some of the most influential representatives of present-day psychiatry and psychology saw development as occurring in this way. For example, Sigmund Freud, the founder of psychoanalysis, saw children as passing through discrete stages of emotional development. Jean Piaget, the father of much of contemporary developmental psychology, believed that intelligence develops as a continuing creative interaction between the child and his environment. According to both theories, children who have not mastered an elementary developmental stage are unlikely to do well in the following, more advanced levels of development.

In contrast to the stage-oriented theories, which assume an uneven or discontinuous pace of development, some learning theorists claim that development is a continual process that shows no variations over time. They maintain that experiences, and hence learning, occur at all times and that the learning of complex behaviours is, in its simplest form, merely the forming of simple connections in response to experience. As these connections are seen as the building blocks for all complex behaviours, the need to think in terms of specific age-related structures, such as the capacity for abstract reasoning, is considered unnecessary.

Present State of Knowledge

The previous deliberations have made it clear that child development is a complex process. They have also shown that representatives of various emotional and cognitive theories have tried in different ways to conceptualize and explain general laws that govern the development of children. What, then, should the student believe, and how should he orient himself?

While the following principles may not be accepted by every expert in child development, they do represent a consensus of most contemporary scientists.

1. *No single concept of development does justice to all the phenomena that we observe in a developing organism.* Some functions, such as body and cell growth, occur continuously throughout development. The acquisition of other functions, such as the use of language or particular ways of thinking, proceeds in stages. This latter means that there is a lower age limit for the appearance of certain combinations of developmental phenomena, referred to as a "stage". These lower limits are primarily determined by the maturation of the central nervous system. For example, no amount of stimulation will lead to speech within the first six months of life. On the other hand, verbal stimulation during this period does play an important role in preparing the ground for the later acquisition of language. What is not known is whether there are upper time bounds for the acquisition of a given ability, such that if the appropriate stimulus conditions are not provided within a given interval the ability will never appear. Despite the common assumption that this is true, convincing evidence in the area of human development has not yet been provided.

2. *The child is an important shaper of his enviroment.* Children do not merely react to their environment; the environment reacts to them as well. Parents have their own needs, and whether or not their particular infant meets these needs will affect the parents' response and therefore the environment in which the child grows. An active, exploring, aggressive infant may prove a delight to parents who value such qualities but

may arouse anxiety, frustration, and annoyance in parents who would have preferred a more passive and non-challenging child. The first parents might have had equal trouble accepting the passive child whom the others would have found much easier to enjoy. Thus the parental feelings and responses will be influenced by the degree to which the child meets their pre-existing needs. The more these are satisfied, the easier they will find it to accept and value their child and the greater their ability to provide the environment their child needs for optimal growth.

Another consequence of this principle suggests that a specific developmental level can be reached by different routes. As the new level will allow for extensive reorganization of behaviour, past tendencies may not persist in present psychological functioning. For example, the feelings and behaviour of a person who, because of doubts and anxieties, avoids marrying until the age of forty, may, by age forty-five, be indistinguishable from those of someone who married without obvious conflict at twenty.

This principle also makes it difficult to predict accurately the final outcome of a child's development because reaching a particular stage such as adolescence can provide a second chance, permitting a revision of earlier adaptations to life. For example, the boy who at age ten was unpopular because he lacked athletic abilities may, in adolescence, be admired for his success in heterosexual relationships, thereby gaining the confidence, self-esteem, and poise he needs for social success.

Only persistent and recurrent deviant transactions between the child and his environment will produce predictable later abnormalities. These abnormal transactions can be due to a severe defect in the child's integrative mechanism (e.g. childhood schizophrenia or severe brain damage) or to very abnormal environmental forces such as severely neglecting or battering parents.

3. *Development is not a phenomenon that affects only one particular sphere of life, such as emotions or intelligence, but is the sum total of various interlocking forces that embrace changes in biological, intellectual, emotional, and social behaviour.* These forces constantly interact and influence their mutual progression. Therefore, development in all areas should be examined in any assessment of possible emotional and intellectual deviations in either children or adults. Table 1-1, at the end of this chapter, may help the reader by demonstrating the syn-

chronized emergence of some developmental functions in children and adolescents. In the Table a number of age-dependent stages are arbitrarily established. During each of these stages, development proceeds simultaneously along biological, cognitive, language, social, and emotional lines. Along with each stage is provided a summary of the level of achievement in each of these major areas normally attained within it.

Patterns of Child Development

At this point we define in general terms each of these five major developmental parameters. This done, we examine in chronological order a number of age-related stages, describing in more detail the usual level of development attained within it for each of the basic parameters. To illustrate the process in more concrete terms, we use the example of two normal, healthy, but very different eleven-year-old boys. We begin by introducing them as they are now. Then we return to them following the discussion of each chronological stage, observing how each boy appeared at that particular level and noting how their personalities took shape as their development proceeded.

> William, called Bill by everyone, has a mass of dark brown curly hair, a pleasant round face and sturdy frame. Bill is in grade six, an average student who prefers gym and math. He is the goalie for the second-string school team, and plays league hockey on the team for which his father is assistant coach. Bill has six really close buddies but no one special friend. All the guys say Bill is okay. He has never gotten into any real trouble, but recently was caught with three other boys climbing on the roof of the recreation centre after a Scouts meeting. His dad seemed quite angry and hit him, but that was the last heard of the incident. Over the past year, Bill has taken an increasing interest in his appearance. He now insists on accompanying his mother on shopping trips to carefully select his jeans, T-shirts, and jean jackets. All Bill's friends are dressed practically identically. They kid one another about girls, and their interest in rock music is second only to their enthusiasm for hockey and football.
>
> Kristian, called Krissie since birth by his mother, is also in grade six. Krissie is a tall, lean, pale, blond boy. A bright, attentive

student, he is well-liked by his teachers, performing better than his classmates. Krissie and his best friend, Peter, are inseparable. They build models of cars, trains, trucks, and airplanes. Although they feel it is babyish, they even "play" with their car collections at times. Krissie enjoys reading, particularly science fiction, and reads at a grade ten or eleven level. Krissie is considered by everyone to be very artistic and creative. He has a good imagination. His art teacher at school has been especially encouraging, although this embarrasses Krissie, who rather shyly avoids praise. He thinks such accomplishments are sissy, but he is proud of his ability in electronics. He just finished building a radio and would like to be a space pilot.

THE BASIC DEVELOPMENTAL PARAMETERS

1. *Biological development* might be thought of as motor maturation or the development of bodily control. It also includes the physical, observable expression in the child of the genetic and familial background. Sometimes whole families tend to be active, outgoing, busy people. In other cases, one particular individual within a family may carry these traits or tendencies from birth. Some authors include such physically linked predispositions as general activity level, degree of passivity, reaction to change in the environment, and adaptability under the heading of temperament.[19] They consider temperament—at times the term "constitutional trait" is used—as a basic biological given, which can later be modified by environmental influence. A child may be born more or less passive, but interaction with the environment may either reinforce the constitutional tendency towards passivity or, alternately, modify this basic trait, allowing him to become more active and assertive. In keeping with Gesell, who in 1940 first developed adequate tests for gauging the level of physical functioning, adaptive tasks (i.e. the child's response to novel situations) are included in Table 1-1 under this heading.

2. *Cognitive development* refers to the development of intellectual processes or mental structures and schemata for comprehending the physical environment. "Human beings do not just passively 'receive' the world; rather they actively structure it," Robert Case notes in describing the basic hypothesis of Piaget, the major contributor to our present understanding of cognitive development. Piaget's theory is

basically epigenetic or stage-oriented. A child's rate of intellectual development may vary, but must always follow a certain sequence. A later stage cannot be accomplished without prior acquisition of all previous ones. For example, the age at which a child learns that an object weighs the same if nothing is added or subtracted may vary, but this concept never occurs before the child has achieved the concept of object permanence. (The term "object permanence" will be defined in some detail later in this chapter.)

3. *Emotional development* refers to the child's intrapsychic development as reflected in his interpersonal behaviour. The infant initially is in a self-interested state, intent only on preserving his own physical comfort, which is disturbed when he is hungry or cold, etc. As he first becomes aware of a world beyond himself, it probably exists only to fulfil his wants; he cries and milk comes, or he is cuddled and burped, etc. But after about six months of age, he gradually becomes aware that there are external forces and people, including his primary caretaker, whose wishes may be contrary to his own. Even though he cries, milk may *not* come, he may *not* be picked up, etc. Thus he gradually realizes there is someone or something out there separate from him with a will of its own. At the same time, the child begins to develop a sense of reassurance, of caring, even of trust in those who he learns are available consistently to respond to his needs. Later, he will try to subject his will to that of his caretaker or parents, and the process of socialization will have begun. Still later, usually between the ages of four and six years, he will begin a process of identification with the parents, as a result of which their standards and expectations will become his. This process will provide the basis for conscience development.

Emotional development can be partially arrested (i.e. fixated) at any stage. While the child may go on to a later stage without having solved the problems of an earlier one, there is usually evidence in subsequent development of the failure to complete the earlier tasks. Such disruptions and distortions of psychological development result in the various disorders discussed in Chapter 6.

4. *Personal/social and language development* are clearly related to biological and cognitive maturation. Verbal speech and later communicative language are most important in our present culture with its emphasis on prolonged education. But man is not necessarily phylogenetically equipped to cope with our type of culture or society. Our level of evolutionary adaptation has prepared us to grow up in a

nuclear family within a small tribe of hunters and gatherers.[4] But most of the world's population must learn to adapt to different environments. Infants are affected by social pressures from the family, the family's culture, and society at large. For example, a child whose family strongly adheres to the rights of the individual and is prepared to fight to maintain these if necessary may have difficulty in kindergarten, where democratic socialization is espoused.

SURVEY OF DEVELOPMENTAL PROGRESS AT VARIOUS AGES

Birth to One Year

Development in the first year of life really begins twenty to thirty years before. Parents tend to repeat patterns of parenting they experienced in their childhood, since they have little else to draw on. Parenthood, and specifically motherhood, is the only profession where one is expected to plunge right into practice without prior training or experience. Occasionally a parent is offered a partial apprenticeship through doll play, babysitting, or an occupation dealing with children. The myth is that somehow through the experience of pregnancy and delivery one becomes a mother. The psychological demands on a new mother are many. She must at some point have felt cared-for, usually by her own primary caretaker, at times by a member of the extended family, a friend or her husband. This person serves as a model, and through identification she develops the capacity for caring. She must also feel secure and confident enough that she does not resent the baby's demands. At the same time, the father must feel secure enough in his relationship with his wife that he does not feel severely deprived by the time and attention she must give to the infant. He must have identified with his own father or some surrogate figure to take on a parental role, while still remaining free to identify with the child sufficiently to tolerate the baby's crying, waking at night, and demands for attention and care. Often these pressures are not even recognized by the parents, much less reported to a physician, but they can prove psychologically stressful for one or both parents and may cause disharmony in the marriage or dissatisfaction or resentment of the child. (For a discussion of the results of inadequate and inconsistent parenting, see also the discussion of Privation and Deprivation Syndromes in Chapter 5.)

Biologically, during the first year the infant gains control over his body: in the first quarter his eyes; in the second, his head and arms; in the third, his trunk and hands; in the fourth, his forefinger and thumbs.

Thus, even from birth the child is ready to begin acquiring the motor skills essential to his development as an independent, autonomous being. The first of these is achieving full control of his arms and hands, which can then be used as tools to begin to explore and understand the world.

Cognitively, during the first year the child can be described as being in a stage of sensori-motor activity. He is born with a number of basic reflexes—sucking, grasping, tracking an object in his field of vision—and with an innate tendency to respond to all forms of sensory stimulation. From reflexes such as grasping when a rattle is placed in his hand, he advances to repetitive voluntary actions such as putting his thumb or fist in his mouth, removing it, and reinserting it. Later the child purposefully reproduces repetitive actions; for example, by kicking his legs, he can make the mobile above the crib jangle. Gradually, he becomes aware that pushing a block with his hand can change its position, thus providing a different view, which helps him recognize that different visual perspectives can refer to the same object. With this recognition comes the first element necessary to the understanding of object permanence, Kagan[11] suggests that the child develops a particular cognitive set, which he then attempts to match with the sets that he observes in the outside world. For example, if the outside face does not correspond with his internal concept of face, he does not smile. Kagan hypothesizes that much early cognitive development occurs as the child seeks to integrate internal and external sets to form a single gestalt.

Object permanence is vital to cognitive, emotional, and social development. It first becomes possible when a child has developed a memory map. Then, for the first time, he knows that something removed from his direct line of vision still exists even though he cannot see it. In contrast, for the infant the object ceases to be once it is out of sight. The child develops the concept of object permanence over a period of time, while gradually learning a series of related but increasingly complex differentiations. At about one year, most children appear to understand that inanimate objects stay put, so that if a toy is hidden under a pillow they will uncover it and regain it with delight. If, however, the task is complicated by moving the toy without his knowledge and hiding it again, the child cannot yet follow the manoeuvre and will continue to look for it in the original hiding place. Between the ages of eighteen months and two years, even if the toy is moved the child will not be thrown by the shift, but will find it under the correct pillow.

The achievement of object permanence has an important effect on the child's relationship with his mother and his emotional responses to separation from her. By one year of age, if the mother leaves the room and he is free to follow, the child usually is not distressed. He understands that she exists beyond the doorway, so that he has only to follow to find her. By fifteen to eighteen months, he is more likely to show some distress at her leaving, partly because of ongoing emotional development, which, as we will see, features at this age increased anxiety in response to separation, but also partly as a result of the achievement of object permanence. He knows that his mother exists outside the door, but he also knows that she may move on to another area of the house. Therefore he must follow her in order to keep some visual or auditory trace to correspond with his memory map of the house and her possible location within it at any one time.

From birth the infant shows a preference for the familiar. Some time between two weeks and two months he begins to smile socially in response to the human voice, and very shortly thereafter the primary caretaker, usually the mother, notices that she is more able to elicit this smile than other people. By six months of age he has good discriminatory vision. As his ability to discriminate his surroundings and recognize his mother increases, the infant is more comfortable and satisfied with her than with strangers. Some time after six months of age, he is noted to "make strange" and may look impassively and directly at a stranger or, if being held by his mother, may hide his face in her shoulder when a stranger approaches him.

In the area of language development, the vowel sounds typical of the infants' squealing and cooing are increasingly interspersed with consonant sounds and babbling by about six months of age. In the first several months the infant's cooing appears independent of environmental factors, but by about the third month the child coos and squeals when stimulated either by his caretaker or by his perception of his own voice. New sounds result more from neuromuscular maturation and the effects of postural changes, such as sitting up, than from imitation of adults. By six months of age, infants are producing most vowel sounds and about half the consonants, and in the latter part of the year babbling that features an increasing number of one-syllable repetitions has replaced cooing. By the end of the first year, words such as "mama" and "dada" are occurring, and the child shows definite signs of understanding some words and simple commands such as, "show me your eyes."

Bill, at a year, was already a sturdy little tyke. Shorter than Krissie, he had trouble standing or walking, but that did not stop him from creeping about and getting into things or trying to get up the stairs when no one was looking. His parents considered his behaviour a great joke. Bill could say a great many things without words and was very clear in his wants. Like Krissie's father, Bill's dad was not much involved with his early care, but he began to enjoy playing as soon as Bill was old enough to toss about, laugh with, and play peekaboo. Bill was frequently cared for overnight by both sets of grandparents from an early age, becoming happily excited if a visit to his "Bopa's" was suggested. He could be comforted by his mother, father, or grandparents, although he had a slight preference for his mother.

Krissie, at a year, was especially shy with strangers. From about eight months of age, he had been able to pull himself up and move about in his walker. By a year he was tall, already wearing an eighteen-month size. His mother had been the only one to look after him except for the odd babysitter in the evening. His family took vacations together at the cottage. Krissie's father, a town planner, was busy at work or making repairs and improvements to the house. He never considered it his role to participate in the direct care of his son. Krissie had two quite severe colds during his first year, and his mother often worried about his becoming ill. When he was distressed, his mother seemed to be the only one who could comfort him.

This bonding of the child to the mother that develops over the first year is called *attachment*.[4] Attachment is the development of a give-and-take relationship between parent and child that brings them together, keeps them interdependent, and maintains them close to each other. One might equate the development of attachment with the growth of love. Neither love nor attachment can be measured, but the nature, strength, and quality of the behaviours that bring about and maintain attachment can.

Even at birth, an infant has a repertoire of built-in behaviours he can utilize to manipulate his environment. Over the first six months, crying, along with smiling, sucking, clinging, and stroking, are actively used to keep his caretaker, usually the mother, close to him. The cry appears hereditarily designed to attract adult attention, to protect the infant from harm, and to provide for his needs. Adults may find it irritating, but they are not able to ignore it, possibly because of an instinct towards species preservation. The closeness that develops between mother and child becomes a mutual attachment when the child recognizes the mother as important beyond all other adults. Once established, usually around eight months of age, attachment makes it extremely difficult for one of the pair to give up the other and endure a separation. This is slightly after or concurrent with the development of stranger-anxiety. Future relationships to some extent depend on the quality and strength of this early attachment. Attachment behaviour strengthens from nine months to eighteen months and then declines to four years, as self-regulating and independent behaviours become increasingly important.

Ages One to Three

During these two years, the child perfects his locomotor skills, learning to move about freely and independently. The child of fifteen months runs away from his parents with apparent delight. Able to manage stairs, he generally has free run of the house and sometimes the yard. Fine motor development is so improved that he can hold a crayon to produce a letter or picture on his own. He has started to develop his own creativity.

Intellectually, he has begun to deal with his world through play. He is beginning to order and group objects. For instance, he may line up all his cars, putting a toy animal in each. Possibly the greatest area of progress in the second year is that of language development. By eighteen months, the child has a vocabulary of between three and fifty words, and while he may have learned the occasional two-word phrase such as "thank you", he shows little ability to join words into spontaneous phrases. Understanding is progressing rapidly, however, as by about two years his vocabulary is markedly increased. The child by this time extemporaneously combines words to form two-word phrases and is showing an increased interest in language as a means of communication. Much of his vocabulary develops out of his ordering and grouping. As he increasingly makes his wants known through language, words become tools. Learning his name, he develops a sense of himself through language. He uses language to group objects together to form categories, to define the nature of categories and the relationship existing between them. In this way, he develops a growing awareness of himself, organized around language-lined concepts.

He learns that he belongs to the category "boys", and that certain things are true of all those belonging to this category: when they grow older, they become men; they may someday be daddies, but they will never be mommies, nor will they bear babies; they have penises and urinate standing up, unlike girls who lack them and sit down to urinate; boys don't wear dresses as girls do (except, of course, when they are dressing up and pretending to be girls or ladies); they may be taught that it is better to be "tough" or "brave" than timid or sensitive, and that it is more acceptable to play with cars than with dolls. Thus learning what is expected of one as a boy or girl requires a prior knowledge of the concept of categories and the characteristics of each. This knowledge can only be acquired when cognitive and language development are sufficiently advanced.

The child's emotional development in this stage is intimately connected with the ongoing motor and language development that accompany and facilitate it. Emotional development goes through three important phases during this period. First, the child begins to separate himself from his parents. As his motor and language skills increase, he develops a sense of himself as separate from his mother. Whereas up to this point he has been closely bound to and dependent on her, he is now able to do some things for himself, such as choosing what he wants to play with, assisting with his dressing, or regulating his toilet activities during the day. Initially, he seems to enjoy intensely this separateness without fear of loss of his parents, either physically when he runs from them or emotionally through abandonment. This first phase is followed, at about fifteen months of age, by an intense reunion or "rapprochement". At this time the child returns to an intensified closeness with his parents, experiencing real separation anxiety if they leave the house for a few hours. He becomes whiny and demanding, reverting to some "baby" behaviours. Third, one sees the early development of independence (autonomy) and self-regulation, usually fostered by the parents. These stages of development have been well described by Margaret Mahler.[13]

At this point, parents often note an intense attachment to a special toy or blanket, often seen as the child's "security" object. He will not go to sleep without it, dragging it everywhere, but clinging or holding on to it particularly in unfamiliar situations. One explanation is that this object, because of its texture and shape, reminds him of the soft, familiar, safe, secure world of his first year. It is like having a part of his mother and all she represents to take with him everywhere. This is referred to as a *transitional object*, a stepping stone from the relationship with mother to relationships with other people, sometimes referred to as "object relationships".

At this time, too, the child is beginning to differentiate his wants and needs from those of his parents. These may come into conflict, especially as the parents begin to establish limits and controls. During the second year of life, the child struggles against these, but generally by age three he subjects his will to that of the parents. At this early stage of moral development, the child behaves not because he wants to be good, but because he fears the loss of his parents' love or their anger should he displease them. Toilet training is the classic example of the child subjecting his will to the parents' wishes. The child must first have matured to the point where he is able not only to place his excreta in the appropriate place but to signal his desire to do so sufficiently in advance. The parent who has patience and who responds appropriately to the child's signals will have no difficult in training him within a few weeks, once he is ready. This may be at any time in the second or third year; soiling is unlikely to persist beyond age three in the normal child.

Some children of two or three invent an imaginary playmate, generally one who is larger than life. This playmate has the dual function of acting as a protector against monsters or the dark, but just as important, of taking a subservient role to the child. This allows the child who feels constantly at the mercy of authority and rules to have someone over whom he is boss.[9] In general, children of this age play almost continuously. Their play has four important functions: it permits a discharge of energy; it allows the child to practise new skills; it helps master anxiety about feared situations; it provides an opportunity to practise behaving like the caretaker or other adult, either fantasied or real, whom he sees himself as being most like (i.e. the role model), thus providing the child an opportunity to feel similar to the model.

> Bill, who according to his parents had always had a mind of his own, certainly began to show this at about a year. His father announced proudly that Bill had never walked, but that once he got the idea at around fourteen months he always ran. Bill's

father played baseball with some friends every Sunday. Bill loved to go with his mother to watch, chanting "play ball" over and over. Bill was into everything at home, emptying drawers and cupboards. At eighteen months, toilet training was tried for the first time with no success. Bill had the idea; he would smile and say "put poopy in potty" but he never performed. At twenty-six months, however, he learned within a week. As a special treat, Bill loved to stay with his grandparents for the weekend. But when his parents went away on vacation and left Bill, then twenty months, with his grandparents for two weeks, he became withdrawn and played quietly by himself on the floor, not the usual Bill at all. When his parents returned, he acted as if they had never been away but for three days after behaved very badly. At two, Bill's favourite word was "no" and he wanted only trucks for presents at his birthday party.

Krissie was quite sickly in his second year. His mother was constantly on the phone to the doctor. An early walker, he was able to go up and down stairs well by sixteen months, but although he was able to do a number of things for himself he preferred to have his mother do them for him. He did enjoy the mastery of certain skills. He was quick at manipulating toys, working with plasticine, Playdoh, and crayons. His mother, a sculptress, was proud of his primitive creative abilities, spending long hours helping him make things. Krissie's father also enjoyed his son's creative ability, but even though Krissie wanted to join him, he felt it was too dangerous for Krissie to be around where he himself was building.

The Pre-School Years: Ages Three to Six

During these years further motor skills develop. The child can hop and skip, and his minor muscle co-ordination allows him to draw a circle and later a square. He has both the co-ordination and the observational skills to draw a man having six parts. The child's thinking is still very bound to the physical world that he continues to explore. As objects are seen as entities and named, the child begins to group objects together, naming the whole group. Learning is around action-linked concepts. For example, apple is eaten but it is also grouped with foods. In addition, it has a shape and a red colour that can be crayoned. It begins with the letter "A" and is an "A-word". Thus the original action-linked concept is extended by a series of associated images, which in turn lead to the acquisition of words and the expansion of vocabulary.

By age three, the child has a vocabulary of one thousand words, and about 80 per cent of his verbalizations can be understood even by strangers. Between the ages of three and five, the child adds an average of fifty new words to his vocabulary each month. While errors still occur, the general complexity of his grammatical constructions compares roughly with colloquial adult speech. By age four, language is so well established that deviations from the adult norm are more frequently differences in style than defects in grammar. At about four years, the child begins to use complete six-to-eight-word sentences that are complex in their organization and notable for the increased use of relational words and for the child's mastery of vocal inflections. The child is now able to use language to instruct himself and to negotiate with the environment.

At this age, the child also gradually develops the ability to enter the community, learning to cross the road safely to a friend's house and eventually to walk to school by himself. By now he can completely dress and undress himself. Children in these years become aware of their peers and begin to play together. While not yet ready for true co-operative play or complicated games with rules, they can interact with one another as they play or follow a parallel symbolic theme.

Up to this time, the child controls his behaviour because of outside intervention, but about age five he begins to develop a conscience and his own inner controls. His actions start to be regulated not only by the fear and shame of getting caught, but by the guilt associated with what he himself now sees as wrong. At about the same time, the child begins to think of growing up. He takes on a value system, deciding what he wants to be like and how he wants people to see him. These ideals are usually in line with the parents' expectations. He takes pride in activities that his parents admire, playing out long complicated fantasies on these themes.

Part of this process of becoming aligned with parental expectations involves sex-typing, that is, learning to see oneself and behave in a manner appropriate to one's biological sex. The attitudes of one generation about what constitutes sexually appropriate behaviour are passed on to the next. Children increasingly avoid behaviour that they consider more appropriate to the other sex. As the child grows, he begins to imitate, not always consciously, the same-sexed parent. This parent then acts as a model, showing the child what to be, while the opposite-sexed parent allows and encourages this identification.

Faced with a newly developed conscience, numerous new expectations, and the need to be like the same-sexed parent, children in this age group often experience severe anxiety. These transitory and relatively normal fears may appear as nightmares, night terrors, fear of bodily harm, bed-wetting, or fear of the dark or monsters. For further discussion of sex-typing and transitory symptoms occurring in response to developmental stress, see Chapter 5.

> When Bill was three and a half, his new baby brother was born. Although at first Bill was pleased because he had wanted a brother, after a while he came to resent the time his parents spent with the baby. At this point, his speech became less clear and he reverted to baby talk and wetting his bed. On their physician's advice the parents, particularly his father, spent more time with Bill and soon he was his old self again. Bill was always covered with bruises from falls, not that he was clumsy but because at four and a half he was rather aggressive and trying everything. His father built a rink in the backyard, so Bill could skate sloppily by four and fairly well at five. Bill didn't go to nursery school or junior kindergarten, but looked forward to half-day kindergarten. After two weeks supervision, he walked to the school three blocks away by himself. He enjoyed playing with boys his own age, but at times would leave them to do something on his own. He tended to play by the rules, waiting for outside authority to step in to settle a dispute.

> Krissie made a friend of a little girl down the street. Although she was about five months younger and shorter by a head, she tended to dominate their play. At first, Krissie could not tolerate his mother leaving him at her house to play. Later he became willing to stay and play with her for short periods. When he started nursery school, Krissie had to have his mother stay with him for about the first month. Later he enjoyed all the activities, particularly the group singing. He had a series of repeated colds and was absent more than he was there. As his mother still worried about his health, she kept him away from children on

the street if they seemed to have colds. At five, Krissie still had difficulty sharing his toys with the neighbourhood children. He was a faster runner than any of the others, and he loved riding his two wheeler with training wheels. He would act sullen and angry if his mother worried over him, but he looked forward to being with his father on weekends and helping him build a new porch.

The School Years: Age Six to Ten

Compared with the strong drives, motives, and curiosity experienced by the three-to-five-year-olds, this period, sometimes referred to as latency, is often less stressful for parents and children alike. It continues until just prior to the resurgence of sexual and aggressive drives that initiates adolescence. (See Chapter 2 for a discussion of the continuation of the developmental process during the adolescent years.)

That is not to say that further development ceases or that the child is free from anxiety. With entry into school and the emphasis on continued socialization, the child is confronted by his peer group. He begins comparing himself to his peers. Can I run as fast, climb as high, read as well? Am I stupid or smart? From this point on, his self-image is no longer just a reflection of his parents' perception of him, but of that of his peers and teachers as well. A child, no matter how much he denies it, is keenly aware of whether he is accepted or rejected by his peers and of his place in the pecking order.

The child may handle this anxiety about acceptance either by withdrawal or by retaliation. Withdrawal can take several forms. The child can withdraw physically, sitting on the sidelines instead of attempting to answer for fear of being wrong. He can use denial, stating that he did not want to play even though he really did. Another way of denying strange or stressful situations is by forgetting them. For example, he may forget his homework to avoid the possibility of making mistakes. Alternately, he can steer entirely clear of threatening situations.

Other children may attack anxiety-provoking situations and attempt to conquer them. Success breeds further success, though failure may aggravate the difficulties. A child who feels unsuccessful may act up in class or clown around. Through continued and repeated experiences in school, on the playing field, and at home, the child reaffirms and cements his own self-image, and with this his sense of self-esteem.

While generally boys show more resistence to leaving home and entering school than girls, most children eagerly anticipate school. It is clear, however, that social and cultural factors are important influences on a child's adjustment to school. Sesame Street, designed for disadvantaged youngsters, has become the watchword of the middle class. Middle- and upper-class families generally support education. On the other hand, many lower-class children enter school poorly prepared for academic success. They lack many of the experiences, concepts, and skills possessed by their middle-class peers, and teachers frequently react against the action-oriented behaviour and values appropriate, and even essential, for success on the streets. Their parents, instead of acting as models for intellectual achievement, mistrust the school system and do little to encourage their children to persevere in the face of initial difficulties.

During the early school years, the child's typical manner of thinking develops from a concrete ordering and grouping of objects to a stage of understanding concepts that allows him to begin working with ideas with less need for concrete objects to serve as visual props. True abstract reasoning, that is, the ability to go beyond the concrete and to conceptualize changes without any reliance on visual props, is not achieved until adolescence.

During these years, children begin to develop moral standards concerning their and others' behaviour, identifying what they themselves regard as right or wrong. They also begin to understand nature's laws and to discuss moral issues in a general or abstract way. Their imagination continues to be strong, centring around themes of universal good and bad; fairy tales and monsters give way to cowboys and Indians and Kung Fu. Sex-role formation, which began at age four to five, continues throughout middle childhood.

> Bill had no trouble entering school, but he seemed more anxious before he got on the hockey team. When the team lost a game he tended to be sullen and angry, but he very rarely talked back to either of his parents. His teachers thought he could probably do better than average at his studies. Bill himself, although not afraid of success, preferred to be one of the boys than to stand apart by seeming outstanding. His father admired this in Bill; although he would, at one time, have wanted his son to be a star, he was pleased to see that Bill had friends, was well

liked, and played fairly. He was not terribly concerned about Bill's schoolwork, rarely inquiring if he had any homework. He considered that Bill's responsibility.

Kris, who insisted everyone stop calling him Krissie, was pleased by his progress in school as were his parents. Always marginally ahead of his classmates, he could read and print at home before he went to grade one. Although quick to grasp concepts, Kris always preferred not to compete openly with other students. Learning for him has been more a personal challenge, not unlike his parents' striving for individuality. His mother is now a nationally known sculptress. Kris, who still enjoys working with his father, is getting to be almost as good a skier as he. They often kid one another about their ability. Kris is very close to his friend Peter, with whom he shares everything. They have been friends since nursery school, their interests having grown together as they matured.

Thus, despite apparent similarities in age and family background, Bill and Kris have both developed as normal, healthy boys with rather different personalities. This divergence seems to have resulted partly from inherited (constitutional) differences and partly from ongoing interaction with the environment and its effects on the biological, cognitive, language, emotional, and social aspects of their development.

Table 1-1 Age and Development Correspondences

At completion of	*Biological*	*Language*	*Cognitive*	*Personal Social*	*Psychological*
2 months	Develops eye, head control —looks at rattle in hand —chin and chest held up. Real binocular colour vision.	Impassive face—considerable crying.	Basic reflexes: sucking, grasping, tracking object in field of vision.	Number of feedings reduces from 7–8 to 5–6. Spontaneous reflex smiling (12 hours). Unselected social smile at human voice (14 days). Smiles at face in motion (5 wks). Smile at face with some detail e.g. eyebrows and eyes (2 months).	1. Primary caretaker's bond to the child forming: caretaker responsive to child's needs. 2. Infant aware of this responsiveness: develops sense of predictability of his surroundings—begins to develop sense of security. 3. Infant biased towards the familiar from birth—settles into routine of home.
6 months	Vision: depth perception. Sits bending forward, uses hands for support, bears weight when put in standing position but cannot stand without holding on. Reaches and grasps toy —transfers toy from hand to hand.	When talked to smiles, squeals, and coos. Consonants begin to be interspersed with vowel-like cooing. Cooing changes to babbling resembling one-syllable utterances.	Co-ordination of basic reflexes e.g. can look at toy, reach for it, grasp it, mouth it. Grasps for rattle, but if hidden forgets it —unable to retrieve rattle if even partly hidden from view. —significance: part is not yet indicative of the whole.	Smiles selectively to mother's face. Plays with feet. "Teething".	Begins to distinguish between himself and others, with discriminatory vision able to distinguish visually faces and people. Reacts to the strange, unfamiliar with apprehension: "makes strange".
8–9 months	Sits well. Pulls self to feet at railing. Plays with 2 toys: picks up pellet with thumb and index finger.	Reduplication (more continuous repetitions) utterances can signal emphasis and emotions.	Recognizes top and bottom of baby bottle as belonging to some object —presented with bottom will rotate it to get nipple.	Taking fine solids and rusks, feeds self cracker. Smiles only to whole familiar face.	Links good things (warmth, food) with the familiar —links security with caretakers. Has developed special *Attachment Bonding* with significant adults —anxious or disturbed when separated from them.

Table 1-1 (con't)

15 months	Crawling, climbing stairs. Walks alone. Toddler builds tower with 2 cubes —puts 6 cubes into cup Imitates vertical stroke.	Says Dada, Mama, and a vocabulary of between 3 and 20 words. Responds to "Give it to me", "Show me your eyes." Little ability to join words into spontaneous phrases. Pronoun "I" and "mine" understood.	*Object permanence* —hidden object can now be removed to new hiding place and child will follow the progression, searching appropriately. —significance: object has permanence, independent of child's perception.	Toilet regulated during day, carries and hugs doll, assists and co-operates in dressing.	Demonstrates a sense of self separate from mother. —begins to individuate, i.e. do things adults used to do for him —seems to enjoy separateness *Rapprochement Phase:* (15-18 months) —returns to close, intense relationship with primary caretaker —appears more vulnerable to separation than previously —attachment bonding at its peak. *Transitional Object:* behaves as if favourite toy or security blanket can protect him from harm. —object appears a substitute for contact with primary caretaker.
3 years	Runs, rides tricycle, up and down stairs alone with alternating feet, tiptoes, jumps 12 inches, stands on one foot momentarily. Builds tower 6–7 cubes. Imitates circular scribble, imitates + o	Vocabulary 1000 words, 80% of utterances intelligible even to strangers Grammatical complexity roughly that of colloquial adult language. Gives full name and sex.	True symbolic play —continues exploration of the world. —objects seen as entities and named. —child begins to group objects together, naming the whole group.	Puts doll to bed, feeds self well, puts on socks, unbuttons, asks for toilet during day, begins to want to play with peers. Interested in difference between boys and girls.	Parents expect some obedience and socialization. —child establishes "self" by opposing will of parents: the "terrible twos". By age 3, child subjects his will to wishes of parents: —often experiences anger at having to give up own wishes. —fear of punishment, imaginary dangers, and monsters common: fears physical injury through play. —may defend against these dangers via imaginary playmate or animal who, while ferocious and larger than life, is subject to child's whims.

Table 1-1 (con't)

6 years	Hops on one foot, stands on alternate feet with eyes closed for 10 seconds, jumps 12 inches high landing on toes, can throw a ball. (age 6) Imitates (age 7)	Language well-established —deviations from adult norm tend to be more in style than grammar. Can name values of coins, all colours: Can give description of pictures.	Builds on objects to form concepts and on concepts to form classes of concepts —continues grouping, regrouping, naming and exploring.	Ties shoelaces. Can walk to school by self, crosses road at lights safely, plays co-operatively with peers. Can play simple game by rules without adult supervision.	Acceptance of parents' morals and wishes. Child "identifies" with parent of same sex, taking on that parent's values, sex-role behaviour. —conscience and value system develop. Child increasingly behaves as if controlled and regulated by own internal standards and ideals. —not as influenced by external punishment or reward.
8–10 years	Can tap either foot on floor and right or left finger on table at same time maintaining rhythm for 20 seconds. By age 10, good fine-motor control. Can balance on board, standing with arms out in front, palms down, eyes open.	Good understanding of general language and its rules —e.g. knows plural of man is men. —gives 3 rhyming words for "map" or "cat" within 30 seconds. By age 10–11, can express self in abstract concepts —e.g. can name 10 wild animals in one minute.	By age 9, can group objects in 2 categories simultaneously. e.g. bead is both red and wooden —this is still a building process on reflexes and grouping. True abstract reasoning (i.e. the ability to go beyond the concrete and envision changes without visual props) does not occur until adolescence.	Uses knife at table, combs and brushes hair. Catches a baseball, plays complicated games by rules.	School involves: accepting rules and regulations; adapting to others; competing with others; possibility of defeat, ridicule, humiliation; persisting at task even if unpleasant until it is complete. Child's self-image and self-esteem are cemented by sense of own accomplishments and feedback from others.

RECOMMENDED FOR FURTHER READING

1. ARIES, P. *Centuries of Childhood.* New York, Alfred A. Knopf, 1962.
—a book that gives a good historical review of the role of children in various societies.

2. BAYLEY, N. "Research in Child Development: A Longitudinal Perspective". *Merrill-Palmer Quart. Behav. Dev.* 11: 184-90, 1965.
—a short summary of this author's enormous contribution to the longitudinal observation of children's physical and emotional development.

3. BIRCH, H. G., and GUSSOW, J. D. *Disadvantaged Children.* New York, Harcourt, Brace and World, 1970.
—an extremely scholarly and emotionally moving review of the world literature on the impact of institutional and other psychosocial insults on children.

4. BOWLBY, J. *Attachment and Loss.* Vol. 1: *Attachment.* New York, Basic Books, 1969.
—the classic text on attachment theory.

5. BRODY, S. *Patterns of Mothering.* New York, International Universities Press, 1956.
—a review of thirty-two mothers and infants in the first year of life, which concludes that maternal skills can be learned.

6. CASE, R. "Piaget's Theory of Child Development". *Orbit.* 3,4: 8–11, 1972.
—a brief, excellent review of Piaget's stages of development.

7. ERIKSON, E. H. *Identity and the Life Cycle.* New York, International Universities Press, 1959.
—the classical volume, describing Erikson's developmental theory.

8. FLAVELL, J. H. *The Developmental Psychology of Jean Piaget.* New York, D. Van Nostrand, 1963.
—a very concise summary of Piaget's theoretical concepts. Fairly hard reading.

9. FRAIBERG, S. *The Magic Years.* New York, Scribner's, 1959.
—a psychoanalytic approach and beautifully descriptive book of the early pre-school years.

10. GOLDFARB, W. "Emotional and Intellectual Consequences of Deprivation in Infancy: A Re-Evaluation", in Hoch, P. H., and Zubin, J., eds., *Psychopathology of Childhood,* pp. 105-8. New York, Grune and Stratton, 1955.

—a review of the outlinés and other studies on the impact of institutionalization on childrens' later emotional and cognitive development.

11. KAGAN, J., and MOSS, H. A. *Birth to Maturity*. New York, Wiley and Sons, 1962.
—a classical volume introducing modern concepts of cognitive development.

12. KNOBLOCH, H., and PASAMANICK, B. *Gesell and Amatrude's Developmental Diagnosis*. 3rd ed. New York, Harper and Row, 1974.
—the definitive description of Gesell's stages of psychomotor development.

13. MAHLER, M. S.; PINE, F.; and BERGMAN, A. *The Psychological Birth of the Human Infant*. New York, Basic Books, 1975.
—the text of Mahler's theory of development from the symbiotic phase through separation-individuation, rapprochement, and beginning of later separation with complete research data.

14. PASAMANICK, B., and KNOBLOCH, H. "Retrospective Studies on the Epidemiology of Reproductive Casualty: Old and New". *Merrill-Palmer Quart. Behav. Dev.* 12: p. 7, 1966.
—a review of the outlines and classical studies on the possible impact of later behaviour in children.

15. SEARS, R. R.; MACCOBY, E.; and LEVIN, H. *Patterns of Child Rearing*. New York, Row, Peterson, 1957.
—of historical interest, a learning-theory approach to child development.

16. SKEELS, H. M., "Adult Status of Children with Contrasting Early Life Experiences: A Follow-Up Study". *Monog. Soc. Res. Child Dev.* 31, serial no. 105, monograph 3: 1966.
—a study describing the twenty-five-year follow-up of children initially institutionalized, some of whom were given special stimulation.

17. SPITZ, R. A. *The First Year of Life*. New York, International Universities Press, 1965.
—a psychoanalytic description of the first year of life, relying on direct observation of infants.

18. THOMAS, A.; BIRCH, H.; CHESS, S.; HERTZIG, M. E.; and KORN, S. *Behavioral Individuality in Early Childhood*. New York, New York University Press, 1965.
—the standard work describing the authors' concept of temperament and its effect on the later development of behaviours.

19. THOMAS, A.; CHESS, S.; and BIRCH, H. G. "The Origin of Personality". *Scientific American*. 223, 2: 102-9, 1970.
—the classic article describing genetic and constitutional theories of development, inborn traits, and temperament.

20. MUSSEN, P. H., and CONGER, J. J. *Child Development and Personality*. 4th ed. New York, Harper and Row, 1974.
—a recent updating of a well-organized and highly readable general textbook of child development. Presents and integrates a variety of developmental theories along with a summary of supportive research findings.

HARVEY GOLOMBEK
JAMES WILKES
ARTHUR P. FROESE

2. The Developmental Challenges of Adolescence

Adolescence is a period of major change. Ushered in by the hormonal activity associated with the growth spurt of puberty and by changing environmental expectations, it is a stage of rapid though uneven biological, psychological, and social development. The rate at which individuals progress through adolescence varies widely. Psychological development may lag behind physical development by years. For example, a youth of sixteen may leave home, establish himself on his own, and be fully self-supporting, while a nineteen-year-old student may remain much more dependent economically and emotionally on his family. There does exist within this stage, however, an orderly sequence of physiological and psychological developments through which different adolescents pass in their own time and at their own rate.

Normally, puberty occurs between the ages of ten and eighteen years in girls, and twelve and twenty years in boys. So marked is the variation in age of onset and rate of growth that one teenager may have completed his biological maturation while another of the same chronological age is just beginning it. Biological maturation includes increases in height, weight, and strength, and changes in body proportion, as well as the development of secondary sexual characteristics and the accompanying awareness of heightened sexual urges.

Psychologically, adolescence has been defined as the period from the youth's first asking, "Who am I?" to his arrival at the answer,

"This is me." To find this answer and attain maturity and independence, the adolescent is confronted with a series of developmental tasks. At the same time, continuing intellectual maturation increasingly allows for the development of rich abstract reasoning, which Piaget terms "formal operations".

Adolescence can be divided conveniently into three sub-periods:

Early adolescence includes the developmental changes and the onset of puberty initiated and indicated by the growth spurt. During this early period, the adolescent remains home-centred. His behaviour may temporarily show a disorganized, erratic quality along with a decreased willingness to accommodate the expectations of his parents and others, while wide mood swings and periodic bouts of feeling ill-treated and unloved may dominate his emotional life. His group activities are primarily with members of his own sex.

Mid-adolescence follows puberty by about one to one-and-a-half years. At this time, the first tentative interest and approach towards the opposite sex usually takes place. This awakening of heterosexual interest often disrupts previous peer groupings and intimate friendships. Characteristically, this is the stage when adolescent rebellion starts, a period of irritability, wide mood swings, and rapidly changing feelings. Obedience to parental dictates is replaced by conformity to peer-group standards and loyalties. Early sexual explorations begin.

Late adolescence is a period of transition as the young person consolidates his identity and comes to grips with his future. He is more able to be selective and discriminating in his relationships. Feeling himself a more complete and separate person, he is more able, by this stage, to form and maintain truly intimate relationships with others whose beliefs, ideals, and motives he can see and respect as clearly as he does his own. As a result, his relationships show a greater variety than is typical of those of the mid-adolescent. Each of these sub-phases has its characteristic problems and demands, and each requires a different approach.

1. Developmental Tasks

a) BIOLOGICAL MATURATION

Early adolescents are preoccupied with adjusting to their new physical growth and developing sexuality, with the inevitable effects on body image and self-concept. Adolescents, typically, are extremely self-conscious and sensitive about their physical appearance and any deviation from "normality". Even moderate acne, unflattering nose shape, obesity, or gynecomastia can cause exquisite, though apparently quite needless, distress. The comparison is always with others of their own age.

Early maturers generally have the advantage over late maturers. While they may be under stress from undue expectations placed on them because of their mature appearance, they have the strength and height to enforce their place in the pecking order. Later maturers, on the other hand, are forced to compete athletically and socially with peers who surpass them in size, stature, and strength. The early developers' pride in the development of their bodies only emphasizes lack of maturation. Their sexual interests and activities leave the late developers feeling alternately envious, inadequate, confused, and excluded. They know their day will come, but they surely wish it were here to let them be at least part of the gang if not the leader.

b) PSYCHOSOCIAL DEVELOPMENT

Adolescence may be an upsetting period not only for the adolescent but also for his family. The process of growing and groping towards maturity and of integrating powerful but conflicting biological and social demands may generate confusion and upheaval within the adolescent. Parents may respond to this confusion as if it were adolescent rebellion. The nature of parental response may either assist or impede the resolution of the conflicting demands the adolescent is struggling to integrate.

For a detailed look at this period, let us examine first some of the tasks to be confronted during adolescence, and then explore the difficulties presented to the adolescent and his family in the achievement of these tasks.

i) *Independence and Psychological Separation from Parents*

One of the major achievements of adolescence is emotional independence. This occurs through the continuing process of individuation, that idiosyncratic synthesis of individual hopes, desires, attributes, skills, and defences. Most adolescents approach independence with considerable ambivalence. They long to be self-sufficient and resent those on whom they depend. Yet they are loath to trade the security and comforts of continued dependence for the uncertainty and responsibilities of independence. They need to feel that they are gaining their independence without being overwhelmed by too much too soon. The inner struggle between these strong and antagonistic sets of drives generates within the adolescent confusion and anxiety, which are, in turn, reflected in behaviour and attitudes as intense as they are inconsistent. All too often the upheaval aggravates parental anxieties and precipitates ambivalent and exaggerated reactions, which complicate the movements towards independence. The more parents perceive normal adolescent behaviour as evidence of pathological rebellion, the more difficulty they will have in tolerating that behaviour and the harder they will make it for adolescents to achieve mature independence without unnecessary trauma and continuing alienation.

> The mother of Joan, age seventeen, was concerned about changes in her daughter's behaviour, and unsure of how to respond to her confusing demands. In her earlier years Joan had always been willing, compliant, and helpful. Now, in late adolescence, she began alternately involving her mother in her own affairs and then complaining bitterly that she was treated like a "little girl". She complained about her mother buying clothes for her and about the way her bedroom was decorated. Yet when her mother suggested that Joan make her own choices, Joan retorted bitterly that her mother was not helpful and cared less about her than the two younger siblings. Joan complained frequently of recurrent headaches. Her mother repeatedly suggested that she see their family physician. When Joan failed to do so, her mother, because of her difficulty in allowing Joan to face the consequences of her own behaviour, took over and made the appointment for her. Joan, at that point, bitterly resented her mother's repeated butting into her affairs. Her parents, faced with one such situation after another, found that Joan's irritability and her demands for independence alternating with accusations of overinvolvement left them feeling inadequate, confused, upset, and resentful.

ii) *Development as a Mature Heterosexual Individual*

The hormonal changes of early and mid-adolescence lead not only to the development of secondary sexual characteristics but also to an accompanying increase in sexual drives. Parents have become less permissible as love objects, and the early adolescent fills the void by involving himself in intense friendships, or "crushes", which may be with members of either sex. The early adolescent typically finds and relates intensely to others who, he feels, have some quality he himself needs. The crushes of the mid-adolescent are highly narcissistic and are frequently one-sided and intense. The object of the crush is idolized and admired, even loved, at times passively and yet passionately. The idealization serves temporarily to keep the adolescent unaware of the erotic, and frequently homosexual, component of the friendship. The eventual recognition of this element often contributes to the sudden disruption of these relationships. As sexual interest and fantasy are intensified, they may be accompanied by sexual explorations, which are often more concerned with breaking through inhibitions and testing capacities than with any interest in intimacy. For some adolescents, sexual acting-out can become a problem, but for the most part love and sex are kept quite separate. Whereas boys tend towards discussions of exaggerated sexual feats, girls are typically more taken up with romantic fantasies of love relationships. Throughout this period, both boys and girls are often concerned, to the point of preoccupation, with their acceptability to members of the opposite sex. A capacity for mature heterosexual relationships and true intimacy may develop in late adolescence, as the self-preoccupation that is characteristic of early and mid-adolescence gradually recedes.

> Nancy, age fifteen, had developed a casual relationship with her favourite disc jockey. Periodically she and her friend would visit the local radio station to chat with him over coffee or a Coke. Nancy became increasingly infatuated with him while he for his own reasons encouraged the crush. She began calling him at home and making a nuisance of herself to the point where he finally told her he did not want to see her again. Nancy dealt with her subsequent sense of abandonment, affront, and depression by becoming increasingly dependent on her best girl friend. It was not too long before she became anxious and threatened by the unrecognized homosexual aspects of this relationship. As her anxiety increased, the friendship suddenly terminated, following an argument which Nancy unconsciously precipitated. Her need to depend on someone

led her once again to set up a "special" relationship, this time with her history teacher. He, too, abruptly withdrew his offer of special tutoring when he realized that in her fantasies their relationship had gone well beyond that of student and teacher. In desperation, she became dependently attached to an older married cousin who, because of his needs, saw himself as the only person who could rescue Nancy. Before long these attempts at help developed into a passionate sexual relationship. Her cousin, realizing the possible complications of such an involvement, terminated it abruptly. Nancy then threw herself into a series of sexual relationships, attempting to improve her own immature image of herself by proving she could be desirable to boys. Through therapy she gradually developed some insight into this immature and self-defeating pattern of relating, and began for the first time to develop more stable relationships with boys. Two years later she was involved with a boy in a relatively mature, intimate friendship which had been maintained for over a year.

iii) *Acquisition of Moral Values*

The value system of the pre-adolescent largely imitates that of his parents. As adolescence proceeds, the increased influence of the peer group leads to experimentation with an initial incorporation of values that are distinctly the adolescent's own. This process usually involves modifying, giving up, and derogating from some firm parental precepts, a move that may cause considerable anxiety and friction within the family. Whereas previously the parents were regarded with awe and assessed unrealistically, they are now undervalued and subject to the adolescent's inflated evaluation of his own ideas, values, and experiences.

The mid-adolescent is typically intolerant of ambiguity; consequently, he is attracted to moralistic and simplistic positions on highly complex issues. He thus invites polarization by his manner, which, while at best naïvely idealistic, is frequently arrogant and abrasive. This, combined with the adolescent's typical intolerance of shortcomings, especially in parents, creates a stage difficult for parents to weather. This existential polarization may lead to an irreversible weakening of the bond between parent and child if these experimental dialectics are not understood as a necessary step in defining and consolidating the adolescent's feeling about himself as a separate and unique individual.

> Scott was the second of five children in a rigid, fundamentalist, religious family. Scott's father was a strict disciplinarian with high moral expectations. The other children followed in father's footsteps in a compliant manner, while Scott began questioning some inconsistencies he had observed over the years in father's behaviour. Often when travelling on the highway, for example, his father would ask the children to be on the lookout for possible police patrol cars, and around income tax time he would brag about how he had out-foxed the income tax department again.
>
> Whenever Scott openly questioned the contrast between his father's stated moral positions and his actual behaviour, his father, who was not consciously aware of the inherent contradiction, became defensive, angry, and threatening. Scott, in return, became disillusioned and resentful, convinced his father was a liar and a hypocrite. Increasingly alienated, he withdrew from their relationship and became belligerent and resistant to adult authority within or beyond the home. His behaviour became increasingly antisocial but, when confronted with evidence of car theft, breaking and entering, or assault, he could see nothing wrong in what he had done, other than the fact that he had been caught.

iv) *Educational and Vocational Choices*

During middle and late adolescence, a number of key decisions of lifelong importance must be made. These will be very much affected by the adolescent's earlier school and vocational achievement—or lack of it—but will also be influenced by pressures from parents and by pervading social and cultural values. Particularly if the attitudes and aspirations of his parents are in marked conflict with those of his peer group or if his parents are seeking to live vicariously through him, considerable confusion and conflict may be generated. As a result, key decisions may be influenced more by powerful but unrecognized emotional factors than by rational evaluation.

2. Developmental Problems

a) FAILURE TO PROGRESS DEVELOPMENTALLY

Such failure may result from some distortion or pathological influence during childhood. Excessive rejection or deprivation, for example, may result in an individual who is seriously and chronically limited in his capacity for forming successful relationships, in his self-esteem, and in his ability to establish successfully his independence and to avoid a pattern of antisocial behaviour. (For further description of the long-term effects of deprivation, see the discussion of Deprivation Syndromes in Chapter 5.) On the other hand, excessively solicitous or overprotective parents may inadvertently encourage other forms of developmental arrest. Their adolescent children may continue to be excessively dependent, remaining "good", submissive, and considerate throughout adolescence, showing little or no behavioural evidence of inner unrest. Although convenient, this type of behaviour may indicate a serious delay of normal development. These adolescents during childhood established a pattern of defending excessively against their biological drives. The intensification of these drives during adolescence is countered by an increase in their defences crippling enough to block the normal maturation process. Burdened by strong feelings of inadequacy, they are frequently unable to persevere in any activity in the face of initial difficulty or frustration. Therapeutic intervention may help remove the inner restrictions and free the path for normal development.

> Dennis was two years younger than his brother Scott, whose conflict with his father was outlined above. He found their repeated battles extremely upsetting, and he determined, not entirely at a conscious level, to avoid all similar confrontations. With so rigid a father, he could achieve this only by totally suppressing any aggressive, hostile, or self-assertive tendencies. This he did, becoming a pleasant, passive, conforming, and considerate boy with few interests and little ambition. "Getting along" became an end in itself for him. Even his choice of a career and a wife were based primarily on their predictability and freedom from challenge. Whenever in his work or his marriage he faced stress he could no longer avoid acknowledging, he would try desperately to placate everyone involved at whatever cost. Should this prove impossible, he

would become increasingly anxious, depressed, and withdrawn, the long-repressed rage breaking through only occasionally. As years went on, while remaining as pleasant and considerate as when he was a teenager, he gave up most of his former interests, becoming increasingly passive and restricted. Only his chronic pessimism and lack of energy gave any suggestion of the subclinical depression lying just beneath his pleasant exterior.

b) EXAGGERATION OF THE USUAL BEHAVIOUR PATTERNS

All adolescents show mood swings of some degree, but some experience these much more markedly. Constitutional factors may make their first appearance here, carrying ominous predictions. Mood swings may indicate an inner clash between newly intensified drives and the augmented defences called into play against them. Such struggles may occur in any area of the adolescent's emotional life. For example, the need to be cared for and looked after is opposed by the drive to gain independence and control over one's life. Any experience or expression of normal sexual interest may be smothered in a cloak of rigid asceticism. Alternately, sexual drives may break through tenuous controls to produce a riot of indiscriminate and exploitative sexual gratification. In all such cases, the behaviour reflects the exaggerated struggle, as periods of extreme constriction alternate erratically with phases of extreme impulsiveness.

c) TRANSACTIONAL DIFFICULTIES WITH PARENTS

Adolescence frequently stirs up unresolved feelings and conflicts in parents, who may react to their child with extreme, inconsistent, or other unusual behaviour. Parental stress is most likely to occur around three main areas:

i) *Sexuality*

The adolescent's sexual development and behaviour may provoke strong sexual attitudes and feelings in the parents. Repressed attitudes may be activated so that the parents respond too harshly and puritanically, or they may be excessively permissive or overly involved in the adolescent's dating behaviour or sexual practices. In such situations, the adolescent frequently tunes in to and complies with the parents' underlying expectations rather than their spoken admonitions, which often contradict the former.

> Alice, a fifteen-year-old adopted girl was referred by her mother because of increasingly rebellious behaviour. Alice constantly defied her mother's requests or else responded with a string of four-letter words often followed by physical attacks. Their relationship worsened to the point where Alice repeatedly stayed away overnight, once approaching the children's aid society asking to be placed in a foster home.
>
> Unusually attractive and physically mature, Alice was always surrounded by several boys three to five years older than she. Her behaviour was obviously seductive, yet she felt confident that she could handle their sexual advances. Her mother, however, was less sure, and in their battles repeatedly called Alice a slut, letting her know that she did not trust her and did not believe she was still a virgin. Her father, too, frequently became involved in these arguments, telling Alice on several occasions that if she ever did get pregnant he would make her have an abortion.
>
> Examining the mother's background in more detail, it became evident that she grew up in a controlling family. She had greatly admired her older sister, who had had a rebellious adolescence, yet she herself had remained very compliant. She was now threatened by Alice's attractiveness and apparent closeness to her father. Unconsciously she encouraged Alice's seductive behaviour, envied her, and was reliving her own adolescence vicariously. By the time Alice was fifteen, she was sexually active. She was twenty-four weeks pregnant before her parents realized it consciously. Thus Alice lived up to her parents' expectations, and at the same time won the abortion issue by hiding the pregnancy until it was too late.

Confronted with the burgeoning and often intense sexuality of their adolescent son or daughter, some parents may become concerned about their own (real or apparent) diminishing sexual capacity or attractiveness. This may precipitate clinical depression or attempts to seek affirmation in extramarital affairs, or even competition for the attention of the adolescent's friends.

ii) *Authority*

It is appropriate that parental authority gradually recede and that the adolescent develop greater autonomy. Parents who have precarious or incomplete control over their aggressive or antisocial tendencies are particularly likely to be threatened by the expression of similar tendencies in their adolescent. They may respond with rigid authoritarianism or, paralysed by indecision, they may abdicate their parental role. Alternately they may belittle or plead ineffectually with their adolescent in a frequently futile and always destructive attempt to cling to the vestiges of their control.

> Doug, at fifteen, was the third of five siblings, the rest of whom were very compliant and accepted the rigid expectations of their authoritarian parents. Doug, on the other hand, repeatedly struggled with authority figures, taking on not only his father but also his teachers and the law. He had several arrests for thefts of minor objects for which he had no use. His father responded to his rebellion at times with threats he was not willing to carry out and at others by throwing up his hands in helpless disgust. Even when Doug's behaviour was more acceptable, both parents would rant on about what a bad influence he was on his younger siblings or, alternately, would plead ineffectually in a futile attempt to regain some control. Doug responded to his parents' anxiety, ambivalence, and inconsistency by alternating between being a compliant "good boy" and a rebellious delinquent. This only added to the parents' confusion and feelings of inadequacy, contributing to the ineffectuality and vacillation that in turn perpetuated Doug's reliance on acting-out behaviour as a means of dealing with his inner anxieties.

The adolescent, even under ordinary circumstances, has mixed feelings about parental authority and is sensitive to parental anxiety and inconsistency. He may veer towards rejection of parental control at one time, while at another time using it gratefully to make decisions he cannot make for himself. As a result, adamant demands for autonomy may alternate with regression to childlike dependency. These vacillations in the adolescent's responses to parental authority may do much to compound parental confusion, anxiety, and resentment.

iii) *Values*

The adolescent's stated moral, religious, educational, and vocational choices may stir up parental anxiety, criticism, and hostility, especially if the parental positions are precariously or ambivalently held. Direct opposition to parental values and positions may lead to hostility and alienation which will induce feelings of guilt and inadequacy in parent and child. Parental opposition may extend to such areas as choice of friends, recreational interests, dress, and music. Occasionally, in a misguided attempt to maintain closeness, parents may become overly involved in the adolescent's life-style, thus depriving him of the authority figure he requires who can oppose and reward at appropriate times.

> Jane was a pseudo-mature fifteen-year-old who had recent arrests for shoplifting and possession of marijuana. She had grown up in an average middle-class religious family. Both her parents were university graduates. Her relationship with her father, a probation officer, had always been a close one from which her mother was consistently excluded. The interaction between father and daughter was mutually seductive. Father frequently commented on Jane's physical maturity and about how there had been a gang of boys hanging around her ever since age eleven. Jane had rejected her Roman Catholic upbringing and was involved in an Eastern religious movement together with her nineteen-year-old boy friend. She was sexually active and planning to move in with him as soon as she turned sixteen.
>
> Jane's father responded to her acting-out by attempting to "understand her", taking a great interest in her new-found religious beliefs, discussing her marijuana experiences, and initiating long discussions about the liberal sexual mores of today's youth. Jane sensed that the only way she could deal with the hostile component of her ambivalence towards her father would be to become involved in delinquent behaviour. It was this which led to her father seeking help for the family.

The issues cited above may not be evident in such a clear fashion, but may be shifted to the usual instrumental battlegrounds of everyday family life, such as cleanliness, neatness, dinner, hours of coming and going, chores, and use of cars.

d) DIFFICULTIES WITH COMMUNITY

The task of making the transition from family to community is complicated today by a pervasive disenchantment with society. The adolescent is expected to find his place in a society marked by increasing social isolation and an unparalleled rate of technological change ("future shock") of which he may be at least as aware as his parents. This changing world makes it difficult to anticipate, let alone plan for, adult life. Many of the traditional values around which our society has been organized—the work ethic; material success; competitiveness; the supremacy of law; concepts of sex roles, sexual morality, and family life; religious beliefs—are under constant attack and, in the eyes of a well-defined and articulate minority of the adolescent's peer group, have already been discredited. Where does he stand and where is he to go in the midst of all this uncertainty? This dilemma can precipitate a crisis of social identity. If conflicts with his family have led to a severance of family ties and significant alienation, the parents will not be available—or cannot be used—to provide even minimal orientation or support during this crucial period of transition. Some adolescents, overwhelmed by demands for adaptation beyond their capacity to cope, respond by dropping out; they withdraw into a non-demanding, non-working world, retreating to the refuge of subjective reality for pleasure and satisfaction.

3. Important Tasks in Dealing with Adolescents and Their Families

a) ASSESSING DEVELOPMENTAL LEVEL

The physician, counsellor, or worker who recognizes that the adolescent is not an adult is less likely to set excessive expectations. By also recognizing that the adolescent is not a child, he avoids being patronizing or authoritarian. Different circumstances call for different strengths and abilities, and consideration must be given to the adolescent's ability to cope with the particular situation.

b) MAINTAINING OBJECTIVITY

The adolescent's problem frequently presents itself in a dramatic fashion that may challenge the value system of the adult attempting to counsel him. When tensions exist between parents and child, it is easy to get caught up in the situation and to side with one or the other. A thorough understanding of the situation before judging or acting assists in maintaining objectivity. Information from outside the family—for example, from schools and social agencies—will help in making an accurate and balanced assessment.

c) AVOIDING OVERINVOLVEMENT

The adolescent tends to involve adults in situations from which they will have difficulty extricating themselves. The physician (or worker or counsellor) may end up being manoeuvred into doing things or negotiating concessions for the adolescent who is quite capable of handling the situation on his own. Should this occur, the dependency of the adolescent is unnecessarily and inappropriately increased. Such overinvolvement or excessive closeness on the part of the physician may threaten the adolescent, who will then frequently withdraw and become hostile. If the adult, hurt, responds with anger or attempts to force his help on the adolescent, the situation may be aggravated by the overly zealous attempt at intervention.

There is an invitation, too, for the physician or other counsellor to identify with the parents against their adolescent son or daughter. Overinvolvement—where one emotionally takes sides and assumes someone else's problem as one's own—runs the risk of aggravating disruptions in family life or interfering with programs of intervention already instituted by school or social agency.

d) DEVELOPING TRUST

Trust is built on clear and matter-of-fact communication. One cannot be vague or misleading or talk down to adolescents. Arrangements regarding plans, visits, and appointments must be clear and the adolescent notified promptly about unavoidable changes. If the physician expects respect and trust from the adolescent, he must first give it.

e) ESTABLISHING CONFIDENCE

The adolescent must be treated as the situation demands. He will reject unnecessarily authoritarian or dogmatic attempts to direct him. On the other hand, he will have no confidence in the adult who allows him to behave in a manner he knows is destructive, under the guise of allowing him to make his own decisions.

The adolescent expects adults to be appropriately firm and to have the courage of their convictions. Often he tests adults with outrageous requests or protests, hoping to meet the strength he needs to give him a sense of security. An openness and willingness to listen without judgment will bolster the adolescent's sense of confidence and trust. One must realize that while decision-making ultimately is the responsibility of the adolescent and his family, the physician may be in a position to help them recognize important factors or potential consequences that should be considered in understanding a problem and in arriving at a course of action.

f) FACILITATING INDIVIDUATION

Psychopathology within the family system may make it harder for the adolescent to achieve successfully the goals of emotional independence and the formation of individual identity (a process termed "individuation"). If either the adolescent or the parents seek to avoid these conflicts by an abrupt, unilateral decision to live separately, especially if the decision is made at a point of crisis or in frustration and anger, a lasting guilt may result, which will leave both adolescent and parents with damaged self-esteem. For the physician or counsellor to propose geographical separation as a solution to the difficulties of adolescent individuation would be naïve. He should rather attempt to help both the adolescent and the other family members to identify and resolve the tensions they are seeking to bypass. In attempting to counsel the adolescent and his family, one may be under major pressures, either from the family or from the adolescent, to make the decisions for them. But the appropriate role for the physician and counsellor is that of helping the family define as clearly as possible the sources of their distress and of providing them an opportunity to work towards a constructive resolution. Clearly he must be prepared to accept their decision if they cannot or will not use this opportunity.

g) CLARIFYING CONFIDENTIALITY

The degree of confidentiality the physician will allow his adolescent patient will vary with the adolescent's age, with the nature of the relationship between the adolescent and his family, and with the subject under discussion. Wherever possible, and adolescent's request for confidentiality with his physician or counsellor should be respected. Sometimes, however, it is in his own best interests that an issue be raised with his parents. Should this be the case, this should be discussed with him fully and frankly, leaving no doubt that unless he is prepared to raise the matter with them the counsellor will. It can be extremely difficult to decide which issues must be shared, and this decision can reflect more the value system or anxiety of the counselling adult than the needs of the adolescent. Nevertheless, it is essential that anyone treating or counselling adolescents be aware of the need to allow each adolescent that degree—and only that degree—of confidentiality consistent with his well-being, and that he recognize the danger to his relationship with his patient of promising and allowing more or less.

4. Problems of Drug Use and Abuse in Adolescence

Drug use in adolescence may range from harmless, transitory experimentation to persistent use with physical and psychological dependence. Depending on the pattern, the drug use may indicate a social phenomenon of no medical or psychological significance or it may be symptomatic of serious emotional disturbance. This topic is discussed in more detail in Chapter 14.

5. Principles of Management

a) GENERAL PRINCIPLES

i) Adolescents are often psychologically ill and not just "going through a phase".

ii) Parents, family, and involved members of the community are important in assessment and treatment.

iii) Any adequate assessment of an adolescent must evaluate:

a) his biological maturation and associated feelings (including his self-esteem and body image);

b) his intrapsychic conflicts, in all areas listed above;

c) where he stands in relation to his developmental tasks;

d) his relationships with his family;

e) information from outside the family (e.g. schools, social agency, etc.).

iv) The goals of treatment are the attainment of independence, emotional health, and orientation to reality.

b) IMPORTANT GUIDELINES IN DEALING WITH ADOLESCENTS

i) The first contact is important. Who made it? How? How calm or upset was he? These questions provide clues to the resources available and to the strength and the manipulations of the people concerned.

ii) Adolescents often do not present themselves or their concerns willingly. The important point is that they come. To save face, they may need to protest that help is not needed, but unless they come nothing can be done.

iii) Observe physical appearance and dress, noting change on future occasions.

iv) Never promise a relationship of complete confidentiality. What you tell anyone else will depend on your judgment. Consider the adolescent's wishes in this regard but do not be bound by them.

v) Be prepared to inquire into all areas of the adolescent's life, his school, clubs, sports, and dating, etc.

vi) Deal with manipulation as it arises. The adolescent may count on parents' reluctance to use existing agencies such as police and court. The adolescent may initially have trouble distinguishing between an attitude that is easy-going and relaxed and a permissiveness that derives from weakness or indifference. The former is a distinct asset, while the latter will inevitably prove to be a liability.

vii) Remember that teenagers may not be able to handle adult obligations and responsibilities.

viii) Recognize that argument and challenge are part of how the adolescent relates. Do not be so preoccupied with the chip that you lose sight of the shoulder—and the teenager—beneath it.

ix) Be prepared to work with school teachers, clergy, athletic instructors, agency workers, etc.

x) Be prepared to share some of your personal values, ideas, and morals, but do not assume these have any value or relevance for the adolescent patient. What you *are* in your dealings with him will prove more important than what you *say*.

xi) In all cases it is probably useful to have at least one family interview. For further treatment, the family approach seems more fitting for the younger adolescent, while group or individual therapy fits later adolescence.

These are some of the major developmental tasks confronting the adolescent and his family. The manner and success with which they are handled may do much to determine both the continuing nature of family relationships and the character of the adolescent as he enters adult life.

Issues related to treatment and the role of the primary physician in the total program of management will be discussed further in Unit Five.

RECOMMENDED FOR FURTHER READING

1. AICHHORN, A. *Wayward Youth.* New York, The Viking Press, 1971.
—classical monograph describing a therapeutic approach to delinquency.

2. ANTHONY, E. J. "Psychotherapy of Adolescence", in Caplan, G., ed., *American Handbook of Psychiatry,* 2nd ed. Vol. 2: 234-49. New York, Basic Books, 1974.

3. BALSER, B. H. *Psychotherapy of the Adolescent.* New York, International Universities Press, 1957.
—comprehensive description of different levels of psychiatric practice, with special emphasis on the role of the school.

4. BLOS, P. *On Adolescence.* New York, The Free Press of Glencoe, 1963.
—most authoritive statement of the psychoanalytic position.

5. EASSON, W. M. *The Severely Disturbed Adolescent.* New York, International Universities Press, 1969.
—a description of in-patient, residential, and hospital treatment of severely disturbed adolescents.

6. ERIKSON, E. H. *Identity, Youth, and Crisis.* 1st ed. New York, W. W. Norton, 1968
—a fundamental contribution to understanding growth and development.

7. ERIKSON, E. H. *The Challenge of Youth.* New York, Basic Books, 1963. Anchor Books edition, 1965
—provides a good sociological perspective.

8. GINSBURG, H., and OPPER, S. "Adolescence", in Ginsburg, H. and Opper, S., eds., *Piaget's Theory of Intellectual Development: An Introduction.* Englewood Cliffs, New Jersey, Prentice-Hall, 1969.
—good description of cognitive development in adolescence.

9. HOLMES, D. J. *The Adolescent in Psychotherapy.* Boston, Little, Brown and Company, 1964.
—clearly written description of therapeutic technique with adolescents, using many examples.

10. HOWELL, M. C.; EMMONS, E. B.; and FRANK, D. A. "Reminiscences of Runaway Adolescents". *Amer. J. Orthopsychiat.* 43: 840, 1973.
—reports on experiences of teenage runaways: their reasons for leav-

ing home, problems encountered when away, effects of leaving and future plans. Offers recommendations for management of adolescent runaways.

11. LEVINE, S. V., and SALTER, N. E. "Youth and Contemporary Religious Movements: Psychosocial Findings". Paper presented at the Annual Meeting of Canadian Psychiatric Association, Banff, Alberta, 1975.
—explores the involvement of youth in contemporary religions and cults, discussing what the youth involved are seeking and what they feel they are getting from their religious involvement.

12. MEEKS, J. *The Fragile Alliance.* Baltimore, Williams and Wilkins, 1971.
—a good introductory textbook in adolescent psychiatry.

13. MUHICH, D. F., and JOHNSON, B. J. "Youth and Society: Changing Values and Roles". *Pediat. Clin. N. Amer.* 20, 4: 771-77, 1973.
—an up-to-date commentary on some sociological factors affecting youths' changing values.

14. NICHOLI, A. M. "A New Dimension of the Youth Culture". *Amer. J. Psychiat.* 131: 396–401, 1974.
—discusses the recent religious preoccupation among youth. Describes the social and psychological determinants of religious conversion; its relationship to drugs, sexual and social behaviour; existential despair; results of conversion on adolescents' attitudes towards drugs, self-image, parents, sexuality, and relationships.

15. OFFER, D. *The Psychological World of the Teenager.* New York, Basic Books, 1973.
—study of the "normal" middle-class American adolescent.

16. PHILIPS, I., and SZUREK, S. A. "Conformity, Rebellion, and Learning: Confrontation of Youth with Society". *Amer. J. Orthopsychiat.* 40: 463–72, 1970.
—suggests that satisfaction associated with early successful learning is reduced and distorted during each developmental phase, and that during adolescence this often results in rebellion, alienation, or nonconformity.

17. RAVENSCROFT, K. "Normal Family Regression at Adolescence". *Amer. J. Psychiat.* 131: 31–35, 1974.
—clear discussion of the process set in motion by puberty that initiates a family developmental epicycle featuring a temporary regression in sibling, marital, and family functioning to earlier modes of behaviour, and provision of a normal framework for family members to share and to facilitate adolescent development.

18. ROBINS, L. N. *Deviant Children Grown Up.* Baltimore, Williams and Wilkins, 1966.

—interesting life-history approach to studying antisocial behaviour.

19. SCHAFFER, C., and PINE, F. "Pregnancy, Abortion, and the Developmental Tasks of Adolescence". *J. Amer. Acad. Child Psychiat.* 11: 511–36, 1972.

—views pregnancy followed by therapeutic abortion as resulting from and heightening conflicts already present during that developmental period.

20. STEINHAUER, P. D. "Abruptio Familiae: The Premature Separation of the Family", in Tulipan, A. B.; Attneave, C. L.; and Kingstone, E. eds., *Beyond Clinic Walls,* 204–11. Univ. of Alabama Press, 1974.

—discusses sociological and psychological factors leading many youth to leave home prematurely in a misguided attempt to solve conflicts around the establishment of independence.

21. WERKMAN, S. L. "Value Confrontations Between Psychotherapists and Adolescent Patients". *Amer. J. Orthopsychiat.* 44,3: 337–44, 1974.

—explores differences in life-style and values between adolescents and their therapists, which can complicate treatment, suggesting appropriate modifications of treatment.

22. WERKMAN, S. L. "Psychiatric Disorders of Adolescence", in Caplan, G., ed., *American Handbook of Psychiatry.* 2nd ed. Vol. 2: 223–33. New York, Basic Books, 1974.

—the clinical disorders of adolescence are listed and related to the development challenges characteristic of the period.

23. MASTERSON, J. F. "The Symptomatic Adolescent Five Years Later: He Didn't Grow Out of It". *Amer. J. Psychiat.* 123: 1338–45, 1966–67.

—disturbed behaviour in adolescence cannot be dismissed lightly as "just a phase". Disturbed adolescents frequently go on to become disturbed adults.

PAUL D. STEINHAUER

3. The Child and His Family

Until recently (the mid-1950s) psychiatrists rarely treated the families of their patients. Until that time, any intensive and direct involvement with families was seen at least as undesirable, if not as incompatible with good psychiatric practice. The reasons for this lay in the fear that family contacts would undermine the patient's trust in the psychiatrist, as well as complicate and contaminate the doctor-patient relationship, which plays such a key role in successful psychotherapy.

Sometimes, however, it was realistically impossible to treat one individual without involving his family in some form of therapy. This was the case when a family sought treatment for a child. It was recognized, of course, that the child's problems both contributed to and were aggravated by other tensions within the family, particularly within the marital relationship. Furthermore, it was appreciated that direct treatment of the child for one or two hours a week was likely to have limited value as long as the family environment, which often contributed so much to causing and maintaining his difficulties, remained unchanged. When a child required treatment, it was provided by a team of therapists who collaborated with one another. Someone, usually a psychiatrist, treated the child who had originally been identified as the patient. Meanwhile someone else, usually a social worker, met with the parents for the sake of the child. The social worker, usually accepting the parents' definition of the child as the patient, worked to help the parents understand the nature of the child's problems and to recognize and deal constructively with the upsetting feelings that the child and his behaviour stirred up in them. Between treatment sessions, the therapist of the child was expected to collaborate with the therapist of the parents. This collaboration process was as effective as the time available and the freedom of communication between members of the therapeutic team permitted. Incomplete or distorted communication was not infrequent, leading at times to a failure to integrate the two streams of therapy and to overidentification on the part of each therapist with his or her members of the family. When the collaboration was successful, the therapeutic team functioned as an effective unit, and collaborative therapy was the treatment traditionally employed in child guidance clinics since the 1930s.

More recently, however, there has been an increasing unwillingness to consider the family member originally referred (labelled) as the patient. Rather, he is termed the "identified patient", meaning: *You* (the family) consider him the patient (sick one); *I* (the therapist) do not. To those who think this way (i.e. family therapists):

1. The unit of pathology (the patient) is no single individual but the family *as a unit*.
2. The member originally referred (the identified patient) is demoted (or promoted, depending on one's point of view) and seen as the *symptom-bearer* for the family. Satir has referred to him as the scab on the family sore, meaning that his symptoms are merely the obvious part of a pathological process involving the family as a unit.
3. If this is so, it follows that the *aim of treatment* becomes not merely the removal of the symptoms of the identified patient but a modification of the pathological structure and equilibrium of the family unit.

The Family as a System in Equilibrium

The family can be understood as a system in equilibrium at three interrelated levels (see Fig. 3-1).

1. At an *intrapsychic* level, each person must reach a balance between biological, psychological, and social demands (for further discussion, see Chapter 6). The dynamic tension between these compelling and often contradictory sets of forces, along with the ways in which the individual defends himself from the anxiety it generates, constitutes the *intrapsychic level of equilibrium*.

2. At an *interpersonal* level, all members within the family system affect and *are affected* by one another, even if their influence on one another is not readily apparent. Symptomatic behaviour in one person almost

Figure 3-1 The Family as a System in Equilibrium

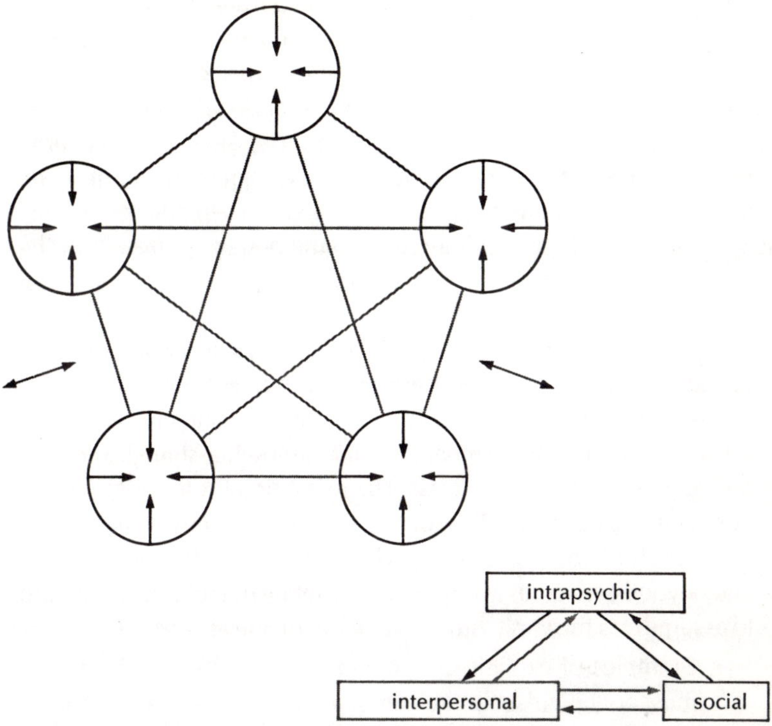

invariably elicits a response from other family members. A child's misbehaviour evokes parental discouragement, anger, and rejection, which in turn feed in a circular manner the feelings of deprivation and rage that contribute to the child's misbehaviour. This is but one example of the *interpersonal level of equilibrium*.

3. At a *social* level, all members of the family—and the family as a unit—are constantly exposed to, and in continual interaction with, the standards and influences of the social environment: this is what is referred to as the *social level of equilibrium*.

Since these three levels of equilibrium are interrelated, stresses or events occurring at one level will inevitably reverberate through other levels of the family system. For example, a child's failure in school (event at the social level) will likely produce conflict between him and his parents (effects at the interpersonal level) and these together may combine to produce feelings of depression and low self-worth (effects at an intrapsychic level).

In another instance, severe and chronic marital conflict may originate from personality problems that husband and wife brought into marriage (liabilities at the intrapsychic level). These may be aggravated by the stresses and strains of living together (interpersonal level) so that neither parent is free to meet the children's emotional needs (interpersonal level). If the children respond to the resulting feelings of insecurity and rage (results at the intrapsychic level) by aggressive or antisocial behaviour in the community (results at the social level), the community (neighbours, school, police) may react to the behaviour (results at the social level), bringing pressure on the family and producing effects at all three levels of equilibrium.

There are six basic principles governing family equilibrium:

1. For any family, all members *are assigned* and *assume* roles, and relate to one another in repetitive and highly characteristic ways. Thus the roles family members assume are both assigned by others and assumed by the individual. The question of roles, their definition, and role conflict will be discussed later in more detail.
2. Each family has a *set of rules* (some overt and explicit, others implicit and beyond conscious awareness) that define the roles members are to assume and the ways they are to relate to one another.

   Examples of explicit rules could include: boys in this family must not hit girls; children are not allowed to swear at parents; when I tell you to go to bed, you must do as I say promptly.

   Examples of implicit rules might include: we don't discuss sex at the dinner table (never stated in words, but conveyed by a frown, a change of subject, by telling the child not to yell—even though he's talking quietly—or to sit up straight every time the subject is introduced). I say your bedtime is eight o'clock (but your *real* bedtime is when I get angry and holler or hit, which may be at any time between eight and ten, depending on whether or not I'm too harassed and tired to follow through).
3. The roles and rules govern the behaviour acceptable within a given family and define the characteristic structure of that family.

   When we say that a family has a typical structure we mean that given a task, whether it be deciding on where to go out for dinner or how to explain a given proverb, they will approach it in a highly characteristic manner; the same members will dominate, the same ones will withdraw, the same ones will agree to anything, and the same members will disrupt, etc.

4. Within that structure, family members are in equilibrium with one another. Thus each is constantly responding to—and being responded to by—others in a manner that is repetitive and characteristic for that family. This equilibrium is not static, but dynamic. The equilibrium typical of a given family is not defined once and accepted for all time, but rather is constantly being challenged and redefined by the ongoing interaction of daily living. This is the source of much of the normal and inevitable tension of family life.
5. The family equilibrium is a *self-regulating* or *homeostatic* equilibrium. Thus any attempt to shift that equilibrium either from within (e.g. change in a member) or from without (e.g. input from a physician) may be expected to evoke a reaction opposing the change and maintaining the status quo.

   This homeostatic principle operates largely beyond conscious awareness. The strength of the resistance to change may vary from family to family. In general, the better the mental health of the family, the more open it will be to respond successfully to demands for change. Similarly the less adaptive the family, the greater its homeostatic resistance to change.

   > Families may ask for help and express a desire for change while continuing to resist any measures likely to produce it. Thus parents may take a child out of psychotherapy just as he is beginning to improve. Or a husband who once complained of his wife's sexual frigidity may accuse her of being too aggressive or develop impotence as she begins to respond to or initiate sexual relations.

6. The family equilibrium is a *shared defence* against what the family sees as the threat of pain (e.g. anxiety, depression, rage, sexual feelings, and fantasy) or disruption. No matter how destructive or unsatisfying that equilibrium may appear to the outside observer, it represents that particular family's attempt to minimize the threat of disruption and pain. Thus any forcible attempt to alter it (such as when an overly zealous physician seeks to direct a family as to how they should live their lives) will evoke shared (i.e. group) as well as individual resistances to change.

Family Roles

To understand the role of any family member (e.g. father) one must know:

1. How does *he* see himself functioning as a father?

2. How do *other* family members see him functioning as a father?
3. How does he *think* others see him functioning as a father? (This may be quite different from the way he *does* function or from the way others *see him* as functioning.)
4. What is expected of a father in this family and in its particular subculture, and how does this jibe with what father feels he can and will give?
5. What other roles does the father fill, and to what extent are these compatible or in conflict with his or others' expectations of him as a father? For example, he is also: an individual (a self) with needs of his own; a husband; a man; a doctor, mechanic, salesman, a welfare recipient, a machinist, etc.; one of the boys, a member of his lodge; a compulsive sports (or bridge, or theatre) fan; a member of his religious group; etc.

There is no single "best" or "right" way to define the roles of various family members. What matters is not how roles are defined; what matters is that within the family there be *internal role consistency*—that is, each member sees himself in a way that is consistent with the way others see him and that there be general agreement on what is expected of him. It is also important that there be sufficient complementarity of roles to allow for successful *role integration.*

> For example, if a particular father feels that his contribution to the family consists of earning the living and making the major decisions, while housework and parenting are exclusively the responsibility of his wife, this will not present major problems provided that his wife is content and feels fulfilled within this definition of their respective roles. If, however, she finds housework and child-rearing less than satisfying, any attempt to force his role definition on her leaves her just four basic choices: she can submit (remaining unfulfilled and probably becoming depressed), fight (chronic conflict), escape (alcohol, promiscuity), or separate.

It is also important that family role definitions be consistent with actual role performance, since when they differ significantly, confusion, disharmony, and disequilibrium that can shatter a family may result.

Both husband and wife, for example, can agree intellectually upon the wife's having a career outside the home. Should, however, the husband's behaviour betray an unrecognized hostility to his wife's working that is incongruent with his stated position, the resulting inconsistency is bound to arouse both confusion and disharmony until clarified and resolved, either one way or another.

Ideally, role definitions will allow the psychological needs of each family member to be met. Members will be frustrated if continually expected to perform roles that neglect their own social, emotional, and psychological needs, even if these are consistent with their own expectations and those of other family members. What matters, therefore, is that the family arrive at some definition of roles that works for it, allowing enough flexibility so that each individual member's needs are respected and that the family is prepared to respond appropriately to demands for change, while, at the same time, providing enough cohesion to maintain the stability of the family as a unit.

FAMILY TRANSACTIONS AND ROLE DEFINITION

In any transaction between two people, a *subject* initiates the transaction, inviting the object to respond. The *object* reacts to the communication received from the subject. How he reacts will depend both on the nature of the stimulus (the communication from the subject) and on how it is perceived and interpreted (which may be incomplete or distorted, depending on the expectations and internalized psychopathology of the receiver).

The healthy person is sometimes the subject, at other times the object, of transactions. A need to fill permanently the subject role would involve constantly needing to dominate and control others and an inability to meet the needs of others. Such people use others in a parasitic manner, sucking them dry and wearing them out. On the other hand, permanent acceptance of an object role means that one constantly allows others to use him to meet their needs, while abdicating his right to demand that his needs be met too.

In many dysfunctional families, one or more members *are assigned* and *assume* the role of permanent object. To say that they are assigned this role means that pressure is put on them by other family members to accept it. To say that they assume this role indicates that no one is trapped permanently in an object role (giving up his right to demand that his needs be met) without some degree of collusion on his part. Such a person, if his adjustment suffers, is said to occupy the *scapegoat* role. The scapegoat, often a child, is selected because he is in a powerless position. His well-being is sacrificed so that the family as a whole can continue to function. Others (e.g. Epstein) refer to him as being in the binder role, as he seems to bind the family together.

> The family martyr (usually the mother or an older sister), for example, is a scapegoat who constantly sacrifices her own needs in order to meet the needs of others or to keep the peace. This may provide a degree of cohesiveness for the family as a unit but at the expense of the martyr's becoming increasingly unsatisfied, depressed, frustrated, and—often indirectly—resentful.
>
> The child who behaves aggressively or in an antisocial manner, often serves as a lightning rod, drawing onto himself (and away from each other) the hostility of other family members. Sometimes this person is described as being in the *discharge* role; that is, he discharges hostility and antisocial and sexual drives for the entire family who then (a) derive vicarious pleasure from his behaviour by identifying with him; (b) support their own defences (repression and reaction-formation) by punishing him for his badness and lack of control.

In working with a family that scapegoats one or more members, one runs the risk of siding either with the family or with the scapegoat. This risk can be magnified by feelings left over from our own earlier family experience stirred up by our contact with the family (countertransference). If one identifies with the family and against the scapegoat, one joins the scapegoating process. If, on the other hand, one over-identifies with the scapegoat, one may interpret the child's behaviour as *purely* reactive to the family situation. Taking such a position absolves the child of any responsibility for his behaviour, encouraging an "it's all my parents' fault" attitude. This is rarely entirely true, and runs the risk of the therapist unwittingly encouraging further symptomatic behaviour by the child while alienating the parents, who frequently withdraw from therapy to avoid his critical attitudes. The therapist who emotionally aligns himself or takes the side of any member (e.g. the one he sees as "the victim") against other family members ("the victimizers") has lost his objectivity and is in serious danger of losing perspective and compromising his potential usefulness to the family.

Family Communication

Any message sent is a message at at least two levels: (a) the *content* level, that is, the subject matter of the communication; (b) the *metacommunicative* level, that is, the manner in which the message is communicated. This latter level includes tone of voice, facial expression, choice of words, etc., and defines the way the sender is feeling and the relationship between sender and receiver when the message was sent.

The reaction of the receiver will depend on both of these, but also on the way the message is received and interpreted, which may be either incomplete or distorted, depending on the clarity and directness of the sender and the freedom to hear and interpret accurately on the part of the receiver.

Epstein divides communications into three basic categories:

1. *Affective communication:* communication in which the message transmitted is basically emotional in character, e.g. "I hate you."
2. *Instrumental communication:* communication in which the message is related to ongoing tasks of family living, e.g. "Pass the bread, please."
3. *Neutral communication:* communication involving the transmission of information that is neither related to affect nor to the instrumental processes of family living, e.g. "It's raining today."

For each of the above, there are two other sets of variables to be considered:

1. Is the message *clear* or *masked* (i.e. disguised, ambiguous)? The greater the lack of clarity, the greater the ambiguity, the more confusion and anxiety one can expect, and the greater the likelihood of distortion by the receiver.
2. Is the message *direct* or *displaced* (i.e. is it delivered towards the person for whom it is intended, or is it deflected to someone else)?

For example, consider a situation where a husband is reading his newspaper after work as his wife talks on the phone while their three-year-old wanders in with a runny nose. The husband could, of course, merely tell the child to wipe his nose or wipe it for him. But if he were angry with his wife, he could express this anger in a variety of ways:

1. With a *clear, direct* message: "For Pete's sake, Mary, will you get off the phone and wipe Johnny's nose."
2. With a *direct* but *masked* message: "What the devil's the matter with you, Mary!"
3. With a *displaced, masked* message: "What the hell's going on around here?" *or* "Suzy, turn off that damn radio!" *or* slamming down his paper, he might stamp upstairs and bang the door of his room.

Epstein postulates that the more disturbed the family, the more likely there is to be distortion in the affective (emotional) level of communication. Thus what we usually term a "breakdown in communication" is usually symptomatic of a problem in relationships. The more severe the disturbance, the more likely the feeling will spill over to contaminate the instrumental and neutral communications as well.

> In a well-functioning family, for example, a request for a drink of water is merely that (i.e., an instrumental communication) and is responded to as such. In a dysfunctional family, however, such a request may either *be* or *be interpreted as* an attempt to dominate or manipulate (i.e. a masked, hostile communication). In some families, members are so frequently anticipating—and therefore resisting—domination by others that instrumental and neutral communications are frequently misinterpreted as attempts to dominate and control. So hypersensitive are such families in the area of control that differences, disagreements, or common problems are resolved not on the basis of *what fits* (i.e. what is appropriate) but on the basis of *who's right* (i.e. who dominates). Is it any wonder that in such families the clear definition of a problem and the finding of an appropriate solution are severely impaired?

One cannot fail to respond to a message he has received. Silence or pretending to ignore a message merely indicates that one is avoiding a direct and clear response. Thus we cannot choose the messages to which we will respond. We can, however, learn to choose (i.e. control) the nature of our responses.

In some families, members frequently project onto others disowned aspects of their feelings and the responsibility for their own behaviour. Such people have trouble distinguishing their own feelings from those of others (i.e. they have poorly defined ego boundaries). As a result, they imply that the reason they act as they do is determined *solely* by the behaviour of others.

> DOCTOR: Johnny, why did you hit Jimmy?
> JOHNNY: Because he took my truck.

In this example, Johnny implies that Jimmy is responsible for his aggressive behaviour. Actually, Johnny could have responded in a number of ways:

1. He could decide to allow Jimmy to play with his toy.
2. He could ask Jimmy politely to return the toy.
3. He could angrily demand that the toy be returned.
4. He could ask a parent to have Jimmy return the toy.
5. He could grab the toy from Jimmy.
6. He could take something of Jimmy's.
7. He could hit Jimmy.
8. He could hit another sibling who is smaller than he, etc.
9. He could burst into tears.

Thus Johnny's response was determined *not just* by Jimmy's behaviour but by the way Johnny, with his particular personality and his characteristic ways of handling such situations, reacts to stress. The choice, of course, is not always conscious or deliberate. In demonstrating to a family the ways in which the members influence one another's behaviour, one must carefully avoid unwittingly reinforcing anyone's attempts to absolve himself of the responsibility for his own behaviour by projecting it onto others.

> A therapist, addressing a boy who had been repeatedly stealing, said to him during a treatment session, "If your mother hadn't been so angry at you, you wouldn't have had to steal to get even, would you?" The above statement suggests not only that the mother's behaviour *explains* the child's antisocial behaviour (which in part it may) but also that it *excuses* it (which it does not).

It is useful to distinguish between *ambiguous* and *paradoxical* (incongruous) communications:

1. An *ambiguous communication* is one in which the message sent is

confused, but not contradictory. What does it mean, say, if father arrives home from work and slumps down on the couch without a word? Has he had a bad day at work? Is he angry, and if so, at whom? Is he sad, worried, or tired? Has he a headache or heartburn?

2. A *paradoxical (incongruous) communication* (mixed message) consists of messages at two different levels which contradict or are incompatible with each other—for example, the statement (made in a quivering voice), "Of course I'm not angry, I just can't be bothered wasting any time discussing it!"

The effect of such a mixed message on the receiver is to induce confusion. To which level is he expected to respond? He can't respond to both. This dilemma is most marked in what Jay Haley has termed the *double bind,* in which:

a) No matter how the receiver attempts to respond to the mixed message, he will be wrong and criticized.
b) The receiver cannot either escape from or clarify his confusion, because the sender will not allow clarification of the intended meaning (checking out), and the receiver cannot afford to break off the relationship or antagonize the sender because their relationship is too important to him to risk alienation.

Several authors (Bateson, Lidz, Wynne, Jackson) have commented on the frequency with which double binds occur in the families of schizophrenics. At one time, the "double bind hypothesis" of schizophrenia held that schizophrenia results from a defensive withdrawal in the face of the extreme anxiety generated by a long-term exposure to massive and continuous double binding. More recently, there has been general agreement that the double bind hypothesis was originally oversold. Current thinking holds that the use of the double bind is neither confined to the families of schizophrenics nor specific to any single form of mental illness; rather, it is seen as an interference with successful communication and relationship and as a source of chronic tension in families where it occurs frequently.

The more disturbed the family, the greater will be the *inadequacy* and *distortion* of communication within that family. Family therapists assume that if a family can reach the point of communicating successfully it will have no further need for therapy. This implies both that the improved communication will allow for the effective identification and resolution of those pressures inevitably generated in the course of living, and that the family (as individuals and as a system) has reached

Table 3-1 Comparison of Functional and Dysfunctional Families*

	Dysfunctional Family	*Functional Family*
Communication:	unclear indirect non-specific incongruous	clear direct specific congruous
Individuality (autonomy):	thwarted, at least in the identified patient	guaranteed for all. Individual differences are not just tolerated, but serve as a stimulus for growth.
Decisions:	made on the basis of a power struggle: *who's right* is more important than *what fits*.	made on basis of the problem at hand: *what fits* is more important than *who's right*.
Outcomes:	chaotic & unpredictable	orderly & predictable
Response to demand for change:	all demands for change tax a rigid/unyielding system. The result is stress, symptom formation, and decompensation.	the family system is flexible enough to change in response to environmental demands for adaptation. There is no need for cramping, symptom formation.

*adapted from Satir.

a point of health that will allow its members to maintain open channels of communication, which can then be used to keep pressures from building up again.

Symptoms as an Expression of Family Dysfunction

The symptoms of the identified patient may play a central role in attempts by family members to influence one another and in maintaining the equilibrium of a dysfunctioning family. Freud acknowledged that symptoms at times prove useful in an individual's relationships with others. This he called secondary gain, emphasizing that, while such symptoms offer fringe benefits to the individual, the primary gain—the main purpose of the symptom—is the defence against neurotic anxiety. The family therapist, however, feels that neurotic symptoms, regardless of their origin, are to a major degree maintained by the response of the environment. As long as symptoms pay off, the individual may be encouraged to rely on them to manipulate the environment. When symptomatic behaviour no longer works for him, the individual is forced to reappraise the situation. This is part of what happens in psychotherapy: the therapist, ideally, does not respond to, and is not manipulated by, symptomatic behaviour. Instead, he merely focuses on what the patient is trying to do and reflects how he is using his symptoms to control their relationship. When the usual distortions, threats, attacks, hysterical outbursts, attempts at emotional blackmail, etc., do not succeed, the patient is left more aware of his manipulative manoeuvres and of the fact that these are not working. The therapist can then help the patient recognize the degree to which he relies on similar devices in his attempts to manipulate and control others.

In certain families, for example, any attempt to discuss the behaviour of a certain member results in an outburst of tears, accusations of being picked on, etc. One soon learns that this happens at home whenever anyone tries to confront that member with undesirable aspects of his behaviour. The result, typically, is that either the family members learn to put up with the symptom to avoid a scene *or* they end up forced to justify their complaint against the accusation that they are being unfair *or* the discussion shifts to the method by which the member is defending himself (i.e. the unreasonableness of the scene). In any case, the original issue has been successfully deflected—and, therefore, defended against—by the defensive manoeuvres of the member whose pathology was under discussion. But if this member is in an interpersonal situation where his typical defence will no longer work—for example in therapy, where the therapist refuses to be intimidated, deflected, or diverted—the patient can learn to recognize the nature of his defensive manoeuvres. Only then can he be helped to achieve more direct, more rational, more mature methods of dealing with his problems. Let us list some characteristics of symptomatic communication.

1. The symptoms of a particular family member may have considerable communication value. For example, a statement of how miserable, lonely, hurt, or helpless one is may communicate: (a) a plea for support and/or pity; (b) an implied reproach (e.g. "look what you've done to me"); (c) an attempt to control (e.g. the martyr-mother who uses her weakness to keep her family in line).
2. Other symptoms may constitute a more direct attack. The child who vomits when angry not only demands attention but punishes mother by making her clean up. Similarly the rituals of the obsessive compulsive may enable the psychologically crippled wife to dominate

totally a rigid and authoritarian husband. (See description of obsessive neurosis in Chapter 6.)

3. Symptomatic behaviour may mask a demand that the environment relax expectations that would be made of others on the basis that the patient is not up to them. It is as if he said, "How can you expect me to be pleasant and to carry my weight in the family when I'm so nervous, depressed, or crazy?"
4. Finally, some symptoms can be seen as taking the place of sudden, intense feeling outbursts: for example, the increased disorganization of thought processes in the schizophrenic as an anger equivalent; an increased stutter at times of emotional tension and anger; psychosomatic symptoms (asthma, migraine, ulcer flare-ups) in moments of repressed rage or grief.

The Family as the Unit of Treatment

Pathological or symptomatic behaviour, then, is maintained both by internalized (intrapsychic) and by interpersonal factors. One can treat a family equilibrium that is contributing to distress or dysfunction in one or more members by intervening at a number of levels.

The individual psychotherapist (or counsellor) chooses to intervene at the intrapsychic level. Defining his task as that of helping his patient see clearly the way his difficulties are related to his own not fully recognized conflicts and his role within the family environment, he then attempts to help him use this knowledge to deal with his conflicts more successfully.

In contrast, the family therapist chooses to intervene primarily at the interpersonal level. He assumes that if the family can learn to identify and resolve its interpersonal difficulties, members can function more successfully both individually and collectively without further help. Thus, while to some extent dealing with the psychopathology of individual family members (i.e. the intrapsychic level of equilibrium), his prime concern is with the relationships between members and the pathological structure of the family system itself. Family therapy implies that if the pathological structure of the family can be modified, the psychopathology of individual family members will in turn be improved, even without having been confronted primarily and directly. In order to do this, the therapist must first make family members aware of the gaps and distortions in their communication.

The therapist can accomplish this awareness in the following ways:

1. By the way he responds to the members, by establishing rapport, empathy, and communication between himself and the family.
2. By providing an atmosphere in which issues can be examined and discussed rather than argued. This family therapist listens to everyone and helps family members hear one another. By encouraging silent members to speak up despite discouragement or resentment, he tries to encourage ventilation of negative feelings, serving both as a safety valve and as a source of encouragement. He encourages the clear, direct expression of both positive and negative feelings, avoiding scapegoating and transforming concealed conflicts into open expressions of feeling, which, if denied an outlet, would instead build up only to be discharged periodically in an indirect, masked, explosive, and destructive manner.
3. He can often help family members identify the basic nature of an issue around which they are struggling in a confused, frustrating, and non-productive manner. He provides this assistance by locating and counteracting the various barriers, sources of confusion, and defensive manoeuvres, so that he and the family arrive at a mutual definition of what is really wrong. In so doing he will use confrontation and interpretation to undermine resistances and to reduce shared conflict, guilt, and fear.
4. By serving as an educator and as a reality-tester, focusing the family members' attention on the ways they communicate with one another—and especially by making members aware of covert levels of their own communication—thus helping members learn to communicate more fully, more directly, and more clearly with one another. To the extent that this can be achieved, it will provide the family with a safety valve, that is, an apparatus for identifying precisely areas of conflict and for working together to find appropriate and generally acceptable solutions.
5. By making the family aware of power struggles within the family, and the covert and frequently pathological ways in which members manoeuvre to dominate one another. This will help family members recognize (a) why others react to "innocent" requests or remarks as they do; (b) why minor incidents are continually being inflated into major ones; (c) the degree to which issues are settled on the basis of *who is right*, rather than *what is appropriate*.

6. By helping the family members become aware of how and why so little true communication occurs: for example, the degree to which they talk, but don't listen (i.e. two monologues, rather than one dialogue); the degree to which they battle over irrelevancies, upsetting one another but never identifying or resolving the basic issues; the degree to which disagreements, rather than being resolved, are merely sidestepped by a form of pseudoconsensus in which one member appears to give in to keep the peace, only to sabotage the false agreement later on.

Some families will respond readily to attempts of a therapist to clarify the nature of their difficulties and will, with relatively little resistance, be able to use what they have learned to find newer and more effective ways of communicating and problem-solving. In other families, the homeostatic principle may evoke considerable resistance to any proposed change. These are families who may demand more time and involvement than the primary physician has to give and who might be considered for a referral for psychiatric consultation and psychotherapy.

CONTRA-INDICATIONS TO FAMILY TREATMENT

Treating the family as a unit almost inevitably results in an intensification of ongoing family interaction. This tendency, which contributes so much to the potency of family therapy when properly selected and applied, can be destructive and may even contribute to family breakdown if used inappropriately or ineffectively.

Contra-indications to treatment of the family as a unit include:

1. Evidence of a malignant and irreversible trend towards break-up of the family, except where "separation counselling" is indicated.
2. Unwillingness or inability of the family as a unit or of key family members (especially the parents) to tolerate open discussion of contentious issues in a manner that allows all family members and the therapist the right to question, to disagree, and to express how they feel.
3. An inability to obtain the presence of all family members whose presence is considered essential to the success of treatment.
4. An inability on the part of the therapist to avoid being drawn into the transactional games according to the family's rules, thus causing him to lose objectivity and perspective and to behave as a part of the

pathological family system, rather than as a neutral and separate observer.

5. Should the family situation or the behaviour or adjustment of any individual member continue to deteriorate in spite of ongoing family treatment, psychiatric consultation is indicated.
6. Earlier, scapegoating was discussed as a symptom of family disturbance. Nevertheless, severe and chronic scapegoating that does not shift in response to confrontation contra-indicates family therapy, at least initially. When fixed scapegoating persists or is intensified as the examiner tries to explore other sources of family tension, members are utilizing it to avoid other, often more significant, sources of distress. If one is unable to stop the blaming of the youngster or is repeatedly forced into the position of defending the scapegoat against a fixed alliance, one should shift to a collaborative approach. This way identified patient and parents can be treated separately, avoiding the aggravation of existing psychopathology until the parents are able to begin dealing with their contribution to the total problem, at which point a return to family therapy could be reconsidered.

RECOMMENDED FOR FURTHER READING

1. ACKERMAN, N. W. *The Psychodynamics of Family Life*. New York, Basic Books, 1958.
—the original, definitive textbook in the area of family theory.

2. ACKERMAN, N. W. *Treating the Troubled Family*. New York, Basic Books, 1966.
—a more recent work directed more towards issues of therapy than towards basic family theory.

3. ADAMS, P. L. "Functions of the Lower-Class Partial Family". *Amer. J. Psychiat. 130: 200*—03, 1973.
—clear description of effects of social class on family function. Compares complete and partial (i.e. fatherless) lower-class families as to physical health, social control, status, acceptance of the prevailing culture by the children, emotional maintenance.

4. BANK, S., and KAHN, M. D. "Sisterhood-Brotherhood Is Powerful: Sibling Sub-Systems and Family Therapy". *Fam. Process.* 14: 311-38, 1975.
—many patterns of family behaviour and aspects of individual de-

velopment result from autonomous activities within the sibling subsystem. Suggests that understanding sibling sub-system structure and dynamics can lead to more flexible therapeutic interventions.

5. BARTEN, H. H., and BARTEN, S. S. *Children and Their Parents in Brief Therapy*. New York, Behavioral Publications, 1973.
—illustrates how to "think deeply but act superficially" in dealing with the family in crisis.

6. BATESON, G., JACKSON, D. D., HALEY, J.; and WEAKLAND, J. "Toward a Theory of Schizophrenia". *Behav. Sci.* 1: 251-64, 1956.
—a classic paper introducing the concept of the "double bind" and hypothesizing its role in the development of schizophrenic symptoms.

7. BOWEN, M. "Family Therapy after Twenty Years", in Freedman, D. X., and Dyrud, J. E., eds., *American Handbook of Psychiatry*. Vol. 5: *Treatment*, pp. 367–92. 2nd ed., New York, Basic Books, 1975.
—a current review of the field by a pioneer in the area.

8. BOYD, E.; CLARK, J.; KEMPLER, H.; JOHANNET, P.; LEONARD B.; and McPHERSON, P. "Teaching Interpersonal Communication to Troubled Families". *Fam. Process.* 13: 317-36, 1974.
—describes an approach to family intervention directed at ways in which information is exchanged in troubled families.

9. COHEN, C. I., and CORWIN, J. "An Application of Balance Theory to Family Treatment". *Fam. Process.* 14: 469-79, 1975.
—reviews Heider's Balance Theory and demonstrates its application to the diagnosis and treatment of family dysfunction.

10. EPSTEIN, N. B. "Family Psychiatry: Comments on Theory, Therapeutic Technique, and Clinical Investigation". Paper presented at Conference on Multiproblem Families sponsored by Laidlaw Foundation, 60 St. Clair Avenue East, Toronto, 1963.

11. EPSTEIN, N. B.; RAKOFF, V.; and SIGAL, J. J. "Families Categories Schema". Monograph prepared by the above authors and the Family Research Group of the Department of Psychiatry, Jewish General Hospital, Montreal, in collaboration with the McGill University Human Development Study; revised 1968.
—a systematic approach to the analysing and classifying of patterns of behaviour, relationships and communication within the family system.

12. EPSTEIN, N.B., and BISHOP, D.S. "Family Therapy: State of the Art". *Canad. Psychiat. Assoc. J.* 18: 175-83, 1973.

—a second review of the area by a practitioner and researcher of twenty years' experience.

13. FORD, F. R., and HERRICK, J. "Family Rules: Family Life Styles". *Amer. J. Orthopsychiat.* 44: 61-69, 1974.
—describes five main "rules" or "life-styles" that can be inferred from a family's repetitive behaviour, suggesting how a therapist can help by renegotiating family rules.

14. Group for the Advancement of Psychiatry. *The Field of Family Therapy.* GAP Report, no. 78, 1970.
—a comprehensive review of the field.

15. HALEY, J. "The Art of Being a Failure as a Therapist". *Amer. J. Orthopsychiat.* 39: 691-95, 1972.
—witty and informative.

16. HALEY, J., and HOFFMAN, L. *Techniques of Family Therapy.* New York, Basic Books, 1967.
—interviews with five experienced family therapists discussing the work they do and the strategy governing their intervention. Verbatim transcripts of actual therapy sessions are included.

17. HUBBELL, R. D.; BYRNE, M. C.; and STACHOWIAK, J. "Aspects of Communication in Families with Young Children". *Fam. Process.* 13: 215-24,1974.
—describes a study of interaction in sixteen four-person families, each with one child three or four years old and another age six or seven.

18. JACKSON, D. D. "Family Interaction, Family Homeostasis, and Some Implications for Conjoint Family Psychotherapy", in Masserman, J. H., ed., *Individual and Familial Dynamics,* pp. 122-41, New York, Grune and Stratton, 1959.
—an early formulation of the concept of family homeostasis by one of the earliest practitioners of family therapy.

19. JACKSON, D. D.; BEAVIN, J. H.; and WATZLAWICK, P. *Pragmatics of Human Communication.* New York, W. W. Norton, 1967.
—a technical but authoritative introduction to communication within the family system.

20. LANGSLEY, D. G., and KAPLAN, D.M. *The Treatment of Families in Crisis.* New York, Grune and Stratton, 1968.
—a guide to understanding and management of the family in crisis.

21. LIBERMAN, R. "Behavioral Approaches to Family and Couple Therapy". *Amer. J. Orthopsychiat.* 40: 106-18, 1970.

—suggests that the key to success in family therapy lies in changing the ways members respond to each other. Case examples illustrate this behavioural approach to intervention.

22. LIDZ, T.; CORNELISON, A. R.; FLECK, S.; and TERRY, D. "The Intrafamilial Environment of Schizophrenic Patients. 2: Marital Schism and Marital Skew". *Amer. J. Psychiat:* 114: 241-48, 1957.
—an early paper, one of a series which, by focusing on the family environment of schizophrenics, interested others in the family as a unit of psychopathology. The concepts of "schism" and "skew" are still useful to anyone working with marital couples.

23. McPHERSON, S. R.; BRACKELMANNS, W. E.; and NEWMAN, L.E., "Stages in the Family Therapy of Adolescents". *Fam. Process.* 13: 77-94, 1974.
—outlines the opportunity that crises occurring in the course of family therapy may present for change and growth.

24. MINUCHIN, S. *Families and Family Therapy.* Cambridge, Mass., Harvard University Press, 1974.
—a comprehensive description of a form of family therapy concentrating on change-producing and preventive interventions. A must for the serious student of family therapy.

25. MINUCHIN, S.; MONTALVO, B.; GUERNEY, B. G.; ROSMAN, B. L.; and SHUMER, F. *Families of the Slums: An Exploration of Their Structure and Treatment.* New York, Basic Books, 1967.
—stresses the influence of the slum environment on family structure and functioning.

26. RUSSELL, A. "Late Psychosocial Consequences in Concentration Camp Survivor Families". *Amer. J. Orthopsychiat.* 44: 611-19, 1974.
—this study of the treatment of thirty-four concentration-camp survivor families in family therapy is of particular interest because of the effects of a traumatic experience on the second and third generation.

27. SANDER, F. M., and BEELS, C. C. "A Didactic Course for Family Therapy Trainees". *Fam. Process.* 9: 411-23, 1970.
—describes the rationale, procedures, and reading materials used in a didactic course included in a training program for family therapists. Emphasizes the variety of treatment approaches.

28. SATIR, V. *Conjoint Family Therapy.* Rev. ed. Palo Alto, Calif., Science and Behavior Books, 1967.
—written mainly in point form, this small but useful book is a good introduction to understanding the family as a social system in equilibrium. The chapter on the inclusion of children is particularly helpful (pp. 136-59).

29. SCHEINFELD, D. R.; BOWLES, D.; TUCK, S., Jr.; and GOLD, R. "Parents' Values, Family Networks, and Family Development: Working with Disadvantaged Families". *Amer. J. Orthopsychiat.* 40: 413-25, 1970.
—extensive report and evaluation of a system for working with disadvantaged families whose pre-school children show signs of slow development.

30. SKYNNER, A. C. R. *Systems of Family and Marital Psychotherapy.* New York, Brunner/Mazel, 1976.
—a fine, comprehensive introductory textbook, discussing and illustrating a variety of theoretical approaches, techniques, and procedures.

31. SPIEGEL, J. P. "The Resolution of Role Conflict within the Family", in Bell, N. W., and Vogel, E. G., eds., *A Modern Introduction to the Family*, 391–411. New York, Free Press, 1968.
—a useful discussion of family roles and the part that the resolution of role conflict can play in family therapy.

32. STANTON, M. D. "Family Therapy Training: Academic and Internship Opportunities for Psychologists". *Fam. Process.* 14: 433–40, 1975.
—provides information on both university departments of psychology and psychology internship facilities that include family therapy training in their programs.

33. STEINHAUER, P. D., "Reflections on Criteria for Selection and Prognosis in Family Therapy". *Canad. Psychiat. Assoc. J.* 13: 317-22, 1968.
—one of the early attempts to define criteria for the more selective use of family therapy as a treatment technique.

34. VAN DER VEEN, F., and NOVAK, A. L. "The Family Concept of the Disturbed Child: A Replication Study". *Amer. J. Orthopsychiat.* 44: 763-72, 1974.
—discusses a study that confirms the close association between theories of family pathology and childhood disturbance, shows how the family's concept of the identified patient serves the purpose of the family as a system.

35. WATZLAWICK. P. "A Review of the Double Bind Theory". *Fam. Process.* 2: 132-53, 1963.
—reassesses and reviews the "double bind" theory.

36. WYNNE, L. C., and SINGER, M. T. "Thought Disorder and Family Relations of Schizophrenics". *Arch. Gen. Psychiat.* 9: 191-98, 1963.
—one of the early papers exploring the nature and significance of the family environment on the symptoms of young adult schizophrenics.

UNIT TWO: **Assessment of the Child and His Family**

ELSA BRODER

4. A Guide to the Assessment of the Child and His Family

A thorough assessment of the child and his family forms the foundation on which adequate understanding and effective intervention are based. Without this foundation, therapy proceeds blindly.

> Doreen was a sixteen-year-old girl referred for intensive psychotherapy by her children's aid society worker after the treatment centre where she had been resident closed unexpectedly. The current problems were failure at school, lack of confidence, and a feeling of not belonging. Her life history, which she presented with much psychiatric sophistication, was full of losses, deprivation, and punitive parenting. She appeared to have many serious conflicts, and psychotherapy did indeed seem needed. But, despite her glibness, the examiner began to suspect her understanding and for the first time had her intelligence tested. The result revealed borderline intelligence (IQ 72). This finding resulted in a modified treatment plan including a change from academic school to vocational training, concrete counselling around interpersonal relationships, and support of a placement with an older married sister. At last report, Doreen was happier than ever before, had finished her vocational training, had a job, and was still with her sister.

In this chapter the goals, techniques, and common problems of assessment are discussed. An outline for organizing the data collected in the course of assessment is included. The chapter concludes by discussing how to present findings to the family and issues involved in negotiating a treatment contract.

General Considerations

Children rarely come and ask for help. They are usually brought by others (e.g. parents) who are more concerned than they are about their behaviour. The children may resent or be frightened by being brought for an assessment, which they see as a punishment or as an indication that they are considered crazy. They may have fantasies of "needles" or other painful procedures, of separation from parents by the children's aid society, child welfare association, hospital, or training school. They often feel singled out and vulnerable to siblings and peers. They may mistrust the examiner as another adult brought in by parents to force them to conform to unwanted parental standards or demands. Or they may feel blamed for a situation seen as not of their making, since their definition of the problem may differ considerably from that of the parents.

> Teddy's parents sought help when they could no longer tolerate his bullying of his younger brother, his constant antagonism, and his feeling hard-done-by when asked to do anything around the home. Teddy, however, saw himself as the victim of the younger brother, who continually provoked him, and a mother who consistently favoured the brother and picked on him. Thus to Teddy the assessment was an attempt to blame him for a situation in which he felt entirely the innocent victim.

Instead of seeing themselves as having problems, children and adolescents often project feelings and responsibilities onto others whom they blame for any difficulties they are experiencing. The family, the usual target of their projections, not only becomes the object of their aggression but frequently responds to the child's behaviour and attitudes in ways that intensify the problem. The question of who is the patient in such a situation—child, family, or both—has been explored in the preceding chapter.

The anxiety or resentment with which some children approach an assessment is not the only factor that limits their ability to co-operate with the examiner. Children often find it difficult to express abstract but powerful and disturbing feelings in words. They frequently communicate through behaviour, leaving much to inference. How the child acts, the way he relates to the examiner, and the nature and content of his play may tell more about what he thinks and feels than what he says, which often may be quite unreliable. Fear, anger, or a feeling of being blamed may also block the communication of the older child or adolescent, particularly during family diagnostic interviews. An individual interview at another time, beginning with a discussion of the adolescent's feeling about the assessment and his reasons for non-participation, may help. While an explanation of what will be kept confidential and what will be revealed may be in order, it is a mistake to promise total confidentiality. One should always retain the option to use one's judgment if necessary to protect the youngster or others from harm.

Some older adolescents request that their parents not take any part in the assessment. Although in many cases their wish can be respected, the reason for their request should always be explored carefully. Where there is concern about the adolescent being potentially destructive to himself or to others, professional responsibility demands that one inform the parents about the seriousness of the situation and seek their involvement. In such situations, the adolescent should be encouraged to be the one to contact the parents directly. Should he refuse, he should be informed of the examiner's intention of involving the family, preferably before the contact is made.[26]

Because children and adolescents are so often unable to discuss their difficulties directly, the examiner frequently must rely heavily on others, who may or may not be good observers and reporters, as sources of information. First among these are the parents. But parents often have their own difficulties bringing their child for help, at times doing so only under pressure from school or police. Most parents care about the well-being of their children. When things are not going well, they question themselves and feel guilty, frustrated, and even angry at their child for undermining their sense of competence and self-esteem. At some point, one must evaluate the adequacy of their parental skills and determine whether the child's needs are being met. It requires a clear sense of direction and a delicate touch to explore areas of weakness or difficulty without having the family become defensively and non-productively enmeshed in guilt and blame. It is not surprising that despite their conscious determination to do the best for their child there may be unrecognized resistance to the assessment. This may take the form of coming late, failure of key family members to attend or participate, avoidance of crucial topics, forgetting relevant data, etc.

> Mrs. P. came for the first appointment with her two daughters, expressing concern over the withdrawn, tearful behaviour and lack of academic progress of the elder. She seemed genuinely surprised when the examiner asked where her husband was, explaining that he had been called out of town and had not thought that his absence mattered. At a later interview where the husband was present, it came to light that the parents were in such deep conflict that separation was being contemplated.

In assessing a child and family, three basic parameters must be explored. These include:

1. *The intrapsychic parameter.* This parameter includes the inner conflicts and feelings with which the child is struggling as well as how he is dealing with and defending against the anxiety generated by this inner struggle (see Chapter 6).

2. *The systems parameter.* The child has a role as a member of a family system with its own characteristic structure, organization, and ways of coping with stress and conflict. If the family is faced with more stress than it can handle at a given time, emergency defences are called into play. If these prove inadequate the system will either disintegrate or present one of its members, often a child, as being in need of help.

> Joan, age eight, was referred because of bed-wetting, day-dreaming, thumb-sucking, deteriorating school performance, and difficulty getting along with her playmates. At assessment it became clear that for some time her mother had been deeply depressed, feeling she could no longer cope and contemplating suicide. She had not been able to communicate to others the depths of her distress. Joan sensed her mother's despair and confusion. Not knowing what to do, she feared what might happen and became increasingly anxious. As her mother's

problems responded to treatment, Joan gradually became asymptomatic.

3. *The developmental parameter.* There is considerable variance in the sequence and timing of the stages of growth and development. The examiner needs a sound knowledge of the normal range for each age to use as a yardstick against which to measure what is seen or reported. Development, as Erikson has pointed out, is a lifelong process. Not only are children developing; parents are developing, too. The life tasks that each is attempting to master at a given time may clash, leading to conflict and anxiety.[7]

> Mrs. J., in her late thirties, had for years thought she was infertile. Suddenly and unexpectedly she became pregnant. Fifteen years earlier, she would have been delighted, but after years of unsuccessfully trying to conceive, she finally and not without difficulty had come to terms with her supposed infertility, returned to college, and established herself in a successful and satisfying professional career. Now, however, she was deeply distressed. The child that earlier would have been loved and cherished was, instead, unwanted and rejected because he came at what, for the Js, was the wrong time.

The question of how much data are necessary and what is really relevant merits some consideration. One needs enough information to arrive at an understanding of what has led to the presenting problem and to develop a workable plan for treatment. One should avoid overwhelming oneself with irrelevant details and subjecting the informants to useless, seemingly endless questioning. People seeking help want intervention that seems to go directly to the heart of their concern. They want change quickly and are more interested in relief than in extensive alteration.[13]

The philosophical approach of the examiner and the goal of assessment influence the nature and the amount of information collected. If one is trying just to determine whether there is a problem sufficient to merit referral, then less data are required than if one intends to undertake the therapy personally.

Some authorities contend that an adequate assessment needs only to see how the child is currently functioning in the major areas of his life, arguing that it is the here and now that one uses in therapy, not the past. Others contend that one cannot fully understand the "now" without knowing what has gone before. Studies of how change occurs suggest that both are important.[24, 29] One must know about those factors leading to the development of the problem (predisposing and precipitating causes) as well as those presently contributing to the difficulty (perpetuating causes). Without information about all of these, one lacks the understanding needed to derive a strategy for effective treatment.

In addition, the behaviour(s) in need of change should be identified objectively with data about frequency, conditions of occurrence, factors increasing or decreasing their frequency, as well as knowledge of the consistency, thoroughness, and duration of previous therapeutic measures. Sometimes perfectly reasonable methods have failed because of lack of perseverance or sporadic application.

In assessment there are a series of questions to be answered. Keeping these in mind helps the process become both more goal-directed and, in itself, therapeutic. The purpose of assessment is to define the problems and to develop methods for beginning to resolve the difficulties. How the examiner approaches the task can, for healthier families, provide a model they can use to define and solve problems on their own. Going through the process with an experienced guide, the examiner, may be all that is necessary. Thus for some, assessment can also be treatment. The questions that require answers are:

1. What is the nature of the problem?
2. Is it a problem that requires action?
3. What is the diagnosis? This includes both defining the nature of the problem (i.e. arriving at a diagnostic label) and identifying the factors causing and maintaining the problem (i.e. formulation).
4. What action, if any, is needed, and by what members of the family system (i.e. treatment plan)?
5. Who best can carry out the therapy? Is referral necessary?
6. Will the family accept the treatment plan?

Surroundings and Equipment

Although assessment can be carried out almost anywhere, some surroundings are more conducive to the task than others. Freedom from interruption is essential, as is sufficient time. To provide this time, many doctors, social workers, and counsellors reserve a particular day of the week or a time late in the day for uninterrupted assessments.

The interviewing room should be comfortable and with a relaxed atmosphere, large enough to seat a whole family while allowing a child some freedom of movement. Furniture should be free of sharp or pointed edges and easy to keep clean, so that the parents and therapist need not be concerned if children climb.

For examination of the child, fancy toys in great variety are not necessary. Relatively non-structured ones that can serve as a stimulus for expression of fantasy are best. Basic equipment should include pencils, crayons, paper, several puppet families,* plasticine, a ball, and books suitable for children of various ages. Competitive games, such as checkers or bean bags, may help but are not essential. Little other equipment is needed to complete an adequate assessment unless a neurological or physical examination is indicated. Then the standard "black medical bag" should suffice.

First Contacts

Assessment begins with the first request for help. However, family practitioners, paediatricians, social workers, or counsellors who have known a family over a period of time have a mass of observational data that is extremely valuable when recalled and reorganized. If the patient is new, then one must begin the process of forming a therapeutic alliance, that is, a relationship based on feelings of trust within which patient (client) and examiner (or therapist, counsellor, or worker) can work together.

The first encounter, be it over the telephone or face to face, is very important for the establishment of rapport and for the setting of expectations. Identifying data, including who makes up the family and an introduction to the major parental concerns, can be obtained by telephone. Some examiners use a questionnaire whose purpose they explain at the same time. By supplying basic information, such forms allow a more economical use of interviewing time, requiring the examiner to spend less time in data collection and freeing him to focus more on the interaction between child and family. Having some data before the first appointment allows the examiner to anticipate the nature of the problem, to plan appropriate strategies for obtaining and clarifying data, and, where indicated, to collect reports from other agencies, therapists, or schools.

*In this day of divorce and remarriage, more than one puppet family may be necessary for the child to portray his life experience.

One should determine in advance how the parents are planning to prepare the child for the forthcoming interview. Many parents will need help to tell the child openly why the assessment has been requested and what they hope to achieve. Both parents and children should have a rough idea of what to expect. The appointment times, the duration of the interview, the number of possible contacts, and whom they will meet should all be mentioned in advance. If audio-visual recording or direct observation is planned, the family should know and should give prior consent.

Examiners should introduce themselves and identify their professional background, especially in agencies or clinics where the clients do not select their examiner. Financial arrangements should be discussed no later than the first face-to-face interview. The immediate use of first names for either therapist (examiner) or an adult patient (client) blurs roles, detracts from the professional nature of the relationship, and, for some, may be resented as an intrusion. The request for the use of first names may have a variety of meanings, including an unconscious resistance to the process (Let's pretend this is a social rather than a professional visit) or an attempt to make the situation less frightening. Unless the meaning of the request is clear and one is sure that the change will be helpful, one should remain with the more traditional modes of address. Children should be asked what they wish to be called, and diminutives like "dear" or the adoption of the family's nickname without the child's consent should be avoided.

Written consent is required before any information can be released. It is helpful to have available a standard form requesting release of information that can be quickly completed, signed, and witnessed. At all times, the privacy of those being seen must be respected. The reports one writes may be used by a variety of people over whom one has no control. Diagnostic labels, therefore, can have serious implications. For example, a report to a school mentioning even the *possibility* of schizophrenia or brain damage can have immediate and lasting repercussions on the way the school perceives and handles the child, leading to undue pessimism which can intensify the child's difficulties. In time, children grow up and may request that information be sent to another setting. Such requests do not permit the release of information about the patient's parents or siblings unless they, too, have signed their consent, a point easily forgotten in photocopying reports.

Others in the community are often most helpful. Public-health nurses may provide home visits, help people come for interviews, and, if requested, take part in the process of assessment. Where a language barrier exists there are usually community organizations that can supply interpreters. No one should be contacted unless with the prior knowledge and consent of the family.

Examiner Operations

A proper assessment is the psychiatric equivalent of a thorough physical examination. The examiner, from the start, assumes control of the interview. This does not mean that he asks all the questions or supplies all the answers. Rather, he must be prepared to direct the inquiry along a path that leads to clear definition of problems and points to where solutions might be found. Everyone's expectations of the examiner and the assessment process should be made explicit. People often expect the examiner to find out all the answers by himself, reading their minds to provide a quick, magical cure. But a family with a psychiatric problem cannot merely put themselves in the hands of the doctor and leave the treatment to him as they might if their child had a medical problem such as appendicitis or pneumonia. The examiner must clarify what they can realistically expect of him and, equally important, what is expected of them. Many think the assessment is the therapy and are disappointed when there is not immediate improvement.

There is no single way to conduct an interview. The examiner must develop his own style of interviewing. It is dangerous to follow too mechanically a set line of questioning; the human interaction between the individuals involved will be blocked, leaving one with a great many facts but little understanding of how the people feel about the problems that led to the assessment and about each other. Creativity is essential. A balance must be struck between activity and passivity; between free flow and structure. The family are focused on the task at hand, avoiding chit-chat. Interactions, as they occur, can be explored to see if they are typical of the family's usual pattern of functioning.

> Dr. B. noticed that every time she asked the identified patient a question, there would be a short pause and then his mother would answer for him. When this was pointed out, mother agreed that this was typical of how withdrawn and uncooperative the patient usually was.

Notes should be made during the assessment interview. No one can accurately remember all the information revealed. In some situations, for example, if court involvement is possible, almost verbatim recording is suggested. Most families do not object to the examiner taking notes and may even appreciate it as indicative of a thorough, serious approach. A seating plan detailing where everyone sits and who interacts with whom can be helpful, and may graphically illustrate when someone is being left out or if there is little or no communication between any of the family members.

The therapist must pay careful attention to the comfort level. It is important that all leave the interview feeling that they have not been violated, in control of their emotions, and in general feeling that the experience has been positive enough to make them willing to return. It is up to the examiner to sense the family's anxieties and to allay them if possible. Structuring the interview is often helpful, as is demystification of the process by describing fully the procedure.

Sources of Data

There are two main sources of data in the assessment interview, the *content* (what people say) and the *process* (what people do). The *content* includes not only the information shared but also what is omitted or avoided. It also includes the family's interpretation of what has been said. The *process* is the manner in which people behave and their ways of relating to one another.

In the previous example the content was the mother's statement that "this was a typical pattern", that is, the identified patient often resisted answering questions. The process was that whenever the patient did not reply immediately, his mother would speak for him, showing him that she really did not expect him to answer for himself.

Assessment Format

Various formats are possible, each providing a particular sort of information. The identified patient can be seen alone or with the parents, the whole family, or any subgrouping of its members.

Unless the identified patient is very young or the family refuses to be involved, a family diagnostic interview is a good place to start, as it is helpful to understand clearly the family environment, of which the child is an integral part. Such a beginning often relieves tension and anxiety, making the child feel less singled out by focusing on the family interaction. Adolescents, in particular, respond well to this kind of interviewing, seeing it as an opportunity not only to hear what is being said about them but also to defend themselves and share information about other family members.

After first making the family comfortable, the interviewer begins to explore their expectations and their perception of the problem. A clear picture of the behaviour that concerns them, along with as much data as possible about predisposing, precipitating, and perpetuating factors and a description of the nature and success of earlier attempts to deal with the problem are then obtained. One encourages family members to talk together and comment upon what is said, and, while they do so, the interviewer observes how the system operates, checking with the family to see if observed patterns of interaction represent their typical behaviour. A history of the family can then be obtained, beginning with the childhood of the parents, following through to the present. Even young children will listen to stories of the past. Their reactions can be quite revealing, saying much about the relationships, structure, and problem-solving methods of the family. Broder, Minuchin, and Satir have discussed in more detail the mechanics of such interviews.[5, 16, 23]

Some assessments can be completed with the whole family present, but for most some separate interviewing is required. This is particularly true if the identified patient is very young, where there are family secrets, persistent scapegoating, severe marital conflicts, or fear of speaking out. The parents, in such cases, can be interviewed alone while the child is interviewed by himself, via play or discussion, depending on age.

The younger the child, the more likely one will utilize play rather than just talking as a vehicle for communication. A variety of play materials are made available, and the child is allowed some freedom to explore, play, and communicate spontaneously. Rapport is established, and what the child thinks, what he plays with, and the way he plays and relates to the interviewer are observed. Toys and drawings may be used to explore how the child feels about the problems that led up to the assessment. Some examiners structure the interaction; others allow it to flow freely. Should novice examiners feel unsure of themselves and their skills at conducting an assessment of a young child, a less active, observational stance will be helpful, allowing the child freedom to use the play materials and come to the therapist when ready. For those preferring a more structured format, the following can be used to tap the fantasy life of the child and to outline main areas of conflict:

1. Puppet play.
2. Drawings, along with stories the child makes up about what he has drawn.
3. Three wishes.

    Mr. and Mrs. A. requested an assessment of their ten-year-old daughter Joanne to determine which of them should receive custody. When asked directly with whom she would rather live, Joanne refused to commit herself. Her three wishes, however, included a trip to England, one thousand dollars, and a new house. Asked what she would do with these she said that she wanted the trip to have a holiday with her grandparents, and the money to spend on the trip. When asked about the new house, she replied that she and her siblings would live in it with their mother, far away so that her daddy would not be able to visit.

4. The animal question, that is, "If you were to be turned into an animal, but could choose what kind of animal you would be, which would you choose, and why? Give three choices."
5. The squiggle game, that is, the child is told to complete a meaningless line or "squiggle" into a picture about which he then tells a story.

    Daniel, a bright nine-year-old, was referred because of stubborn disobedience, soiling, nocturnal enuresis, extreme sibling rivalry, and increasingly direct statements that he felt unwanted. During an assessment, he converted a nondescript squiggle into a picture of a Martian. When asked what the Martian was doing on Earth, Daniel replied that he left Mars because nobody there appreciated him, not even his family. When asked why not, he suggested that it was because the Martian had a funny head and was different from everyone else in his family; this was why no one liked him, and why he used to get so angry and get even with them. But all that did was make the other Martians like him even less, so he had decided to leave Mars searching for a planet where somebody would appreciate him.

6. The house—tree—person test.
   The child is given a blank paper and is told only to draw a house, a tree, and a person. Given good dexterity and co-operation, this test is thought to reveal something about how the child views himself (his self-concept), his body, and his relationship with others.
7. Of all the people in the world, which three would the patient choose to take with him to live on a desert island?

More information on the nature of play and on how to carry out diagnostic play interviews has been presented by Allen, Rich, Werkman, and Winnicott.[1, 21, 30, 31]

Adolescents, usually, are able to co-operate during an assessment, if initial apprehensions or resentment at being assessed have been worked through. Only after trust and rapport have been established can one proceed to discuss emotionally painful or conflicted areas. Holmes and Meeks have described in detail the interviewing of the adolescent.[12, 14] (For a further discussion of issues and problems in interviewing adolescents, see Chapter 2.)

While the identified patient is being seen alone, the parents may be interviewed by an associate who attempts to understand each parent as an individual, their marital relationship, and their functioning as parents. Other emotionally laden material or hints of secrets, including discussion of the sexual relationship where indicated, might be explored as well. If the parents have strong feelings about discussing their relationship and, in particular, any differences in front of their children, their wishes should be respected.

Organization of Material

Appendix 4-1 presents an outline for the organization of data collected. It begins with identifying data and moves through the history of present and past difficulties, the history of the family, and development of the identified patient to a recording of the examination. It ends with a formulation, that is, the pulling together of the examiner's understanding, and a proposed treatment plan.

In preparing a written record, one should make clear the source of one's data, indicating which come from direct observation and which from inference or hearsay. Too often inaccurate data are recorded, transmitted, and by virtue of having been written in a record, soon become considered hard fact.

In Appendix 4-2 is an elaboration of the assessment outline of Appendix 4-1. Points may be added depending upon the needs of the setting or the nature of the problem. This is intended merely as a guide. Data may not be available or even relevant for all subsections. An obsessive attempt to fill all sections would sacrifice all spontaneity; clinical judgment and common sense must prevail.

Problems in Assessment

Aside from the already mentioned difficulty of having to juggle many different tasks at one time, there are some specific situations that do arise which can cause problems. It is sometimes difficult to keep younger children involved, as play and other non-verbal behaviours are their major modes of communication.[15] Parents and older siblings have better verbal skills and can give information quickly. It takes practice to actively include young children, remembering to talk *to* them rather than *at* them and to avoid acting as if they are not there.

In individual interviews, younger children may refuse to leave their parents in the waiting room. One can invite the parent into the playroom with the child. When the child is settled and more comfortable with the examiner, the parent may leave quietly. Reassurance about where the parent is waiting, for even a short visit, may be necessary for the very anxious dependent child.

In spite of all attempts to allay fears and establish rapport, some youngsters remain silent and unco-operative. How the family deals with them can be quite instructive. Frequently, however, their resistance cannot be resolved in a single session. Very rarely, admission to hospital with continuous observation may offer the only way to clarify the nature of the problem.

Fear, anger, or a feeling of being blamed may also block the communication of the older child or adolescent during the family diagnostic interview. Scapegoating, almost always an indication of covert conflict between the parents, may be a problem. The examiner can identify and label the process, help other members explore and accept responsibility for their part in the total problem, focus on other areas or move to longitudinal history-taking. Severe scapegoating that persists in spite of the above suggests a shift to individual interviewing to avoid aggravating existing psychopathology.[25] (For a discussion of scapegoating and its role in family homeostasis, see Chapter 3.)

In Canada, one cannot legally examine a child* without paren-

*"Child" is here used in the legal sense, since definitions vary from jurisdiction to jurisdiction.

tal consent. However, a child may leave home at sixteen. Although the legal status between age sixteen and eighteen is not clear, the law generally supports the giving of help even without parental consent to this age group.[28]

On occasion one parent (or sibling) may refuse to be involved. At times, what the family reports as a refusal to participate is, in fact, engineered by the apparently co-operative members. Direct telephone contact with the missing one(s) explaining the importance of their involvement can sometimes solve the problem. Should this fail, one would have the options of working with the members present, of finding other ways of involving the missing member, or of refusing to see anyone unless the family is complete. One would not usually refuse an assessment because one family member will not, or cannot, attend. After assessment, however, one might well consider it destructive to begin treatment with the incomplete family.

> John, age eleven, was brought to the Centre because of rebelliousness, stealing, and truancy from school. His mother refused to allow her new husband to be involved in the assessment, saying that John was her son and hence her problem. It emerged that mother would not allow the step-father to discipline John, protecting and covering up for John should he attempt to limit or criticize John's behaviour. The examiner confronted the mother with how the boy was manipulating and how she was preventing her new husband from becoming a full member of the family. She was told that therapy could proceed only if she would allow John's step-father to participate.

In other situations, one might decide to move on into treatment without the missing member, making the lack of involvement a point of therapy.

> Margaret, at age fifteen, had had a brief psychotic episode after taking LSD at the suggestion of her older brother. Margaret's family was large and chaotic. When the assessment findings were presented to the family, Margaret's mother emphatically refused to participate in the proposed course of family therapy. She recognized the need for change within the family but justified her refusal to take part on the grounds that she was tired of carrying the responsibility for the total family only to be

> blamed when anything went wrong. Her husband, who had indeed tended to leave most of the burden of parenting to his wife, was, on this occasion, prepared to become involved in the treatment. The therapist, therefore, decided in this case to begin treatment without Margaret's mother, defining the family's first task as that of determining why the mother was unprepared to participate and what they might do about it. By the fourth session, the mother had agreed to attend and to take an active part in the treatment.

What the client really wants from the assessment may not be apparent immediately. There may be unrecognized or unstated objectives, such as a desire to place the child outside the home, a wish to obtain evidence for court, an attempt to use the therapist as a judge or policeman. Unless the examiner and client can agree upon the goal of intervention, the patient will leave dissatisfied and the examiner will have wasted considerable time and effort providing one service when another was desired. The process of exploring unrecognized objectives with the family may in itself provide considerable clarification and relief, as it may be guilt about these very issues that keeps members from stating openly and beginning to deal with their major concerns.

As the rights of children are increasingly recognized it is becoming more and more common for courts to seek the advice of expert witnesses in questions of custody. One can usually be most helpful by refusing to align oneself with one side or the other while remaining available to act from a neutral position to advise the court.[6] By so doing, one can assess the total family situation and determine the best interest of the child while minimizing undue influence by one or other parent.[9] (See Chapter 20.)

Probably the most difficult, but least obvious, problem occurs when the examiner's own feelings are touched in such a way that they interfere with the assessment process. This is commonly termed counter-transference, that is, the professional's "partly unconscious or conscious emotional reaction to his patient".[2]

> Dr. K., a beginning resident, was confronted with a cheeky five-year-old girl who began to climb on the desk, throw toys on the floor, splash water and paint. She totally disregarded his pleas to stop and play nicely. With his own rigid, rather punitive

background and his conscious wish to be unlike his father, Dr. K. felt he could not set firm limits on the girl or make her do as he wished.

In dealing with children it may be difficult not to feel strongly for the child and to side with him, ignoring the parents' position. Not only do parents affect their children; children have a major impact on parents. All too often, parents are blamed for the problems of their child by examiners and therapists responding more to unrecognized feelings left over from their own childhood than to the clinical situation they are supposedly assessing.

One cannot work equally well with all kinds of people and problems. One must know oneself well to recognize personal sensitivities and prevent them from interfering. A colleague with whom one can discuss openly one's reactions may be helpful. Indications for referral for mental-health consultation in such cases are listed elsewhere (see Chapter 24).

Contract-Making

Once the data have been collected, analysed, and organized to provide an understanding of what produced and perpetuated the difficulties and what can realistically be done about them, this understanding must be transmitted to the family and the identified patient.

The examiner's major impressions should be presented clearly in simple, explicit terms, illustrated if possible with examples that occur in the course of the assessment. The family should be helped to define concrete, visible, and realistic goals. If some intervention is being proposed, the nature of the suggested treatment, what the family are being asked to commit themselves to and the possible implications should be discussed directly. Practical aspects (e.g. appointment times, work schedules, fees) need to be explored along with more subtle emotional ones. It is difficult to make major decisions and change behaviour when the issues involved are not clear. Ideally, what needs to be said will be stated directly, kindly, and respectfully, providing, wherever possible, a face-saving way for the family to approach and make a commitment to change.

Giving the results of the assessment often produces great anxiety in the family. They may find it shameful and upsetting to admit that they are in trouble and in need of help. No matter how clearly information is presented, their anxiety may so interfere with their ability to listen that little may be taken in. At a later date it is not uncommon for people to claim they were never told the results of the assessment. More than one session may be needed to transmit the findings. At the second, one can assess what has been heard. Things misunderstood or not heard at all can be reviewed and distortions corrected. Then a contract to proceed may be negotiated.

In inherently healthy families, the assessment itself along with concrete suggestions arising from it, possibly including reading material, may be all that is required.[4, 18, 19] A follow-up session is advisable to see what has been put into practice and to ascertain if real changes have been made. One wants to be sure that claims that the problem has disappeared are not just a flight into health, i.e. avoidance or resistance.

If one is planning to work with the family oneself, one proceeds differently than if referral elsewhere is to be suggested. In the former instance, details of time, frequency, payment, format, goals, respective responsibilities, and expectations must be made explicit and agreed upon.[12, 27] In the latter, the family must be helped to accept the rationale of the referral and prepared realistically for what will occur. The referral agency should then be approached, supplied with a summary of the case and the expectations on referral, and asked if it can realistically provide the requested service. If not, one may have to refer elsewhere. There will be a certain duplication of effort, as most therapists like to reassess for themselves to be sure that they could work with the potential patient or client. Families will usually accept this if helped to understand the reasons. It is important to know what resources are available in the community. Whatever suggestions are made must be feasible. One must come to terms with the fact that it may be impossible to offer what is ideal because of the nature of the problem and the paucity of available facilities. It is better to set realistic but limited goals than to attempt the impossible and succeed only in frustrating everyone.

An adequate assessment is an essential step towards effective treatment. It must take into account the nature of the problem, the desires and capabilities of family and child, and the style of the therapist. At its completion, it should provide enough data to formulate a clear understanding of the problem and to suggest realistic plans for future management.

Appendix 4-1

OUTLINE FOR ASSESSMENT OF A CHILD AND HIS FAMILY

1. Identifying Data
2. Presenting Problems
3. History of Current Difficulties
4. History of Previous Difficulties, Reports, and Results
5. History and Development of Family and Identified Patient
   a) Parents' early life experiences
   b) Courtship of parents, marriage
   c) Arrival of children
   d) Growth and development of identified patient
   e) Current status of marital relationship and family
   f) Relation of family to extended family, community and society
   g) Significant medical and psychiatric history
6. Psychiatric Examination of Identified Patient and Family
   a) Biological functioning of identified patient
   b) Psychological functioning of identified patient (includes mental status)
   c) Family functioning
   d) Impressions of parents and siblings as individuals
7. Other Investigations and Examinations
   a) Physical, neurological, and laboratory examinations if indicated, with dates
   b) Psychological testing
   c) Family testing
   d) Social and environmental studies, including reports from schools and agencies
8. Diagnostic Formulation
9. Differential Diagnosis
10. Provisional Diagnosis
11. Management Plan
    a) Investigation
    b) Treatment Plan
12. Prognosis

Appendix 4-2

OUTLINE FOR ASSESSMENT OF A CHILD AND HIS FAMILY—EXPANDED FORM

General Comments

All data should be recorded, making clear the source of information in as succinct a manner as possible. One should not fill all subsections obsessively nor ask questions in exactly the order given here. Clinical judgment and creativity are essential. One should make clear what has been reported, what observed, and what merely inferred. Sections may need to be enlarged according to the needs of the examiner.

1. *Identifying Data*
   Full name, address.
   Date of birth. Natural, adopted, or foster-placed.
   Referral source.
   Current school grade and type of class; type of work where applicable.
   Dates, circumstances of assessment; persons present, duration of each contact, telephone calls.
   Sources of information and reliability.
2. *Presenting Problems*
   A listing in point form, in observable specific terms, of the current difficulties as seen by the parents, the referring agency, and the child, making clear any differences between what various people see as the major problem.
3. *History of Current Difficulties*
   This includes:
   - a description of the nature of the problems;
   - when they first began;
   - the manner in which they create difficulties, and for whom;
   - where and when they are manifest;
   - what triggers onset, makes them better or worse;
   - feelings about the problems and explanations given;
   - what has been attempted; duration, consistency of application and success;
   - what investigations have been done; how they came for help;
   - goals of various family members, referring agency in asking for help.
4. *History of Previous Difficulties, Reports, and Results*
   This includes an inventory of previous problems of the family, its individual members, and/or the identified patient:
   - duration, severity, relationship to current situation;
   - any previous help and attitude towards it;
   - what was done by family to attempt to solve the difficulties;
   - findings, including dates, of any previous tests or examinations.

5. *History and Development of Family and Identified Patient*

a) *Parents' early life experiences*

A brief review of each parent's early life focusing in particular on:
- the emotional tone;
- the quality of relationships within their families of origin and with peers;
- attitudes to conflict, discipline, sex, money, the law;
- affection-giving, fun;
- work experiences;
- dating patterns, including previous liaisons.

b) *Courtship of parents, marriage*

This includes:
- how they met;
- first impressions of each other;
- expectations of marriage and each other;
- early years of marriage, including sexual adjustment and ways of handling difference;
- recreation, work, living conditions, social relationships.

c) *Arrival of children*

Included here is data about each pregnancy;
- adoption or placement;
- personality of children;
- developmental milestones;
- establishment of routines;
- effect of new arrival on the family;
- the quality of the parental relationship.

If children were adopted or foster-placed, what information is available about the number and quality of previous placements, the reasons for adoption or fostering?

d) *Growth and development of identified patient*

An in-depth study is made of:
- the pregnancy, delivery, adoption, or foster placement; responses to loss;
- early constitution, growth patterns, and activities of the identified patient;
- any physiological or emotional insults or losses;
- pre-school personality and play patterns;
- emotional reaction to beginning of school, and development of academic, social, and physical skills;

quality and quantity of peer relationships;
how child spends his spare time;
particular strengths and aptitudes of the identified patient;
academic progress; attitude and success at school;
work history, where relevant.

e) *Current status of marital relationship and family*

Included here are general data about:
the parent couple;
all aspects of their relationship; sex, social life, work, health, economic state, plans for future;
the state of the whole family;
any economic or emotional insults or losses that may have affected all.

f) *Relationships of family to extended family, community, and society*

Data about the interaction of the family with the extended family, community, church and society in general; any contact with the judicial system; what sources of support are available?

g) *Significant medical history and psychiatric history*

Any illness, physical or mental, past or present; the severity, any sequelae, the effect on the individual and the family.

6. *Psychiatric Examination of the Identified Patient and His Family**

a) *Biological functioning of the identified patient*

Listed here are the physical attributes of the child;
his constitution;
development for age;
temperament;
dominance;
co-ordination and any neurological dysfunction, appropriateness of dress and manner to sex.

b) *Psychological functioning of the identified patient*

This heading is of major importance and broader than the usual mental-status examination. It should include:

i) general impressions;

*This outlines the areas that would be covered if the child were to be assessed by a child psychiatrist. This section is included both as an indication of what data the psychiatrist would consider important and as a guide to members of other professions who assess children as to the significance and organization of similar data.

ii) how the child relates to the examiner;
iii) behaviour (general observations, specific patterns and disorders);
iv) cognition (the process of comprehension, judgment, and reasoning; described as to content, function, and language);
v) perception, apperception (ability to receive accurately, store, integrate and retrieve sensory data from outside or within);
vi) sensorium (consciousness);
vii) affect (person's emotional feeling tone and its outward manifestations);
viii) relations to self (regulation of feeling, thinking and behaviour by self and others, plus attitudes towards the self both conscious and unconscious);
ix) insight (understanding of reasons for assessment, admission of difficulties, desire to change self and others).

c) *Family functioning*

In this section one is looking at the whole system of the family and how it operates, not at the individuals making up the system. The relationship between the presenting problem and the functioning of the family is important to ascertain.

The family functioning can be considered under

i) structure and organization (the individuals making up the family, how they relate to one another to form sub-systems, their roles *vis-à-vis* maintenance of homeostasis and the power hierarchy);
ii) decision-making and problem-solving (not only the methods used but who takes part and what and/or who creates a problem);
iii) behavioural control (methods, how applied, consistency and to whom, by whom);
iv) difference and disagreement (effect of variance and difference of opinion on the family and how it is managed);
v) autonomy (questions of individuation and emancipation and their effect on the family);
vi) expression and reception of affect (both positives and negatives are important as well as how they are communicated);
vii) communications (how messages are sent and received—function as well as content is important);

viii) areas of psychopathology or conflict specific to family.

d) *Impressions of parents, siblings as individuals;* their strengths and weaknesses.

7. *Other Investigation and Examinations* (a summary of findings from the past and current special tests done by examiner or others).
8. *Diagnostic Formulation*

   This is the most important part of the assessment as it is the pulling together of the significant findings with an explanation of how they came to be, leading to a diagnosis and workable plan for further management. It is not just a mini-history (summary) but an understanding of what the identified patient is and how he came to be in need of help at this time. It may be organized under

   i) a *brief* statement of the current problem
   ii) predisposing factors
   iii) precipitating factors
   iv) perpetuating factors
9. *Differential Diagnosis*

   This involves listing other conditions to be considered in arriving at a diagnosis. While members of some of the allied professions may consider diagnosis a purely medical procedure, the concept of differential diagnosis is included for a specific purpose. If the examiner, regardless of training or discipline, develops the habit of routinely thinking, "I suspect I'm dealing with, for example, a behaviour disorder, but what else might be contributing to the problem?" he is much less likely to fall into the trap of premature closure by thinking that the most apparent difficulty is the only or even the basic problem.
10. *Provisional Diagnostic Category*

    Which condition(s) mentioned in the differential diagnosis is considered, on the basis of the data available, to be the problem in this particular child and family?
11. *Management Plan*

    This should arise out of the diagnostic formulation and should be feasible and acceptable to the family.
12. *Prognosis*

    This should include a statement about the natural history of the problem as well as the examiner's estimate of what can be achieved if the treatment as outlined is instituted.

RECOMMENDED FOR FURTHER READING

1. ALLEN, F. H. *Psychotherapy with Children.* New York, W. W. Norton 1942.
—classic book on the subject.

3. AXLINE, V. *Play Therapy: The Inner Dynamics of Childhood.* New York, Houghton Mifflin, 1947.
—the point of view of a non-directive (Rogerian) psychotherapist.

4. BECKER, W. G. *Parents Are Teachers.* Champaign, Ill., Research Press, 1971.
—manuals suitable for giving to parents to teach basic behaviour approach to child management.

6. DERDEYN, A. P. "Child Custody Consultation". *Amer. J. Orthopsychiat.* 45: 791–801, 1975.
—this, along with reference 9, provides some basic principles for this increasingly important area.

7. ERIKSON, E. H. *Childhood and Society.* 2nd. ed. New York, W. W. Norton, 1963.
—classic book on personality development—a must.

8. *From Diagnosis to Treatment: An Approach to Treatment Planning for the Emotionally Disturbed Child.* New York, Vol. 8, GAP Publication no. 87. 1973.
—easily understood detailed discussion of the diagnostic process and its relation to treatment planning. Useful clinical examples.

9. GOLDSTEIN, J.; FREUD, A.; and SOLNIT, A. J. *Beyond the Best Interests of the Child.* New York, Free Press, 1973.
—excellent discussion of interactive psychological and legal problems related to child custody decisions.

12. HOLMES, D. J. *The Adolescent in Psychotherapy.* Boston, Little, Brown, 1964.
—a must for anyone working with adolescents—practical, sound theoretically, classic in its area.

13. KLINE, F.; ADRIAN, A.; and SPEVAK, M. "Patients Evaluate Therapists". *Arch. Gen. Psych.* 31: 113–16, 1974.
—interesting look from the patient's side.

14. MEEKS, J. E. *The Fragile Alliance.* Baltimore, Md., Williams and Wilkins, 1971.
—good introductory text to working with adolescents.

15. MILLAR, S. *The Psychology of Play.* New York, J. Aronson, 1974.
—reviews broadly all aspects of play.

16. MINUCHIN, S. *Families and Family Therapy.* Cambridge, Mass., Harvard University Press, 1974.
—comprehensive statement of this group's philosophy and method of family therapy—quite readable and gives clinical examples.

17. MOUSTAKAS, C. E. *Psychotherapy with Children.* New York, Ballantine Books, 1973.
—comprehensive discussion of play therapy.

18. PATTERSON, G. R. *Families.* Champaign, Ill., Research Press, 1971.

19. PATTERSON, G. R., and GULLION, M. D. *Living with Children.* Champaign, Ill., Research Press, 1968.

21. RICH, J. *Interviewing Children and Adolescents.* New York, Macmillan, 1968.
—easily readable, provides an excellent introduction to interviewing and working with children.

23. SATIR, V. *Conjoint Family Therapy.* Palo Alto, Calif., Science and Behavior Books, 1964. Rev. ed. 1967.
—one of the first books in this area and still a gold mine of practical information.

24. SCHWITZGEBEL, R. K., and KLOB, D. A. *Changing Human Behavior.* New York, McGraw-Hill, 1974.
—comprehensive, detailed book giving basic principles of changing behaviour—thorough but not easy reading.

26. STIERLIN, H., and RAVENSCROFT, K., Jr. "Varieties of Adolescent Separation Conflicts". *Brit. J. Med. Psychol.* 45: 299–313, 1972.
—points out that problems of child may in fact be related to those of his parents—has later enlarged this thesis into a book.

27. STUART, R. B. "Behavioural Contracting Within the Families of Delinquents". *J. Behav. Ther. Exp. Psychiat.* 2: 1–11, 1971.
—behavioural approach to working with families that has wide applicability.

29. WATZLAWICK, P.; WEAKLAND, J. H.; and FISCH, R. *Change: Principles of Problem Formation and Problem Resolution.* New York, W. W. Norton, 1974.
—outstanding look at the question of how to produce change—if it is not one already, it will be a classic.

30. WERKMAN, S. L. "The Psychiatric Diagnostic Interview with Children". *Amer. J. Orthopsychiat.* 35: 764–71, 1965.
—good outline of how to conduct the first interview.

31. WINNICOTT, D. W. *Therapeutic Consultations in Child Psychiatry.* New York, Basic Books, 1971.
—delightful book showing the work of a creative therapist.

ADDITIONAL READING

2. American Psychiatric Association, Committee on Public Information, *A Psychiatric Glossary.* 4th rev. ed. New York, Basic Books, 1975.

5. BRODER, E. A. "Assessment, The Foundation of Family Therapy". *Can. Fam. Phys.* 21: 53–5, 1975.

10. GOLOMBEK, H. "The Therapeutic Contract with Adolescents". *Canad. Psychiat. Assoc. J.* 14: 497–502, 1969.

11. GRAHAM, P., and RUTTER, M. "The Reliability and Validity of the Psychiatric Assessment of the Child. II: Interview with the Parent". *Brit. J. Psychiat.* 114: 581–92, 1968.

20. *Psychopathological Disorders in Childhood: Theoretical Considerations and a Proposed Classification.* New York, GAP publication no. 62, 208–69, 1966.

22. RUTTER, M., and GRAHAM, P. "The Reliability and Validity of the Psychiatric Assessment of the Child. I as in title of article: Interview with the Child". *Brit. J. Psychiat.* 114: 563–79, 1968.

25. STEINHAUER, P. D. "Reflections on Criteria for Selection and Prognosis in Family Therapy". *Canad. Psychiat. Assoc. J.* 13: 317–21, 1968.

28. WATT, S. "Adolescent Medical Care: A Legal Denial of a Basic Human Right". *Ont. Med. Rev.* 38: 623–27, 1971.

UNIT THREE: **Common Syndromes in Child Psychiatry**

GORDON WARME

5. Childhood Developmental Problems

Normal childhood development proceeds through a succession of more or less differentiated phases. Each of these phases confronts the child with specific cognitive, emotional, and social demands. These demands, at times, conflict with one another. The biological urge to satisfy hunger by grabbing food with the hands, for example, conflicts with the social demand that the child learn a set of table manners in order to please his parents. The psychological drive to stay close to mother conflicts with the social demand that the child separate from her to attend school.

Almost all children at some point in their development experience stress that results from the difficulties of integrating and adjusting to the powerful but conflicting biological, psychological, and social demands specific to their age. At times, this stress may lead to the development of behaviours (signs and symptoms) that are upsetting to the child, the parents, or others. These behaviours, if moderate and transient, may have no real significance. The same signs and symptoms, however, if excessive or prolonged, may indicate that the child is experiencing significant difficulty and is in need of help for what is now termed a *developmental problem*.

One cannot say that a developmental problem exists just from the presence of signs and symptoms. It is neither the presence nor the nature of the symptoms but their duration, their extent, and the degree to which the child's over-all development and adjustment are interfered

Table 5-1

Normal Child	*Child with Developmental Problem*	*Child with Psychoneurosis*
May show signs and symptoms —of moderate degree —of transient duration	Signs and symptoms are excessive and prolonged.	Signs and symptoms may appear the same as those of the child with a developmental problem, from whom he can be differentiated only by the history.
Onset of symptoms is related to accentuation of stresses of ongoing development.	Onset of symptoms is related to accentuation of stresses of ongoing development.	Symptoms do not seem related to a developmental stage.
Symptoms are transient.	Symptoms are time-limited and should recede in response to parental guidance and the passage of time.	Symptoms are persistent and relatively independent of external events.
No intervention indicated.	Assessment is indicated. Minimal, if any, treatment will be required.	Following an adequate assessment, treatment is indicated †

* For further discussion of the child with psychoneurosis, see Chapter 6.
† For further discussion of methods of treatment, see Chapter 22.

with that determines whether or not a problem requires intervention. Furthermore, the signs and symptoms of the child with a developmental problem may be identical with those of the child with a psychoneurotic disorder. An essential feature of a psychoneurosis is the persistence of symptoms that are unrelated to a developmental stage and relatively independent of external events. Developmental problems, on the other hand, are clearly related to critical developmental periods and can be more easily modified by parental guidance and the passage of time. Only after an adequate assessment of the child's symptomatic behaviour, of his general development, and of his over-all adjustment can one determine whether one is dealing with a normal child, a child with a developmental problem, or a child with psychoneurosis.

In general, one can identify two main constellations of factors that may bring about abnormal responses to the stress of normal development:

1. *A sudden increase in routine external demands upon a basically normal child.* An example would be the social demand that a child

control his bowel and bladder function. This clashes with the biological urge for immediate evacuation, leaving the child torn between two contradictory wishes, that is, the desire to empty the bowel and the wish to conform to parental demands. In other words, the child is in psychological conflict. While toilet-training is achieved in most families without major upset, occasionally this normal demand can precipitate a struggle between parent and child that can reach crisis proportions. Similarly, the expectation that a child separate from his mother and attend school is one usually carried out without major difficulties. If either mother or child, however, is not psychologically ready for such a separation when the chronological age of the child demands it, the resulting stress may lead to the youngster showing abnormal behaviour. Additionally, the family may react in ways that can aggravate and fix the disturbance.

2. *The inability of a basically normal child to cope with biological changes.* Developmental problems may originate not from an increase in social demands, but from a child's inability to deal successfully with a normally occurring increase in his internal (i.e. biological and psychological) drives. The upheavals of adolescence illustrate this point well. The primary physiological increase that occurs with pubescence is the upsurge of aggressive and sexual tensions. Simultaneously, the child's psychological need for independence urges him to begin relinquishing his dependency on his parents. Finally, social pressures induce him to assume mature heterosexual and vocational roles. The average adolescent is able to assimilate these overlapping demands without excessive difficulties. Two groups of teenagers, however, may respond to these by developing psychological symptoms. Children who enter puberty never having gained a successful and consistent control over their impulses may show uncontrolled aggressive and sexual behaviour in response to the sudden increase in sexual and aggressive tensions; multiple crises for these children and their families will likely result. In contrast, children who enter puberty with their impulses tightly over-controlled may experience a different sort of crisis. The clinical picture will be dominated by the excessive defences called into play to counter the physiological increase in basic sexual and aggressive drives—for example, a boy who suddenly becomes acutely phobic or an adolescent whose asceticism only partially masks his preoccupation with sexuality.

While the focus in this chapter is on developmental problems of children, similar reactions to marriage, to parenthood, to work promotions, to turning forty, to retirement, etc., are examples of developmental problems occurring in adults.

Classification

In the area that covers the majority of problems presented by growing children, the most useful classification and differentiation of symptoms has been provided by the Group for the Advancement of Psychiatry (GAP Report no. 62). The GAP report divides symptom clusters into three categories:

1. Healthy responses: a) developmental crises,
   b) situational crises,
2. Reactive disorders,
3. Developmental deviations.*

1. HEALTHY RESPONSES

a) *Developmental crises* include reactions of a brief and transient nature related to such normal developmental tasks as mastering motor skills, acquiring a sense of trust, achieving autonomy and industry. Examples would include the "stranger" anxiety of the eight-month-old child, many fears in middle childhood, and the majority of the "problems" of adolescence.

b) Transient *situational crises* are merely the converse of the above. They occur when unusual external stresses temporarily upset the child's psychic homeostasis. Normal but time-limited upsets in response to the death of a parent, to the separation or divorce of the parents, or to the birth of a new sibling are typical examples, and the occurrence of these crises is to be seen as a manifestation of normal psychological functioning.

2. REACTIVE DISORDERS

Reactive disorders are ones in which the response to environmental events or situations extends beyond the line dividing healthy responses from pathological ones. The term implies that the usual coping devices are not working successfully, and that corrective action is required to

*The Developmental Deviations, included in the GAP classification under the more general category of Developmental Disorders, are a separate category additional to the problems encompassed by the introductory remarks.

avoid the likelihood of more permanent disability. Unusually severe and prolonged reactions to the death of a parent or to parents' marital breakdown would be examples.

3. DEVELOPMENTAL DEVIATIONS

Developmental deviations are "those deviations in personality development which may be considered beyond the range of normal variation in that they occur at a time, in a sequence, and in a degree not expected for a given age level or stage of development" (GAP). Developmental deviations are not necessarily fixed; they often respond readily to environmental help or therapeutic remediation. They can also, however, represent the earliest precursors of psychoneurotic behaviour and personality disorders.

Basically most developmental deviations have a strong biological origin. Some affect the total functioning, whereas others apply only to specific areas or single dimenstions. Specific disorders include:

a) *Motor developmental deviations:* hyperactivity; hypoactivity; difficulties in co-ordination. (In passing, it should be noted that some recent work would argue for classifying the "hyperactivity syndrome" as a disorder of attention. For further information, see Chapter 10.)
b) *Sensory developmental deviations:* hypersensitivity or hyposensitivity; hyperreactivity or hyporeactivity.
c) *Speech developmental deviations:* (excluding deafness, psychosis, and deliberate opposition to speech); disorders of rhythm and phonation; precocity of style and content of speech.
d) *Cognitive developmental deviations:* included here are deficits in symbolic and abstract thinking, dyslexia, dyscalculia, limitations in auditory or visual learning, sequencing, synthesis, and production. Clinical examination can detect these difficulties, but appropriate intervention requires precise analysis of the defect through specific psychological test procedures. See Chapter 12.
e) *Social developmental deviations:* these disorders include precocious, delayed, or erratic patterns of social interaction, e.g. marked shyness, dependence, impulsive aggressivity, and separation difficulties. These are contributed to both by constitutional factors (Chess) and by the influence of the environment and its reactions.
f) *Psychosexual developmental deviations:* these disorders refer to delay or precocity in sexual curiosity, sexual identification, and

sexual behaviour. They include problems of sexual identity that encompass mannerisms of speech and behaviour, choice of friends, or interests and activities more usually associated with the opposite sex.

g) *Affective developmental deviations:* these include emotional reactions such as anxiety, elation, depression, apathy, or marked overcontrol when these tendencies exceed the normal response to the environment, yet are not sufficiently marked and fixed to require a diagnosis of neurosis or psychosis.

h) *Integrative developmental deviations:* these include, in the absence of a personality disorder or psychosis, difficulties in impulse control, low frustration tolerance, and uneven or unusually pronounced use of such defences as denial, projection, etc.

In considering these developmental deviations, one must remember that it is the interaction between these innate, constitutional tendencies[13] and the child's environment that determines behaviour and influences personality development. Any given constitutional pattern (e.g. passivity or emotional sensitivity) may be welcomed and encouraged in one family but attacked and rejected in another. At times, psychological factors such as infantile fantasy may affect the child both directly, by shaping his behaviour, and indirectly, as when fantasy-derived behaviour elicits an altered response from the environment.

> Jimmy, age seven, was struggling with intense feelings of resentment and competition with his father. He was so fearful of how his father might retaliate if he were to express even normal aggression that he became timid, inhibited, and effeminate. These fears were greatly exaggerated, rooted in Jimmy's fantasies of punishment for daring to resent his father. Actually, Jimmy's father, who could not understand why his son was so fearful of him, could have tolerated directly aggressive or challenging behaviour much better than he could his son's timidity and effeminacy. These frightened and disgusted him, causing him to withdraw from and reject his son.

These developmental deviations have a number of common characteristics:

1. Frequently they are seen together; for example, hyperactivity, emo-

tional lability, speech problems, and difficulty with abstract thought may co-exist.

2. There is commonly a family history of a similar disorder.
3. Frequently the symptoms improve in adolescence, due to physiological or social maturation or increased coping skills. This is not always so, and at times only part of the problem may remit; for example, the hyperactivity may disappear, leaving a disabling attention disorder.[4]
4. The presenting clinical picture may change; for example, the child who was hyperactive when he was five has a poor prognosis for over-all social adjustment, and many have persisting abnormalities of personality often associated with criminal behaviour.[29]

The more commonly occurring developmental disorders will be discussed within the framework of the major functional area affected, the age of appearance, and frequency.

Feeding Disorders

In the absence of organic causes, most feeding disturbances in the early months of life are due to the interactional problems between child and mother. Feeding disturbances are often seen on paediatric wards. A mother brings her child to the ward for in-patient investigation because of a failure to nurse properly. The mother is concerned because the child fusses, eats little, sleeps poorly, and gains weight very slowly. Many of these infants eat as soon as they are fed by an experienced nurse. In observing the mother's attempts to feed her infant, one can often see that she is tense, awkward, and unable to hold and comfort the child. Such mothers may become tense or inhibited by the child's behaving in ways to which they cannot respond in a comfortable, relaxed manner. Their tension may also be derived from extraneous (e.g. marital or financial) pressures. Alternately, the infant, by demanding mothering, may ignite within the mother psychoneurotic conflicts related to her own feelings about being a mother.

Some mothers are severely limited in their capacity to meet the emotional needs of their infants. When this is so, one often finds that the mother had difficulty having her own emotional needs met during her infancy. The resultant insecurity and feelings of deprivation interfere with her ability to make feeding a relaxed and comfortable situation for her infant. She takes the child's feeding response to her as a measure of her capacity to mother and interprets difficulties that arise as confirming her basic inadequacy. Thus the infant experiences being cared for as tense, frustrating, and upsetting rather than relaxing and satisfying.

Infants with mild feeding disturbances may present clinically with slow, irregular eating or with colic, which may have little long-term significance. Although congenital (temperamental) hyperactivity of the infant may predispose it to colic in any event, most cases of colic that come to the attention of nurses or physicians are clearly related to the "primary anxious over-concern of the mother".[36] This anxiety seems the key factor in determining which children will and which will not show these difficulties. Oldest children are more likely to be affected, as are those who have special significance to the mother by reason of sex, birth rank, difficulties of conception and pregnancy, or relationship to other children, for example, the child conceived in order to replace a child that died. The child who is special is often a source of concern and anxiety. Most feeding disorders are self-limiting, usually disappearing by three to four months of age. One can often avert the likelihood of their becoming permanent as well as other consequences by discussing with the mother her functions as a mother, encouraging her to rock and soothe the infant, demonstrating how this settles the baby, and providing healthy doses of reassurance.

Weaning

Most children wean from breast or bottle with ease. They provide the cues that they wish to drink from a cup or eat with a spoon, and the parents are usually delighted to respond. Only occasionally is weaning delayed beyond the age of nine to twelve months. Prolongation may indicate a pathological need on the mother's part for continued dependency and control. Since children initiate weaning when they are ready, the delay itself may not be a problem, but it can be the first sign of a skewed mother-child bond that will reappear in other areas of development as, for example, a series of battles for control as the child tries to assert his independence.

Pica

Pica is the persistent ingestion of inedible materials after the age of eighteen months. Normal children mouth inedible materials between the ages of five and twelve months, but thereafter the habit wanes. Pica occurs most often in children who have been physically and emotionally neglected, and frequently complicates some degree of retardation or brain damage in the child. In areas of poverty, children mouth and eat such materials to relieve hunger, possibly learning the habit from siblings. Wall plaster and paint, which in older buildings is lead-based, are common materials eaten, and pica is the most frequent cause of this kind of lead poisoning. Theories that pica is the child's attempt to remedy a nutritional deficiency have not been substantiated.

Pica merits a full investigation of the physical, mental, and social health of child and family. Primary preventive efforts directed at improving inadequate social conditions, such as deteriorated housing and overcrowding, are gradually showing an increased effectiveness. Most families of children with pica will require extensive support from social agencies, and occasionally, particularly in older children, psychological or psychiatric intervention for an individual child is indicated.

Sleep Disturbances

Sleep disturbances take many forms. Fears of going to sleep are common in the second year of life, and are often associated with toilet-training conflicts or with fears of separation from the mother. Between the ages of two and five, many children attempt to sleep in their parents' bed for comfort, closeness, and sometimes due to curiosity about what goes on in the parental bedroom. In general, sleeping with parents should be discouraged, but such advice cannot be given lightly. Some parents cannot follow such an instruction and are humiliated by their inability to comply, while others see such advice as preposterous and will not return for further interviews. *Sleep-walking* (somnambulism) can be associated with a developing hysterical neurosis, but more often it has no real clinical significance. *Nightmares* are normal between three and five years, as are night terrors, but they are more common in disturbed children. *Night terrors (pavor nocturnus)* are dramatic and frightening occurrences in which the child experiences terror and cannot be completely aroused for five to ten minutes though seemingly awake. He perspires, walks about in a panicky way, but once wide awake cannot remember what he feared. During the episode, the child seems to have a specific fear, often alternately clinging to and fleeing from his parents. It has been suggested that somnambulism, nightmares, night terrors, and enuresis (bed-wetting) may be associated with abnormalities in the central nervous system arousal function.[27]

Rocking Behaviour and Head-Banging

Infant rocking behaviour and head-banging cause great concern to parents. They have been identified as symptomatic of infantile psychosis and mental retardation. But while such an association does exist, these behaviours are also very common in perfectly normal children.

Breath-Holding Spells

This alarming behaviour can appear in children as young as six months, but is more usual between the ages of one and five. The breath is held in expiration in apneic spells that last about thirty seconds. By this time they are showing signs of apneic distress and, soon after, cyanosis. In a few cases, the breath may be held till some tetanic twitches occur or unconsciousness intervenes to end the episode. Rarely, convulsive episodes accompany the breath-holding attacks.

The child's parents often permit themselves to be blackmailed into great overindulgence in order to prevent further frightening attacks. They should be assured that adverse consequences do not occur and be encouraged to handle the spells with a minimum of fuss.

Enuresis

Enuresis is the involuntary passage of urine in persons over the age of four. 80 per cent of cases are nocturnal only, 15 per cent are both nocturnal and diurnal, and the remaining 5 per cent are enuretic only during the day. The condition is common. One-sixth of all five-year-olds are bed-wetters and the proportion declines with age, although about 1 per cent of the population remains enuretic into adult life. Boys are enuretic twice as often as girls. Bed-wetting occurs more frequently in lower socio-economic classes, and is correlated with speech and learning difficulties, lowered intelligence, and delinquency. Frequently, one of the parents or one of their siblings has a history of bed-wetting. The pattern can limit the child's social activities, interfering with overnight visits with friends or attendance at summer camps. However, bed-wetting at home does not necessarily mean bed-wetting away, nor does the temporary cure, for example, at summer camp, necessarily continue at home. These cases do, however, call into question explanations of enuresis that rely entirely on physiological processes, for example, small bladder capacity. It is common to differentiate between children who have never been dry (continuous enuretics) and those who have begun to wet again after having remained dry for an established period of time (intermittent enuretics). Physiological mechanisms are much more likely to contribute to continuous enuresis while intermittent enuresis is almost invariably of psychogenic origin.

As to management, the factor to which the child is reacting should be identified and dealt with accordingly, as should any major psychiatric disturbance identified.

For the majority of cases the following general measures are recommended:

1. Reassurance and suggestions for the parents about home management.
2. Restriction of fluids in the evening.
3. Awakening the child at night to urinate.
4. Establishing a reward system for dry nights, for example, stars on a chart or calendar, emphasizing the successes rather than the failures.
5. When child and family are concerned and motivated to get rid of the symptom, the conditioning device of "bell and pad" can be used. With this apparatus, the child's urination completes an electric circuit and rings a bell that awakens the child. This device has a high success rate when both parents and child wish to use it, and it usually does not give rise to symptom substitution, that is, the selection of an alternative expression of the psychological conflict. In turn, the success can improve the child's self-esteem and the family's comfort.
6. Imipramine therapy. For children over the age of six years, 25 to 75 mgm of imipramine at 8.00 p.m. are recommended. The drug can be given earlier if the wetting occurs early at night. After a three months' trial, the drug should be stopped, and the child should try without it, at least temporarily.
7. Many other medications have been advocated, including stimulants (to make children sleep less soundly and therefore awaken on signals of bladder fulness), sedatives, anticholinergic drugs, antihistamines, etc. Their success rate is limited and little better than the response to placebos. If medication is to be used, at present imipramine is the drug of choice.

Constipation and Encopresis

These two conditions will be dealt with together, as the factors that contribute to psychogenic constipation are present in an exaggerated form in the etiology and maintenance of encopresis.

Constipation in children is usually not a matter of concern if organic factors can be excluded. It is intermittent, self-limiting, and non-noxious, despite beliefs to the contrary among certain groups in the population. But occasionally younger children may retain faeces to the point where they become bloated and uncomfortable. The lower colon is loaded, and overflow incontinence of faeces may occur. The chief complaint, at this stage, may be soiling rather than constipation, which is discovered only on examination. This "functional megacolon" has to be distinguished from Hirschsprungs's Disease (aganglionic megacolon), in which there is an absence of psychological and family problems, no overflow incontinence, and a different radiographic picture in response to a barium enema. In the extremely rare cases of uncertainty, the diagnosis can be confirmed by bowel biopsy.

Treatment of functional megacolon is still a matter of divided opinion. Many claim success from repeated enemas or from other manipulative techniques that physically evacuate the bowel, combined with threats of similar consequences for any recurrence. More common is the opinion that any such manipulative investigations or procedures are contra-indicated or should be kept to a minimum because of the risk of intensifying the frightening fantasies these children already have about their bowel functioning, thus aggravating and perpetuating the problem. Where there is a full and impacted rectum, however, the use of stool softeners, enemas, or even disempaction are appropriate and necessary, although grossly manipulative procedures should be avoided when possible.

Encopresis is passage of stools of normal consistency at times and places deemed inappropriate by society. The child seems unaware or vehemently denies that he has soiled his clothing, despite the obvious discomfort of bystanders. Some children attempt to mask the fact that they have soiled by hiding the excrement and soiled clothing around the house. They are easily found, and the hiding place may even seem designed to get the maximum reaction of anger and disgust from the environment, for example, in a drawer containing clean clothing or in the mother's purse. Such children frequently remain clean at school but soil immediately on returning home. Associated problems include enuresis, temper tantrums, oppositional behaviour, and learning disabilities. Cumulatively, the behaviour of these children invites hostility and severe rejection. Five times as many boys as girls are encopretic.

Not only these children but their families show obvious psychiatric and social problems. Most frequently, these focus on the issues of control, power, aggression, and rebellion.

Eric soiled many times daily, but only after school and much more frequently when with his mother. She was furious with him, and often beat him and retaliated for his soiling by forcing him to wash, dry, and iron his clothes although he was only six years old. He, in return, attacked her physically, but more recently had simply begun to soil more frequently. He seemed unaware of the soiling, but his "accidents" usually seemed to occur at just those moments that were most embarrassing for his mother.

Investigation revealed that Eric's parents had been through a period of severe marital conflict from which mother had retreated because of fear of her husband's physical brutality. At about the same time, she began bickering with Eric, her oldest son, as though substituting him as a safer person to argue with. Shortly thereafter, Eric's soiling began.

Counselling of the mother quickly enabled her to withdraw from the power struggle with Eric and his encopresis soon disappeared. With support, she learned to deal with her marital problems more realistically and to decrease her arguing in the marriage as well. After a few months, her husband became increasingly anxious and requested referral to another psychiatrist for his own needs, which centred around a long-standing inability to tolerate intimacy and tenderness within his marriage. As he responded to treatment, the marital conflict eased considerably, and Eric, now more secure, was left free to proceed with his development.

Encopresis almost always indicates the presence of significant disturbance in both child and family. Most cases should be referred for skilled psychiatric and psychological assessment. Follow-ups of these children indicate that while the soiling gradually disappears at the time of adolescence, problems in relationships with others and increasingly aggressive and antisocial behaviour continue to cause serious concern in many cases.

Faecal Play and Coprophagia

Occasional faecal play and even coprophagia (i.e. the eating of faeces) occur in some children in the course of normal development. If persistent, however, these behaviours warrant a thorough investigation of the child's and family's functioning. Spitz[36] has reported that faecal play has a significant correlation with maternal depression and unavailability.

Sexual Developmental Deviations

MASTURBATION

If one uses the term to include any casual, intermittent self-stimulation, masturbation is an almost universal phenomenon from the first year of life onward. Masturbation aimed at achieving orgasm is considerably less common in children than in adolescents, but does occur in about 13 per cent of children under the age of ten years.[25] It is thought to be more frequent in boys, but this opinion may simply reflect the fact that their masturbation is more obvious.

In most cases masturbation is of no clinical significance, and parents should be reassured and advised to ignore it. It is only a cause for concern when the child is preoccupied by it, when he fails to develop a sense of privacy about his sexual behaviour, or when the parents are unable to allow the child a normal degree of privacy. In the latter case, the problem is primarily the parents' but, because of their over-involvement, will often become the child's. Rarely, excessively open and highly ritualized masturbation may be associated with other obvious symptoms that suggest the presence of a serious underlying condition (e.g. psychosis).

Sexual curiosity, peeping, mutual exhibition of the genitals, and sex play, both heterosexual and homosexual, are common in children and not unusual in normal adolescents. Unless there is other reason for concern, the parents should be assured that this is normal behaviour.

DISTURBANCES OF GENDER IDENTITY AND SEXUAL ORIENTATION

As early as three or four years of age, some boys show clear patterns of speech and behaviour that are referred to as *effeminacy*. Some girls by the same age are clearly identified as tomboys, although what is considered masculine behaviour in girls does not seem to arouse the same anxiety in parents and others as effeminacy in boys. This is because many parents equate effeminacy with homosexuality, while tomboyish behaviour, unless extreme, is generally accepted as within the range of normal behaviour.

A child normally develops his gender identity by identifying with the parent of the same sex, who serves as a model for sexually appropriate behaviour, which the child unconsciously imitates. Other identification models include older siblings, peers, teachers, and other adults with whom the child comes into repeated contact. The basis for successful identification is a satisfactory and long-term relationship. If the relationship between father and son is poor by virtue of the father's being excessively harsh, punitive, and demanding or extremely passive, ineffectual, and distant, the child may be blocked from identifying with him and may instead turn to and identify with the mother. This is especially likely if, in the absence of mutual love and respect between the parents, the mother turns away from her husband and towards her son to seek the involvement and concern she is not getting within the marriage. Should the child identify across sex lines he will show a disturbance in sexual identity, and his modelling of himself on the mother may lead to the development of effeminate behaviour and speech. Similarly a girl who is blocked from forming a successful relationship with her mother may, instead, identify across sex lines and take on many of the characteristics she admires in her father.

While effeminacy in a boy indicates that sexual development has gone awry, most such boys have a definite male-gender identity (that is, they see themselves as boys), despite the behaviour manifestations of identity disturbance. This behaviour may or may not mean that the child is likely to become homosexual. Homosexuality, by definition, used to be considered a deviation or arrest in sexual development. More recently, however, this definition has been challenged, and the American Psychiatric Association has taken the position that homosexuality, in itself, need not be considered evidence of pathology. While the status of homosexuality is somewhat unclear, the fact remains that many parents are much upset by effeminacy or any suggestion of homosexuality, and other children can be merciless in their teasing of the conspicuously effeminate child or the child who is, or who is suspected of being, a homosexual. Those effeminate children who are seen by psychiatrists are often angry, negativistic, confused, or inhibited, both in the handling of their often intense rage and in the sexual area. Frequently their relationships with their fathers are almost non-existent, while their mothers are overprotective and overinvolved. They are frequently teased and rejected by their peer group. Generally, these are angry and unhappy youngsters who evoke a response from their environment that further increases their distress. A thorough psychiatric assessment is routinely indicated, with the aim of helping child and family correct the disturbance if possible and, in any event, of minimizing the destructive reactions to it.

Transexualism is a more definitive disturbance of gender identity, and its precursors are usually established by eighteen to twenty-four months of age. These children remain convinced that they are members of the opposite sex. The physical evidence of their genitals does not share this conviction, but only serves as a source of deep distress. This condition indicates a serious block in sexual development and requires thorough psychiatric evaluation and early treatment by a specialized team of experienced investigators.

Transvestism, that is, dressing in the clothes of the opposite sex, has increased significance at a later age. Occasional cross-dressing does not necessarily indicate the presence of significant psychopathology since it may occur in the course of normal development. However, where clear evidence exists that cross-dressing is becoming persistent or that it is being used repeatedly as a fetish and associated with masturbation, investigation is warranted, as 25 per cent of such children will go on to become homosexual in orientation. The remainder give up cross-dressing at adolescence.

Tics

Tics are sudden, quick, involuntary movements of related groups of muscles, which serve no apparent purpose. Kanner[24] reserves the definition of a tic for those movements that have become a well-established habit in children over the age of six. Using this definition, he found every case to have associated problems. The grimacing, blinking, nose-twitching, shrugging, etc., commonly seen in pre-school children are, by definition, excluded from the diagnosis of tic, and most subside if not too much attention is drawn to them. Tics must be differentiated from hyperactivity and from chorea (St. Vitus's Dance), in which the movements are variable and there are other evidences of rheumatic fever. Tics are difficult to treat, and drawing attention to them often makes them worse. After investigation, the wisest action is to attend to the tiqueur and his adjustment rather than to the tics themselves.

Maladie de Gilles de la Tourette is a rare condition of multiple tics, explosive outbursts of coprolalia (foul speech), and a bark-like cough. It begins at about age seven or eight, most commonly in children who show other evidence of developing personality disturbances. These symptoms are enormously distressing to affected children and their parents, as they attract almost universal attention to their bizarre and socially offensive behaviour. This disorder is a major source of embarrassment: it interferes with social relationships, elicits widespread misunderstanding and condemnation from the majority of those in the environment (who consider it purposefully offensive), and produces a disastrous effect on the child's self-confidence. Many of the symptoms of this disorder are relieved by the drug haloperidol, but in selected cases psychotherapy for child and family may do a great deal to minimize these psychological and social complications.

Speech Problems

Lisping (Sigmatism) refers to difficulty in pronouncing the sibilants (s, z, sh, zh, ch, j). These are the last sounds to be mastered, and lisping is defined as a persistence of this mispronunciation past seven years of age. Occasionally, like baby-talk, it is considered "cute" and persists because of subtle encouragement by the parents. For younger children, no intervention is required, as spontaneous recovery usually occurs, making speech therapy unnecessary. Speech therapy may prove more helpful for older children who actively wish to give up their lisping.

Delayed speech always has meaning, although the significance and the management may vary depending on the cause of the delay. The differential diagnosis includes infantile psychosis, psychoneurotic conflict (elective mutism), dependency in the overprotected child, deafness, mental retardation, and specific developmental speech delay. In the last of these, usually occurring in boys with a family history of speech delay, normal speech will develop but at a slower pace. They show no evidence of other problems and understand speech well. They do not impress one as refusing to speak, as do electively mute children.

Delays in motor development may result in articulation defects (mispronunciation) and in dysgraphia (poor handwriting). The latter may cause concern in school, but with correct identification of the problem the child's teacher will often prove more patient and understanding, particularly if it can be demonstrated that the child is learning normally despite the dyscoordination (see Chapter 12).

Stuttering is defined as interruptions in the flow of speech with blocking, repetition, explosiveness, and scanning. It appears in 1 to 2 per cent of children, occurring more frequently in the school years but with the incidence decreasing at puberty. There is a definite familial tendency, and boy stutterers outnumber girl stutterers by five to one. It is important to note that the normal repetition of words and phrases common in the speech of three-year-olds is not stuttering. Parents can become very concerned about these normal repetitions, not realizing that the speech of a stutterer is more commonly a repeating of the first sound in a word than of whole words or phrases. Children who stutter often have associated reading and writing problems. Older stutterers may grimace in attempts to force their speech, or the stutter may be replaced by a substitute act like stamping the foot. Still later so-called "hidden stutterers" may disguise their stuttering by acts such as staring into space, long hesitations, etc.

Four out of five stutterers recover spontaneously if not pressured. If they do not, special intensive training methods have been developed that, as part of the treatment, systematically desensitize the stutterer to anxiety-provoking situations that precipitate and perpetuate the stuttering. These methods are taught by speech therapists. Some children have associated psychiatric problems that may benefit from psychotherapy or counselling of child and family.

Nail-Biting

Forty per cent of children between the ages of five and eighteen bite one or more nails, and 18 per cent bite all ten nails severely and persistently. Some authors reserve the diagnostic term "nail-biter" for only the severe cases. Nail-biting can begin as early as one year of age, but the incidence peaks in boys at age twelve to thirteen and in girls at eight to nine.

Nail-biting is usually a simple tension-relieving mechanism that occurs in fidgety, somewhat anxious children. Generally, no intervention is indicated. Severe cases should receive a careful psychiatric assessment. Should one find evidence of significant persistent anxiety or other related neurotic problems, the child and family should be offered treatment for the underlying problem, not for the nail-biting *per se*.

Thumb- and Finger-Sucking

This is a tension-reducing act that occurs normally and commonly in infants. Excessive or insufficient gratification of the infant's oral-sucking needs may predispose the child to seek relief of tensions in this way. Children who suck their thumb and fingers are often serene, contented children. At times, thumb-sucking can become a highly erotized act, often associated with clutching a blanket or toy and occasionally associated with masturbation.

Thumb-sucking itself requires no intervention. When the child is old enough to wish to stop the habit, he often does so spontaneously or can be encouraged to do so by the practitioner and family. Dental consequences (malocclusion) must be watched for and may require treatment in older children.

Privation and Deprivation Syndromes

Children reared under certain abnormal conditions may show dramatic and long-term developmental disturbances exceeding any of those discussed earlier in this chapter. There are three groups of children to be considered under these headings:

1. Those suffering from *parental privation*. While they have never been separated from their parents, the quality of the parenting to which they have been exposed has been so unsatisfactory and inconstant that their ability to form an attachment to parental figures has never developed. This results in a persistent incapacity to form mutual relationships rather than self-centred ones.
2. Those suffering from *parental deprivation*. These are children who have formed a successful attachment to parental figures but were then separated from them. In response to the trauma of the separation, the child is forced into the situation where, until he can successfully mourn (i.e. emotionally give up) the lost parental figures, he will not be ready to fully accept (i.e. form a new relationship with) parental substitutes.
3. Some children, for example many of those who, following family breakdown, become wards of children's aid societies and child-welfare associations, have been exposed to both chronic privation and repeated deprivation. As a result, their ability to relate to and trust others has been grossly impaired. They have major difficulties in social relationships, frequently developing severe personality disorders of an asocial or antisocial nature in addition to chronic intellectual, emotional, and physical deficits.

Spitz[34] was the first to notice and describe the graphic effects on children of consistent neglect of their emotional needs. Infants (from birth to three years at the time of the study) were reared in an institution that met all their physical needs but ignored their need for maternal love, care, and stimulation. On follow-up after two years[34], 37 per cent of this group had died, mostly of marasmus or of intercurrent infections.

Those that survived showed delayed development, both emotionally and intellectually, and profound disruption in their development and capacity for social relationships. His historic and dramatic papers on what he termed "hospitalism" for the first time drew attention to the degree to which failure to meet children's emotional needs can impair normal development and even threaten life itself.

More recently Bowlby[7] has emphasized the long-term pathological consequences of parental loss, particularly between the ages of six months and six years. He has described the process of normal mourning as consisting of three stages: a *stage of protest*, which lasts as long as the child continues to hope that protest may bring reunion with the lost mother; a *stage of despair*, in which the child, having given up hope for the mother's return, slips into a period of sadness or "depression"; a *stage of detachment*, in which the child is able to separate from the lost parent, thus becoming free to form a new attachment with a parental substitute. Most probably, the vulnerability to parental loss in the first two years is not as great as once thought, provided that an adequate substitute parenting figure is provided quickly. Another important contributor, Michael Rutter,[31] maintains that as important as the loss of the parenting figure are the events that led to the loss and the alternatives supplied.

Nevertheless it is important to pay serious attention to Bowlby's contention that young children, by virtue of their immaturity and their inability to tolerate the pain that is so integral a part of successful mourning, often abort the mourning process. As a result, they never resolve their grief and never separate (i.e. detach) from the lost parental figure to a degree that will allow them to form the successful future attachments to parental substitutes essential to recovery, ongoing security, and continued development. The child's style of relating develops no further, and future human interactions remain infantile, narcissistic, and self-centred. In some cases the child may secondarily withdraw, turning increasingly to fantasy rather than to real people for his satisfactions. People to him are objects to be placated, used, manipulated, and discarded before they can discard him; this is the basis of the inability to form satisfying relationships and the asocial and antisocial behaviour. Other workers have questioned the extent of Bowlby's conclusions, but most agree that the young child cannot successfully complete mourning without adult assistance, and that such losses cause serious developmental interference.[37]

Less obvious, but much more frequent, than these dramatic

situations are those of the intact family where parents cannot give adequate emotional nurture to their children. Some parents are so obviously inadequate and helpless and so clearly unable to provide basic emotional needs for children that this emotional deprivation of the children is obvious. However, other parents, for example, those who are extremely narcissistic, can superficially appear quite adequate. But closer review reveals their inflated images of themselves, their constant need to be admired by others, and their inability to give to a child except in so far as it brings praise and reward to them, the parents. Such parents, often successful in the pursuit of the careers so necessary for the maintenance of their own self-esteem, often omit, ignore, or are unaware of their children's needs. While providing most lavishly for the children's physical and educational needs and giving all outward appearances of adequately fulfilling the parenting roles, they can impose a degree of emotional privation and create a vacuum sufficient to distort their children's personality development.

Parental death, divorce, and separation are deprivation situations discussed in some detail in Chapter 20. Battered children and many identified as suffering from "failure to thrive" have suffered such deprivation.

Conclusion

Childhood developmental problems assume protean forms. The most common error is to attribute them all to some form of "neurosis" and to recommend psychotherapeutic intervention. The second most common is to dismiss them as "just a stage—he'll grow out of it". Confidence in human resilience is justified when it is not misplaced. This chapter has tried to emphasize where and when to reassure and where it is right to be concerned. Time and care in interviewing, knowledge of normal child development, and the wisdom of accumulated experience will guide in good judgment for necessary and appropriate intervention.

RECOMMENDED FOR FURTHER READING

1. ANDERS, T. F., and WEINSTEIN, P. "Sleep and Its Disorders in Infants and Children: A Review". *Pediat.* 50: 312-24, 1972.
—relates sleep disturbances to stages of sleep, attempting to distinguish those that represent developmental deviations from those that are psychologically initiated.

4. BAKWIN, H., and BAKWIN, R. *Behavior Disorders in Children.* 4th ed. Philadelphia, W. B. Saunders, 1972.
—excellent, relatively brief descriptions of a very wide range of the disorders encompassed by the terms developmental and behavioural disorders.

5. BEMPORAD, J. R.; PFEIFER, C. M.; GIBBS, L.; CORTNER, R. H.; and BLOOM, W. "Characteristics of Encopretic Patients and Their Families". *J. Amer. Acad. Child Psychiat.* 10: 272-92, 1971.
—description of fourteen "typical" and three "atypical" encopretic cases, and the "pathologic complex" of organic, personality, and familial factors leading to persistent encopresis.

6. BLOCH, E. L., and GOODSTEIN, L. D. "Functional Speech Disorders and Personality: A Decade of Research". *J. Speech & Hearing Disord.* 36: 295–314, 1971.
—clear and comprehensive article critically reviewing research literature (1958–68), relating measured personality adjustment to the functional speech problems of articulation, delayed speech, voice, and stuttering.

7. BOWLBY, J. "Childhood Mourning and Its Implications for Psychiatry". *Amer. J. Psychiat.* 118: 481-98, 1961.
—a briefer review than Bowlby's recent volumes (1969, 1973) of his views regarding the consequences of separation and loss, and the nature of childhood mourning.

8. BOWLBY, J. "Grief and Mourning in Infancy and Early Childhood", in *The Psychoanalytic Study of the Child.* Vol. 15: 9–52. New York, International Universities Press, 1960.
—a technical but definitive statement and development of Bowlby's formulation of the process of mourning in young children and infants, followed by a critical discussion by three distinguished psychoanalysts.

11. BURNS, P.; SANDER, L. W.; STECHLER, G.; and JULIA, H. "Distress in Feeding: Short-Term Effects of Caretaker Environment of the First Ten Days". *J. Amer. Acad. Child Psychiat.* 11: 427-39, 1972.
—part of an extensive investigation into infant-caretaker adaptation in

the first eight weeks of life. Illustrates the effect of replacement of the primary caretaker at eleven days of life on the infants' "distress" or discomfort during feeding.

14. CONNOLLY, K. "Learning and the Concept of Critical Periods in Infancy". *Devel. Med. and Child Neurol.* 14: 705–14, 1972.
—advocates replacing the term "critical period" by "sensitive period". Advances the view that attention should be paid to processes and events of sensitive periods of early development rather than to their temporal characteristics.

15. EVANS, S. L.; REINHART. J. B.; and SUCCOP, R. A. "Failure to Thrive: A Study of 45 Children and Their Families". *J. Amer. Acad. Child Psychiat.* II: 440–57, 1972.
—explores the syndromes of failure to thrive (i.e. infants or children who fall below standard measurements in height or weight without apparent basis). Three groups were isolated, each with distinctive characteristics that could be used as indicators for prognosis and mode of treatment.

18. FRAIBERG, S. *The Magic Years.* New York, Scribner's, 1959.
—an excellent book for parents to read but so charming and full of information that every practitioner will enjoy it and learn from it.

19. FREUD, A. *Normality and Pathology in Childhood: Assessments of Development,* pp. 56–92. New York, International Univ. Press, 1966.
—a fundamental theoretical statement by one of the great contributors to child psychiatry.

20. FREUD, S. "Analysis of a Phobia in a Five-Year-Old Boy", in Freud, S., ed., *The Complete Psychological Works of Sigmund Freud.* Vol. 10: 3–152. London, Hogarth Press, 1909.
—a fascinating and very readable case study by the founder of psychoanalysis. The sexual roots of the boy's fears are dramatically revealed in the child's own words.

21. GRAHAM, P.; RUTTER, M.; and GEORGE, S. "Temperamental Characteristics as Predictors of Behavior Disorders in Children". *Amer. J. Orthopsychiat.* 43: 328-39, 1973.
—assessment of sixty children each with one mentally ill parent shows that certain temperamental characteristics can predict the development of later psychiatric disorder.

22. GREEN. R. *Sexual Identity Conflict in Children and Adults.* New York, Basic Books, 1974.
—presents a more detailed discussion of many of the issues related to sexual identity conflict.

25. KINSEY, A. C.; POMEROY, W. B.; and MARTIN, C. C. *Sexual Behavior in the Human Male*. Philadelphia, W. B. Saunders, 1948.
—this book is the product of an extremely thorough collection of facts about male sexual behaviour and is still an outstanding resource.

28. MAHLER, M. "On the First Three Subphases of the Separation-Individuation Process". *Int. J. Psya.* 53: 333–38, 1972.
—describes research findings from the intensive observation of the first three years of life. Advanced psychoanalytic theories are constituted from the data obtained.

30. RICHMAN, N.; STEVENSON, J. E.; and GRAHAM, P. J. "Prevalence of Behaviour Problems in Three-Year-Old Children: An Epidemiological Study in a London Borough". *J. Child Psychol. Psychiat.* 16: 277-87, 1975.
—discusses the prevalence of such behavioural problems as overactivity, wetting, soiling, and fearfulness in an epidemiological study of the behaviour of a random sample of three-year-olds.

31. RUTTER, M. "Maternal Deprivation Reconsidered". *J. Psychosomat. Res.* 16: 241-50, 1972.
—suggests that acute distress is due in part to a disruption of the bonding process, and that affectionless psychopathy may result from failure to develop family bonds by three years of age. Distinguishes privation from deprivation.

32. SCHWARZ, J. C.; KROLICK, G.; and STRICKLAND, R. G. "Effects of Early Day-Care Experience on Adjustment to a New Environment". *Amer. J. Orthopsychiat.* 43: 340–46, 1973.
—children in day-care from infancy were compared with children entering day-care at age three and four. Ratings of affect, tension, and social interaction supported the view that infant day-care does not lead to emotional insecurity.

33. SPERLING, M. "Sleep Disturbances in Children", in Howells, J., ed., *Modern Perspectives in International Child Psychiatry*. New York, Brunner/Mazel, 1969.
—emphasizes the role of the mother in producing abnormal sleep patterns in children.

34. SPITZ, R. A. "Hospitalism: An Inquiry into the Genesis of Psychiatric Conditions in Early Childhood". *Psychoanalyt. Stud. Child.* 1: 53–74, 1945.

35. SPITZ, R. A. "Hospitalism: A Follow-Up Report". *Psychoanalyt. Stud. Child.* 2: 113–17, 1946.
—these two by Spitz are classical papers which are strikingly con-

vincing in their demonstration of the pathological effects of the institutionalization of infants.

36. SPITZ, R. A., and COBLINER, W. G. *The First Year of Life*. New York, International Univ. Press, 1966.
—very comprehensive review of the first year of life from an ego-psychological (psychoanalytic) point of view. Important is the concept of "organizers" of psychic functioning.

38. WOLKIND, S., and RUTTER, M. "Children Who Have Been 'in Care'—An Epidemiological Study". *J. Child Psychol. Psychiat.* 14: 97–105, 1973.
—describes an epidemiological study of psychiatric disorder among ten-to-eleven year-old children who have histories of short periods in foster care or in a children's home. Suggests the need for preventive intervention for families seeking short-term placement "in care".

ADDITIONAL READING

2. ANTHONY, E. J. "An Experimental Approach to the Psychopathology of Childhood: Encopresis". *Brit. J. Med. Psychol.* 30: 146–75, 1957.

3. ASCHER, E. "Motor Syndromes of Functional or Undetermined Origin: Tics, Cramps, Gilles de la Tourette's Disease, and Others", in Arieti, S. and Brody, E. B., eds., *American Handbook of Psychiatry*. 2nd ed. Vol. 3: 800–807. New York, Basic Books, 1974.

9. BOWLBY, J. *Attachment and Loss*. Vol. 1: *Attachment*. New York, Basic Books, 1969.

10. BOWLBY, J. *Attachment and Loss*. Vol. 2: *Separation: Anxiety and Anger*. New York, Basic Books, 1973.

12. CHESS, S. "Healthy Responses, Developmental Disturbances and Stress or Reactive Disorders. 1: Infancy and Childhood", in Freedman, A. M., and Kaplan, H. I., eds., *Comprehensive Textbook of Psychiatry,* 1358–66. Baltimore, Williams and Wilkins, 1967.

13. CHESS, S.; THOMAS, A.; and BIRCH, H. G. "Behaviour Problems Revisited: Findings of an Anterospective Study". *J. Amer. Acad. Child Psychiat.* 6: 321–31, 1967.

16. FINCH, S. M. *Fundamentals of Child Psychiatry,* 64–93. New York, W. W. Norton, 1960.

17. FRAIBERG, S. "On Sleep Disturbances of Early Childhood". *Psychoanalyt. Stud. Child.* 5: 285–309, 1950.

23. NORNICK. E. J. "Healthy Responses, Developmental Disturbances and Stress or Reactive Disorders. 2: Adolescence", in Freedman, A. M., and Kaplan, H. I., eds., *Comprehensive Textbook of Psychiatry,* 1366–67. Baltimore, Williams and Wilkins, 1967.

24. KANNER, L. *Child Psychiatry,* 4th ed. Springfield, Ill., Thomas, 1972.

26. LEVY, D. *Maternal Overprotection,* 37, 196. New York, Columbia University Press, 1957.

27. LOWY, F. H. "Recent Sleep and Dream Research: Clinical Implications". *Canad. Med. Assoc. J.* 102: 1069–77, 1970.

29. MENKES, M. M.; ROWE, J. S.; and MENKES. J. H. "A Twenty-Five-Year Follow-Up Study on the Hyperkinetic Child with Minimal Brain Dysfunction". *Pediat.* 39: 393–99, 1967.

37. SZUREK, S. A. "The Child's Needs for His Emotional Health", in Howells, J., ed., *Modern Perspectives in International Child Psychiatry,* 157–99. New York, Brunner/Mazel, 1969.

PAUL D. STEINHAUER
GRAHAM BERMAN

6. Psychoneurosis, Behaviour Disorders, and Personality Disorders in Children

The child is born with universal basic needs (for food, sleep, stimulation, etc.) and with innate constitutional characteristics (more or less active, adventurous or timid, big or small, persistent or distractible, etc.). He will develop in a process of interaction with his family and the world.

From birth the child experiences continual bombardment by strong basic biological needs or drives. These include hunger, thirst, the need for elimination, for physical stimulation and pleasure, for aggressive release, for love and security. As long as these drives are left unsatisfied, the child will remain uncomfortable and tense.

Parents, like children, have their characteristic ways of behaving (rigid or flexible, involved or detached, verbal or action-orientated, etc.). The parents have the task of learning to understand and meet the needs of their child. Meanwhile the child is learning to adapt to the characteristics and routines of his family. Sometimes the needs of the child and those of his parents may not mesh; then a mismatch between the parents and child will occur—for example, when anxious, timid parents are blessed with a young Tarzan. Other conflicts may stem from a parent's neurotic difficulties (an obsessive-compulsive parent who cannot tolerate the child's normal messing).

Not too long after birth, usually in the second year of life, the environment, and especially the mother, begins to face the child with another, conflicting set of demands: she begins to insist that the child

Figure 6-1

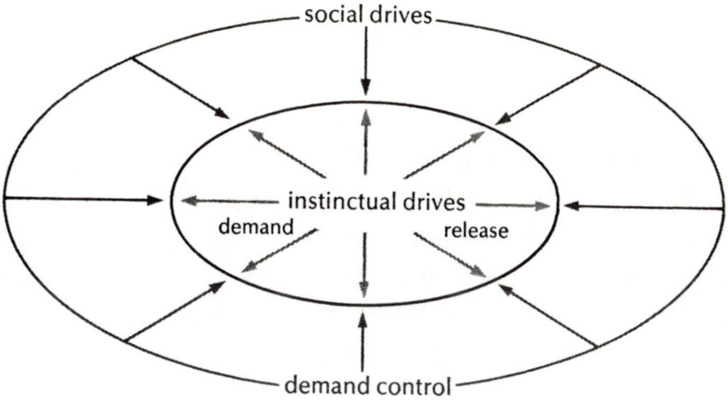

give up or modify the demands of some of his basic drives and endure the resulting discomfort in order to retain her approval and avoid being punished. A toddler's mother may, for example, insist that he remain hungry and uncomfortable if he asks for a snack shortly before supper. She may even become angry or punitive if he takes something anyway or remains annoyingly persistent in his demands. Similarly a two-year-old girl whose mother's enthusiasm for toilet-training greatly exceeds her own is faced with a choice every time she feels a powerful urge to move her bowels. Does she obey her sphincter (i.e. do it now—in her diaper—and feel better) or does she hold back and put up with the resulting discomfort until her mother places her on that cold, white, slippery seat with the hole too big for comfort? When a four-year-old boy sees his favourite toy in the hands of an ambivalently loved younger brother, he knows what he would like to do about it. Past experience, however, tells him that if he follows his aggressive impulses the younger brother will scream and his mother will be at least upset, if not spanking mad.

All of these situations have something in common: in each of them, the young child is torn between two conflicting sets of demands. (See Fig. 6–1.)

From within, the young child is faced with pressures from intense biological drives—hunger, elimination, sex, or aggression—that demand immediate satisfaction. But, increasingly, he is faced with an often incompatible set of social pressures which insist that he repudiate or modify some of the biological demands in order to remain loved and secure. Thus, gradually but increasingly, the child is pressured towards such socially acceptable behaviour as cleanliness, some degree of obedience, etc.

Even the child who feels there is nothing wrong with his demand-dominated behaviour knows he will be punished if he fails to control it. This tension is especially hard on the pre-school child, whose drives are intense and who has not yet brought them under effective control. As a result, the toddler often demands immediate gratification, only to burst with those random, diffuse explosions of frustration and rage we call temper tantrums when the gratification is not immediately forthcoming. Thus the young child's control over his basic biological drives is precarious; he is in constant danger of being overwhelmed at any time by intense drives, which, should they escape his insufficient controls, will threaten his need for love and security by exposing him to attack and rejection.

Between the ages of four and six, yet a third set of forces is called into play as the child begins to identify with the key people in his environment. The term *identification* refers to an ongoing process of imitation that occurs largely beyond the child's conscious awareness. As the child identifies with the parents, their standards of good and bad or right and wrong increasingly become his standards. At first, it is as if he had inside him a tape recording of their voices saying to him, "If you do that, we will be angry." Later, as this inner echo of the parents' values becomes more integrated within his own personality, the child avoids misbehaving not just to placate others but to live in peace with what he is now increasingly aware of as his conscience. Thus by this stage what was once a two-way struggle between biological drives and social demands is now joined by the newly developing conscience, the representative within the child's own personality of the values of the parents and of society. As he grows older and as identification proceeds, what was once primarily a conflict between his biological needs and the demands of the social environment becomes more and more an internal one between the biological needs and the developing conscience (See Fig. 6–2).

The result of the ongoing conflict is the generation of anxiety. Anxiety can be defined as the fear of impending danger. The danger in this case is that the biological drives will prove too much for the child's available controls, causing him to lose control of his impulses. This would be dangerous because it would leave the child vulnerable to attack either from the environment (punishment or rejection) or from the

Figure 6-2

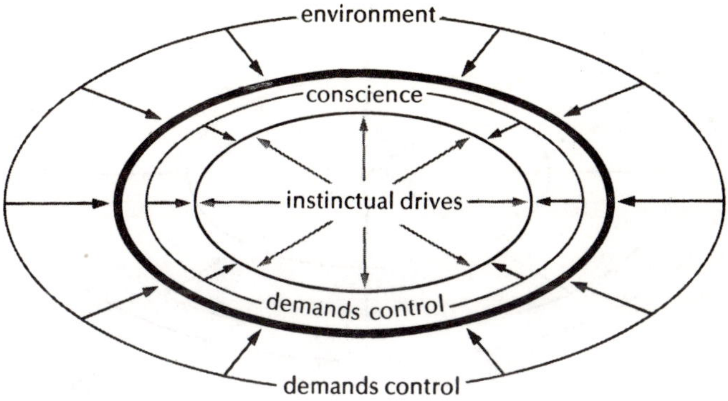

conscience (guilt or shame). No child can totally avoid anxiety; it is constantly being produced by the continual inner conflicts described above, as well as by the inevitable frustrations and disappointments of everyday life. To some extent, particularly as he grows older and is in better control of his feelings, he learns to be more adept at using thinking and talking to anticipate, to avoid, or at least to try to resolve situations that are potentially anxiety-provoking. When this proves impossible and when anxiety cannot be avoided, he develops ways of minimizing his discomfort and containing the unacceptable drives whose presence is generating so much anxiety. These are called *defence mechanisms.*

It is not just the neurotic or emotionally disturbed child who uses defence mechanisms. Since we all have to deal with the anxiety generated in the course of normal living, we all use defence mechanisms every day of our lives to keep our anxiety within tolerable limits.

> Consider the case of the student who, through lack of preparation, fails an examination. An appropriate response might be for him to say, "Boy, an I ever stupid (irresponsible, or lazy). I didn't put nearly the time into preparation that I should have." More frequently, however, the student is likely to soften the blow (i.e. defend himself against his feelings of guilt and shame) by some response such as, "What a stupid (unfair, or excessively hard) exam. . . . With a teacher like that how can anyone be expected to learn mathematics (physiology, or psychiatry)? Besides who cares? Who needs it? It's irrelevant. So let's forget it and get high (on television, alcohol, drugs, or sex)."

Figure 6-3 The Normal Child

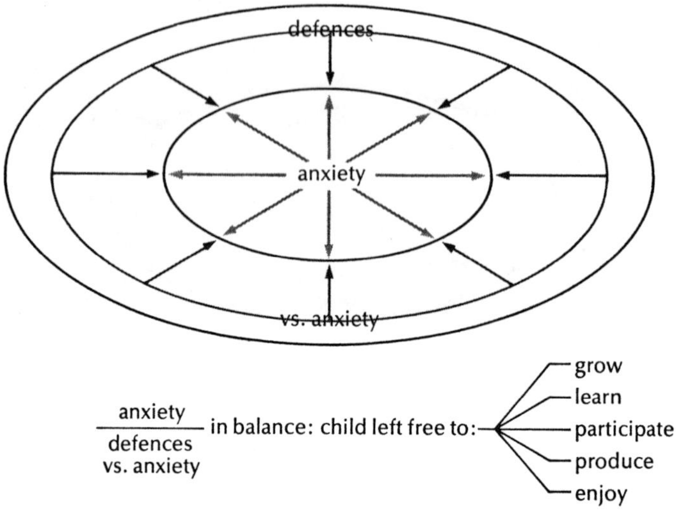

Many of the symptoms of children with a variety of psychological problems are related to their difficulties in dealing with anxiety and the sometimes excessive, and at other times inappropriate, nature of their defences.

In the *normal* child, the defences developed are sufficient to ward off intolerable anxiety without interfering with the child's freedom to grow, to learn, and to live a full, satisfying, and productive life. They neither seriously distort nor rigidly fix the developing personality (See Fig. 6–3). The normal child is not afraid of his anger getting out of control, as he has confidence in his own self-control. Therefore, he is well aware of his angry feelings but is sufficiently in control of them to assess a situation realistically and behave appropriately in response to it. *The psychoneurotic child,* on the other hand, continues to fear that his basic drives (e.g. anger) might get out of control. Much of his energy will therefore be invested in defences against any awareness of drives. Depending on the form the neurosis takes, one of several outcomes might occur:

1. The defences might prove insufficient to protect the child from constant, generalized, intolerable anxiety that results not from a problem with the outside world but from an inner conflict of which the child was unaware. The pervasive anxiety of such children stems from their lacking defences capable of adequately containing the powerful but unacceptable basic drives that threaten to break through into conscious awareness. Examples would include the child with anxiety neurosis, the

Figure 6-4 The Neurotic Child: (a) Defences Inadequate

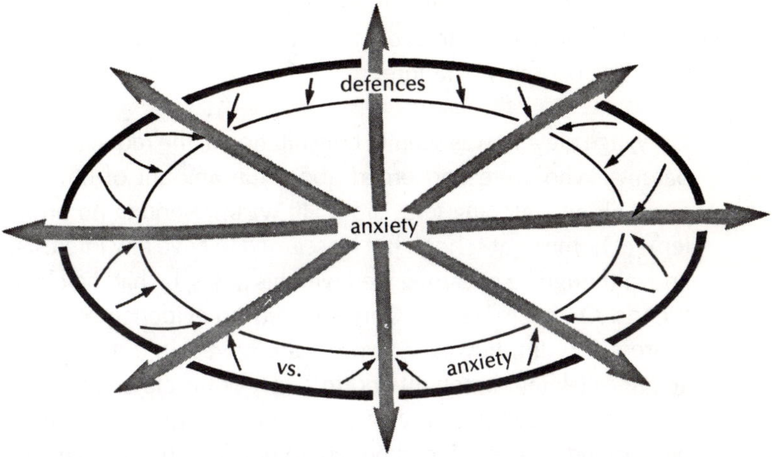

anxiety exceeds available defences

phobic child, or the child with traumatic neurosis (for definitions, see the discussion of Types of Psychoneurosis later in this chapter. See also Fig. 6–4).

2. The defences might succeed in keeping the child free of anxiety, but would be applied so rigidly, would be so limiting, and so draining of energy that the child was not left free to live a satisfying and productive life. (See Fig. 6–5.)

Figure 6-5 The Neurotic Child: (b) Defences Restricting

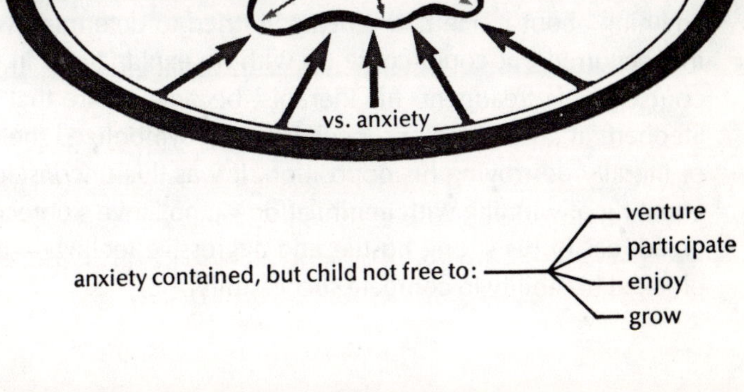

anxiety contained, but child not free to: venture / participate / enjoy / grow

One example would be that of the *restricted* child, who restricts or narrows down the field of his life by refusing to attempt, or participate in, major areas of life in order to avoid anxiety associated with involvement or with the possibility of failure.

> Gary, age eleven, was seen in consultation at the request of his parents, who were concerned about the amount of time he spent alone watching television. He was presenting no problems at home or at school, but he seemed to have few interests, and, although he got along well with his peers, he had no close friends. On examination, Gary showed no evidence of acute distress. He did, however, express an interest in a number of activities (skiing, baseball) and in a few of his classmates. He had never developed any of these interests or relationships because he was convinced he would not be good at them and might make a fool of himself if he tried, so that he felt it was not worth the effort. Thus he avoided the anxiety connected with a variety of activities by staying away from them, thus restricting the scope of his involvement in life.

Another example would be the *constricted* child, for whom not the act of trying but a particular activity has taken on a symbolic significance which, since it is taboo, means the activity must be avoided.

> Stephen, at age fourteen, was a fine natural athlete, a superb skier, and a tournament tennis player. When competing merely for his own enjoyment, he was almost unbeatable within his age group. Whenever he was involved in a major competition, however, he found himself unable to concentrate and to perform at the level he routinely achieved when relaxed. Although he recognized this as a repeated pattern, he was unable to do anything about it. He had repeatedly tried to determine why this occurred but could come up with no explanation. In the course of his treatment, his therapist became aware that for Stephen, at an unconcious level, winning symbolized the act of literally destroying his opposition. It was this unconscious equating of winning with annihilation—and Steve's unrecognized fear of his strong hostile and aggressive feelings—that blocked his ability to compete successfully.

Figure 6-6 The Neurotic Child: (c) Defences Distorting

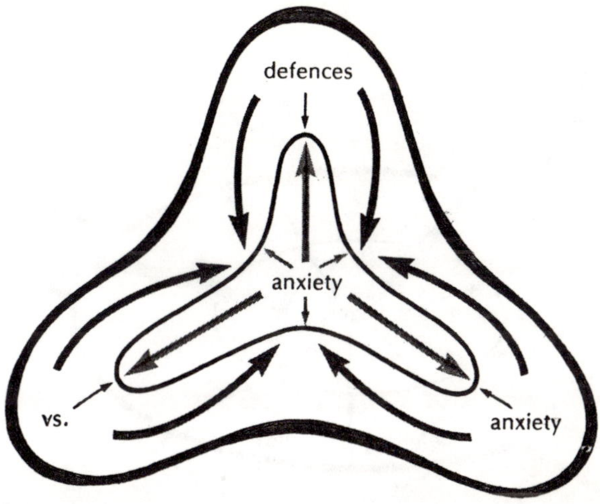

personality distorted by $\frac{\text{over-investment in defence}}{\text{excessive anxiety}}$

3. The defences may keep the child free of anxiety, but may be used so excessively and inflexibly that the entire personality is warped and distorted by the overinvestment in the defence. Examples would include the obsessive-compulsive child and the hysterical child. (See Fig. 6–6.)

In the child with a *neurotic behaviour disorder,* unacceptable feelings (e.g. anger) are expressed through behaviour, although the child is not aware of the origins of the behaviour. (For a definition of neurotic behaviour disorder, see discussion of Types of Personality Disorders later in this chapter.) In all these cases, the behaviour, termed "acting-out", is derived from and takes the place of strong but unacceptable feelings, even though the child is unaware of the intensity of the rage and its connection with his behaviour. (See Fig. 6–7.)

> The parents of Howie, age eight, were at their wits' ends. They could no longer tolerate his continuous disobedience, misbehaviour, and provocation. No matter how they tried, they could not persuade him to obey, and if they attempted to reason with him he either tuned them out or defied or mocked them. When seen together with them, Howie fully lived up to their description. When seen alone, however, he was an angry,

Figure 6-7 The Child with a Neurotic Behaviour Disorder

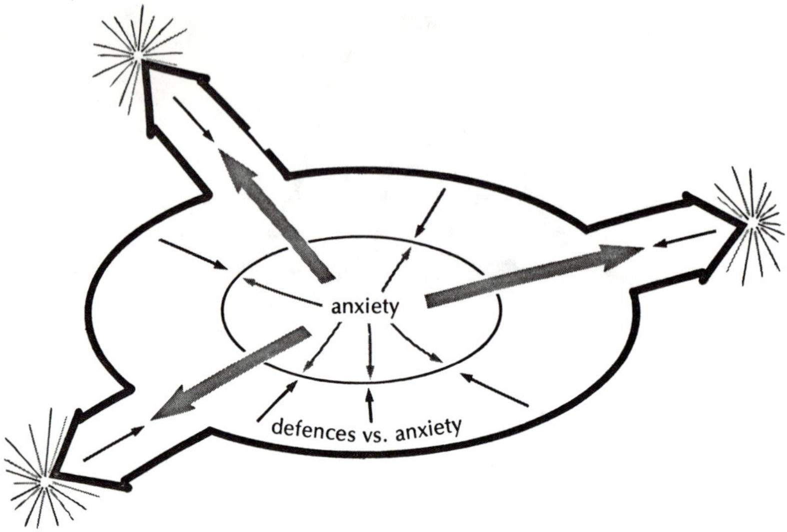

acting-out behaviour —(takes the place of / serves to mask)— anxiety resulting from inner conflict

unhappy little boy. He knew how angry his parents were at him, and felt rejected and deprived. His depression and rage were too intense for him either to tolerate or to control. His defiant and provocative behaviour was derived from and took the place of these feelings, but at the same time served to mask his underlying depression.

The child with a *personality disorder* has a cohesive, well-functioning personality, but his defence pattern, instead of being flexibly available to be used or dispensed with as the situation demands as in the normal child, is a constant and an outstanding feature of his mode of relating to others. Such a child might be so intensely defended against his anger that he was meticulously fair, kind, self-sacrificing, and benign in all his dealings with others. He would never feel or express any anger, and would be unable to be normally assertive or to defend his interests even when it seemed appropriate for him to do so. In such a child the exaggerated defence against the anger has become a personality trait, that is, it is accepted as an integral part of the person. Unlike a symptom, which would be experienced as foreign and distressing, the trait would serve to protect him from his conflict while being seen as a rational and even desirable part of his character.

In the child with a *psychophysiological disorder*, a disturbance in physiological function mediated through the autonomic nervous system may serve to mask and discharge conflict and anxiety that have remained trapped within the child. (For further discussion, see Chapter 9.)

> Jan's parents were concerned about her frequent headaches. In taking a history, the paediatrician soon established that Jan was an intense, self-willed, competitive girl who was frequently involved in conflicts with her mother and older sister. When she realized she could not win, Jan would retire to her room in tears, but soon would return complaining of a headache and asking for medication.

The directions in which a particular child might develop are influenced by the child's basic characteristics (assertive or timid, big or small, persistent or distractible, etc.) and by the parents' behaviour (rigid or flexible, authoritarian or permissive, etc.). As a result, some children respond to the same basic conflicts and anxieties in a totally different way than do others, thus leading to very diverse clinical pictures. Also the same symptom (e.g. stealing, lying, or the inability to make and hold friends) in different children may result from the simultaneous action of a number of constitutional and environmental factors.

> Johnny, who grew up in an area of the inner city where stealing was accepted if not obligatory behaviour, stole for completely different reasons than Jimmy, whose stealing was an attempt to ward off the intense feelings of deprivation which resulted from the break-up of his parents' marriage.

Symptoms may be the outcome of a child's attempts to cope with his feelings, with varying stages of his development, and with the demands of other people. Most people develop symptoms temporarily in times of stress. Many children acquire symptoms temporarily while going through a difficult stage of development, then learn to cope with the situation, and drop the symptom (See Chapter 5). A symptom is neurotic if the child is unable to recognize its connection with the

Table 6-1 Traditional diagnostic categories related to the balance between conflict-generated anxiety and available defences

Defences	*Presentation*
Adequate	Normal child in healthy equilibrium, free to grow
Inadequate	Child with anxiety neurosis; the phobic child; child with traumatic neurosis
Excessive	Child with restricted personality; child with neurotic constriction
Distorting	Obsessive-compulsive child; the child with conversion hysteria
Acting-out Predominates	The child with neurotic behaviour (personality) disorder

internal conflict from which it protects him. As the child progresses through his development, the type of symptom may alter, so that in his handling of the same conflict a given child may show differing symptoms at various ages. Unlike a character or personality trait, a symptom (e.g. tic, phobia, compulsion, stealing, etc.) is regarded by the patient and by his family as a disturbance, something irrational and foreign to his personality.

A child's psychological structure is not entirely intelligible unless viewed as a product of the developing child in a family. Since the child lives and develops as an integral part of the family unit, his interactions with other family members will have a major effect on how he learns to deal with conflict and defend against anxieties, on how successful he will be at this, and, if unsuccessful, on the nature and extent of his symptomatology. Therefore, diagnosis consists not just of naming the symptom picture, but of seeing and understanding how this particular set of reactions arose at this time in this child in this family.

The interaction of the child and family is often clearly demonstrated in the child with neurosis or a behaviour disorder. Here the child may be seen to be struggling against a particular set of parental demands that he can neither accept nor avoid. An example would be that of an angrily soiling child who is struggling against unsuitably timed or excessively harsh toilet-training demands. What may begin as a reaction to child-rearing techniques or parental neurosis may, over a period of time, become internalized and neurotic (that is, a rigid and automatic tendency to oppose and struggle against all adult expectations). By this stage, the child will have lost contact with the reasons for his oppositional behaviour, which, as an internalized part of personality, would colour his responses even in the absence of the family environment to which he had originally been reacting.

The relationship between the diagnostic terms commonly used and the basic model which has been presented is summarized in Table 6-1. Some common neurotic pictures will be discussed. It must be remembered, however, that the specific symptoms of the child are but a small fragment of the total picture of a child struggling to develop in his family setting. To understand, one must learn not just about the symptoms but about the child as a person and about his role within his family.

Types of Psychoneuroses

ANXIETY TYPE

The child is in the grip of generalized intense anxiety that arises not from a problem in the outside world but rather from an unconscious conflict. His defences are not sufficient to contain the impulses that threaten to break through into conscious awareness. Anxiety neuroses are usually relatively short-lived, as defences develop which may lead to the development of a different and more structured disorder. In the following case example, a child's anxiety neurosis is the result of her inability to handle her intense ambivalent feelings towards her mother and father.

> When Ann was three, her father left home to live with his secretary. Ann was upset, but she got over it as her mother came to terms with the situation. Ann visited her father each weekend. When she was four and a half she developed a generalized anxiety, fearing that her mother would disappear or that she herself would die. She had no defences sufficient to ward off her anxiety, but like most neuroses of the anxiety type, it did not last long, instead developing into a different and more structured disorder—in this case, a phobic neurosis.

PHOBIC TYPE

In a phobia, emotions that the child feels too guilty or fearful to accept are projected onto some external situation, which is then fearfully avoided. The phobia may bring secondary rewards, such as additional concern and care from the parents. Ann, the girl introduced in the case example above, provides a clear illustration of this mechanism.

> Ann became afraid that a kidnapper would come and get her during the night. Her generalized anxiety diminished as she structured her neurosis and her life around this one phobia. She protected herself by moving into her mother's bed. In play therapy sessions Ann repeatedly enacted the same fantasy with the doll family. A girl would go away with her father. A robber would kill the mother. Then the girl, who was also a doctor, would revive the mother and look after her.
>
> As Ann reached the Oedipal stage of development (usually around four years of age), she had been faced with a number of feelings she had difficulty handling. She felt in competition with her mother for her father's affections, yet she was also angry at her father, who had, after all, deserted both of them. She was angry at both parents, but she really liked and was dependent on them both, particularly on her mother. Her original neurosis, the anxiety type, was an expression of her inability to handle her ambivalence towards her parents. By organizing the more structured phobia, she was able to confine her anxiety to one area of her life, functioning more comfortably the rest of the time. The unconscious conflict is represented symbolically in Ann's symptoms. Ann would like to be with her father, but she has angry feelings towards him which she cannot resolve within herself. This illustrates the mechanism of the phobia. She handles the anger she cannot accept by putting it outside herself and into the kidnapper, that is, by projecting it. In this case, Ann also reassures herself that her angry feelings towards her mother will not harm the mother by sleeping with her, as a guarantee of continuing safe dependency.
>
> We can also see the phobic mechanism in Ann's play when she projects her angry feelings onto the robber who kills the mother while Ann retains awareness, in the girl representing herself, only of the protective feelings towards her mother.

School phobia

Also termed school refusal, school phobia is a condition in which the child refuses to attend school because of an intense but irrational fear expressed through a combination of frank anxiety and somatic symptoms. Technically, it differs from a true phobia, as defined above, in that the disturbance is often deeply rooted in a pathological mother-child relationship in which the normal development of independence is disrupted due to the mother's need to maintain a continuing attachment. The child is typically symptom-free as long as there is no pressure to attend school, since it is school that serves as the external situation onto which the conflict has been projected and that the child, therefore, seeks to avoid. Sometimes a minor physical illness in the child serves as a precipitant. Most children with school phobia show a number of psychoneurotic features, but they are better than average students and reasonably well adapted socially. A smaller but still substantial number suffer from a pathological distortion of the total personality (i.e. a personality disorder). These are usually older children, more dependent on their mothers and more immature in their social adaptation. In their cases, the onset is often more insidious, as they may have a long record of chronic absenteeism for questionable illnesses. An even smaller group suffer from psychosis; those in this group tend to be older children or adolescents. The sooner the child is returned and maintained in school, the better the prognosis. Persistent inattendance aggravates and fixes the pathology, and may provide considerable secondary gain (that is, additional advantages obtained from the phobic pattern) such as time alone with mother, treats, and bribes, etc. This is particularly true within the neurotic group.

The initial step in the treatment of school phobia involves getting the child back to school as soon as possible. This may be achieved in a variety of ways. One begins with an adequate assessment of child and family to ensure that the child is capable of returning to school (which is usually the case) and to determine factors within both the child and the family environment that are keeping the child from returning to school and those strengths that can be built upon to support the child's return. This done, parents and child are informed that while inability to attend school is symptomatic of an emotional disturbance requiring treatment, an essential part of that treatment is getting the child back to school immediately. From this point on, the treatment may vary. Some therapists merely inform the parents that it is up to them to derive a workable and acceptable method of doing this. Psychotherapy sessions several times a week are then used to identify and help parents and child resolve difficulties that occur as they attempt to implement their chosen plan.

When Kenneth, age fourteen, was first seen, he had been away from school and on home-bound teaching since shortly over a year before when he had developed diabetes. The illness had terrified his already overprotective and overinvolved mother, who became even more smothering in response to the diagnosis. A thorough assessment verified that Kenneth was capable of returning to school, even though he insisted he was too panicky and could not tolerate it. The therapist stood firm with the expectation, making it clear that the primary phase of treatment involved the parents somehow getting Kenneth back to school in spite of his anxiety and protestations. The parents reluctantly agreed, and twice weekly sessions were set up in which the therapist would meet with all three to assist in the process.

By the first session three days later, the parents had not succeeded in persuading Kenneth to go to school. He had complained of a stomach ache. Although they doubted he was seriously ill, as they were unsure they allowed him to stay home, justifying this on the grounds that they did not want to upset him. The therapist reiterated that an important part of Kenneth's learning to overcome his anxiety involved his getting back to school, pointing out that the parents had unwittingly been manipulated into undermining the treatment plan.

In the second therapy session, Kenneth's mother described a scene in which Kenneth had refused to get up and get dressed. His father had announced that unless Kenneth dressed himself he would dress him. Kenneth had refused and provoked a physical battle that ended with the father slapping him and the mother turning on her husband for resorting to violence. The father had capitulated, and again Kenneth stayed at home. The therapist outlined the role of all three in the transaction. Kenneth could have avoided it by dressing himself as he was told, as it was in response to his refusal and his subsequent provocation that the father had intervened physically. The father was supported in his attempt to take a firm stand, and mother was helped to see how her lining up with her son against her husband had the result of colluding with Kenneth in his attempt to remain away from school. Fortunately the mother could acknowledge her collusion, and was subsequently able to point out to Kenneth that the choice was his whether in the future he dressed himself or was dressed by his father, but that if he failed to do so he would be responsible for the consequences and she would not interfere.

The next day, for the first time in over a year, Kenneth made it to school, basically remaining in school despite frequent short absences with which his mother regularly colluded. The psychotherapy sessions were soon decreased to one a week, focusing on trying to improve the relationship between father and son, to help Kenneth separate from his mother, and to help the mother allow him to do so. The family remained in psychotherapy for over a year. Kenneth was by this time attending school regularly and without anxiety. There was some symptomatic increase in harmony within the family, but neither the family therapy nor the individual psychotherapy in which both Kenneth and his mother were concurrently involved succeeded in modifying the excessively close bond between mother and son which was contributing to an obvious effeminacy, which the parents could not acknowledge and left therapy to avoid having to deal with.

An alternate plan of management is illustrated by the case of Alice, age eleven, who had been out of school for a much shorter period of time.

An emergency assessment had established that while there was no reason why Alice could not immediately return to school in spite of her anxiety, her parents seemed to lack the resources to help her do so. Alice's mother, who had never achieved independence from her own mother, found it impossible to stand firm in the face of Alice's clinging and tears. Her father, a highly anxious and passive man, was unable to take any position unless directed to do so by his wife. It was decided, therefore, with the parents' agreement, that a social worker from the clinic would call at the house each morning and take Alice to school, as the parents appeared unable to do so. Along with Alice's principal, her teacher, and the family, the social worker drew up a plan for a gradual reinvolvement of Alice in the school: the first day they would go together just as far as the door at a time when no children were in the schoolyard; the next day they would spend five minutes in the schoolyard during recess; the next they would stand just inside the door of the school; the next they would stand in the hall just outside the classroom, etc. This process of gradually introducing Alice to increasing exposures to school at a predictable rate that she could tolerate while in the presence of a kind but determined adult whom over the two-week period she learned to trust, gradually decreased Alice's anxiety about being present in the school. Twice-weekly psychotherapy sessions were concurrently conducted in an attempt to prepare the parents to replace the social worker in giving Alice clear direction and the support she needed, while helping Alice become aware of and more able to deal with her marked hostility to her parents directly.

After about two weeks, the parents began to feel that Alice was manipulating them, and that anxiety was no longer a major factor keeping her away from school. This, added to their mounting frustration, led them to take and follow through on the position that Alice would be rewarded if she attended and stayed in school but sent to her room if she did not. Once Alice was convinced of the parents' ability to hold to their position, she returned and remained in school. Unfortunately once school attendance was no longer an issue, the parents were not motivated to continue to work on the relationship difficulties that had precipitated the school refusal, and against the advice of their therapist withdrew from treatment.

The latter example is one in which behaviour therapy and psychotherapy were combined in the treatment of the school refusal. The gradual exposure to increasing doses of school was an attempt at desensitization (classical conditioning), while the decision to reward school attendance and isolate Alice in her room for non-attendance in the phase when anger and attention-seeking seemed to be the major perpetuating factors, was an example of operant conditioning[22]. (For a brief description of the theoretical base and techniques of behaviour therapy, see Chapter 22.)

As can be seen from the above examples, the treatment of school refusal usually requires co-operation on the part of the school, the parents, the child, and the treatment team. Both parents and child require immediate psychotherapy aimed at clarifying and resolving the family situation leading to the development of the refusal. Neither simple return to school nor psychotherapy in itself can be considered adequate management. In very severe cases which fail to respond to treatment or where suicide, self-injury or further decompensation are apparent, in-patient treatment may have to be considered. In the majority of cases, it is possible to get the child back to school relatively quickly, but frequently this undermines the parental motivation to deal fully with the underlying psychological and relationship problem.

CONVERSION TYPE

In this form of psychoneurosis, the conflict is first repressed and then converted (i.e. represented symbolically) into a somatic symptom usually involving the voluntary muscles or the somatosensory system. Hysterical blindness, paralysis, pain, or vomiting would be examples. A conversion symptom differs from a psychophysiological disorder in that it involves no physiological dysfunction. A conversion neurosis is more likely to occur in a child with a hysterical personality. (For a definition, see discussion of Types of Personality Disorders later in this chapter.)

> Ten-year-old Nina had one younger brother, who, almost a year before, had been left hemiplegic and aphasic following a sudden and dramatic illness. Needless to say, this had deeply upset the entire family. Every day after work, both Nina's parents would rush down to the hospital, leaving Nina in the care of her aged grandmother. Nina, too, was very upset about her brother's illness, but she also deeply resented it. She felt her parents no longer had time or love for her, but if she complained, she was called selfish and was punished. She stopped complaining but developed pain and a persistent limp in her left knee which defied repeated investigation. During her third appearance in emergency, an intern noted that the brother was paralysed on his left side and wondered if her symptoms represented a conversion reaction. On inquiry, Nina told of a series of repeated dreams. In some of these, her brother had died and was going to heaven. In others—and she broke down and sobbed as she told of these—she had killed him. Further investigations suggested that Nina's intense conflict between feelings of love, hate, and guilt had been converted into the leg

pain and stiffness, which to her symbolized (unconsciously) an identification with the ambivalently loved brother.

DISSOCIATIVE TYPE

In a dissociative reaction, there is a temporary marked personality disorganization based on a neurotic conflict that results in fugue states, amnesia, somnambulism, etc.

> A twelve-year-old girl, who had always been unduly close to her father and to some extent had taken her mother's place in an unsatisfactory marriage, felt greatly upset when the father left home for another woman. In her waking life, the girl quickly regained her composure and continued her academic and social life. At night, however, she had fugue states in which she would wander about, acting out sexually-tinged fantasies that represented unconscious feelings for her father, although she could not recall any of these episodes the next day.

OBSESSIVE-COMPULSIVE TYPE

An obsession is a thought that occurs repeatedly, seemingly against the patient's will. A compulsion is a ritualized act that the patient feels impelled to repeat. Departure from the ritual, which may at times dominate the personality and cripple the child's function, leads to intense anxiety.

> An adolescent girl who was struggling to attain a sense of identity separate from her loving but overpowering mother felt compelled to leave the rotating part of the combination on her school locker set at the number sixteen. She felt that sixteen was nice and rounded, the square of a squared number. Fifteen and seventeen were odd, jagged, and dangerous numbers. She felt compelled to check several times that the lock had not been left at a dangerous number, or she feared for her mother's safety. Sometimes she also phoned her mother to check that she was all right, which annoyed the mother. The girl was unaware of any hostile feeling in herself. She knew only that she was concerned about her mother. She realized this was absurd, but if she didn't check she became unbearably anxious.

DEPRESSIVE TYPE

Children are often depressed in reaction to a loss, a disappointment, or a physical illness. Depression is neurotic when it becomes a chronic condition based largely on internal conflict rather than external circumstances. The depression may be masked, with the clinical picture being dominated by one or more "depressive equivalents", for example, an eating or sleeping disturbance, social withdrawal, antisocial behaviour, academic underachievement. For a more extensive description of depression in children see Chapter 7.

Types of Personality Disorders

In a neurosis, the child or the parents complain of a symptom that seems foreign to the child. In personality disorders, the combination of impulse and defence, rather than producing a circumscribed syndrome, is built into the personality and seems to be a part of the child himself. The complaint is not about a symptom, but about the child.

COMPULSIVE PERSONALITY

The child with a compulsive personality is clean, tidy, respectful, and pseudomature. Compulsive behaviour, representing a successful defence against any aggressive impulses and against messing and untidiness, characterizes the whole personality. But the inability to experiment with noise, aggression, and mess seriously limits the scope of his life experience unless the child manages, as is often the case, to break out in adolescence and discover how the rest of the world lives.

HYSTERICAL PERSONALITY

The child with a hysterical personality is histrionic, emotionally labile, seductive, and manipulative. These children often seem socially skilled and sexually oriented, but in fact they have learned to reproduce whatever behaviour will work in order to bring the attention and support on which they depend for their sense of well-being.

ANXIOUS PERSONALITY

These children are afraid of all new and unfamiliar situations, but with initial support manage eventually to cope with their experiences. The parents often note that the child has been somewhat tense and has avoided new situations from early infancy.

OVERLY DEPENDENT PERSONALITY

These children are characteristically clinging, demanding, and slow to achieve autonomy (independence).

OPPOSITIONAL PERSONALITY

These children resist socializing efforts of parents and teachers, and are unable to merge as a regular group member among peers. Aggressive and difficult, they often show a real wish to be loved but are unable to submerge a strong need for independence and individuality in order to get the love.

OVERLY INHIBITED PERSONALITY

Such children are shy, seemingly passive, and afraid of assertiveness. There may be inhibition of learning at school or elective mutism. They may be more spontaneous and independent at home.

OVERLY INDEPENDENT PERSONALITY

Noisy, active, driven, and difficult to control, these children cannot tolerate being restricted or being looked after.

ISOLATED PERSONALITY

Distant, withdrawn, seemingly uninterested in warm attachments, these children compensate by means of an extensive fantasy life. Their social difficulties tend to remain with them through adolescence into adulthood. One often has the impression of a basic inability to relate closely to others, rather than a defensive inhibition of the function.

MISTRUSTFUL PERSONALITY

Characteristic of these children is their suspicious, paranoid-like attitude, often becoming apparent in adolescence.

TENSION-DISCHARGE DISORDERS

These are the children with behaviour disorders. Their aggressive and sexual impulses are acted out in conflict with societal norms, rather than being inhibited by various defences as in normal or neurotic children. There are two subgroups: 1) impulse-ridden personality; 2) neurotic personality disorder.

1. *Impulse-Ridden Type*

Impulse-ridden children are primitive and unsocialized, with shallow relationships, lack of inner control, and little ability to guide present behaviour according to forseeable consequences. Often they represent a product of deprived and inconsistent backgrounds with multiple foster-placements, family breakdowns, etc. Their symptoms may include stealing, destructiveness, etc., with little apparent anxiety or guilt.

2. *Neurotic Type*
For children with a neurotic personality disorder, antisocial and impulsive behaviour resembling that of the impulse-ridden type arises in an often repetitive way out of the child's relationships. The actions often express symbolically (i.e. act out) an inner conflict or a wish for control by the parents.

SOCIOSYNTONIC PERSONALITY DISORDER
Here, children exhibit behaviour that is unacceptable in society at large but that is normal for the environment in which the child has lived. An example would be that of a child who, having grown up in a neighbourhood in which gang warfare was the norm and in which he fitted satisfactorily, behaves in an antisocial manner.

SEXUAL DEVIATION
Most deviant sexual behaviours or attitudes in childhood are aspects of some other neurotic, psychotic, or personality disorder. Occasionally a specific deviation (e.g. homosexuality) is diagnosed as the main disorder in adolescents.

Management
For a detailed discussion of management, refer to the three chapters in Unit Five. The following general principles may serve as a guide in assessment and management:
1. Assess what the child and family are like generally. What are their difficulties and what are their strengths? What part do the symptoms play in the family life? How did the symptoms develop? Does it seem to be a temporary situation or is it rather fixed?
2. How is the child affected? Consider emotional control and expression, social relationships and school work.
3. Are family relationships and reactions appropriate?
4. If child and family are functioning reasonably well, the problems may resolve themselves. It is as well to wait and watch. If functioning is noticeably disturbed, or if a lesser disturbance is becoming chronic, then referral for psychiatric consultation should be discussed with the child and the family.

RECOMMENDED FOR FURTHER READING

1. ADAMS, P. L. *Obsessive Children: A Sociopsychiatric Study.* New York, Brunner/Mazel, 1973.
—a definitive study of the obsessive child.

2. ANTHONY, E. J. "Psychoneurotic Disorders", in Freedman, A. M., and Kaplan, H. I., eds., *Comprehensive Textbook of Psychiatry,* 1387–90. Baltimore, Williams and Wilkins, 1967.
—a highly condensed presentation.

5. CHESS, S. *An Introduction to Child Psychiatry.* 2nd ed. New York, Grune and Stratton, 1969.
—clearly written, this textbook stresses the classification of disorders and the importance of constitutional and organic factors. The contribution of psychodynamic and environmental (familial) factors is grossly understated.

6. COOLIDGE, J. C.; WILLER, M. L.; TESSMAN, E.; and WALDFOGEL, S. "School Phobia in Adolescence: A Manifestation of Severe Character Disturbance". *Amer. J. Orthopsychiat.* 30: 599–607, 1960.
—an excellent formulation of the dynamics of school phobia, including changes in the dynamic picture as the school refusal becomes chronic.

8. FREUD, A. *Normality and Pathology in Childhood.* New York, International Univ. Press, 1966.
—a more comprehensive approach to a developmental understanding of child psychiatry by the distinguished psychoanalyst and theoretician.

9. *From Diagnosis to Treatment: An Approach to Treatment Planning for the Emotionally Disturbed Child.* New York, Vol. 8. GAP Publication no. 87, 1973.
—easily understood detailed discussion of the diagnostic process and its relation to treatment planning. Useful clinical examples.

10. HERSEN, M. "The Behavioural Treatment of School Phobia: Current Techniques". *J. Nerv. Mental Dis.* 153: 99–108, 1971.
—following a review of case histories, suggests various behavioural modification techniques that were found effective in managing children with school phobia.

11. LASSERS, E.; NORDAN, R.; and BLADHOLM, S. "Steps in the Return to School of Children with School Phobia". *Amer. J. Psychiat.* 130: 265–68, 1973.
—presents eight steps found useful in helping children with school phobia return to school and helping their parents keep them there.

12. LIPPMAN, H. S. *Treatment of the Child in Emotional Conflict.* 2nd ed. New York, McGraw-Hill, 1962.
—a basic textbook of child psychiatry, notable primarily for excellent clinical vignettes, illustrating the common syndromes and children's responses to psychotherapy. Written from the vantage point of the child analyst.

13. LO, W. H. "A Note on a Follow-Up Study of Childhood Neurosis and Behaviour Disorder". *J. Child Psychol. Psychiat.* 14: 147–50, 1973.
—discusses a follow-up of forty-two neurotic children and thirty children with behaviour disorders from one to four years after their psychiatric assessments.

14. MALMQUIST, C. P. "School Phobia: A Problem in Family Neurosis". *J. Amer. Acad. Child Psychiat.* 4: 293–319, 1965.
—stresses the interpersonal (familial) factors contributing to and maintaining the child's school refusal.

15. POZNANSKI, E. O. "Children with Excessive Fears". *Amer. J. Orthopsychiat.* 43: 428–38, 1973.
—intelligent observation of twenty-eight children with excessive fears, discussing demographic characteristics, the nature and content of the fears, their context, symbolization, and displacement.

16. *Psychopathological Disorders in Childhood: Theoretical Considerations and a Proposed Classification.* New York, Vol. 6. GAP. Publication no. 62, 1966.
—a useful succinct discussion and classification of each disorder. Provides a developmental framework around which to organize child psychiatry.

18. ROCK, N. L. "Conversion Reactions in Childhood: A Clinical Study on Childhood Neuroses". *J. Amer. Acad. Child Psychiat.* 10: 65–93, 1971.
—conversion reactions are more common in children than is generally believed. A thorough evaluation, including observation of parent-child interaction and an inquiry into school performance and peer relationships will prove helpful both in establishing a diagnosis and in avoiding further emphasis on the symptom.

20. WHITE, R. B., and GILLILAND, R. M. *Elements of Psychology of Defense.* New York, Grune and Stratton, 1975.
—a brief, clear description of the mechanisms of defence. Excellent clinical illustrations.

21. BARKER, P. *Basic Child Psychiatry.* Baltimore, University Park Press, 1976.

—a good elementary text on child psychiatry of value to anyone wanting an introduction to the subject.

ADDITIONAL READING

3. BAKWIN, H., and BAKWIN, R. *Behaviour Disorders in Children.* 4th ed. Philadelphia, W. B. Saunders, 1972.

7. EISENBERG, L. "School Phobia: A Study in the Communication of Anxiety". *Amer. J. Psychiat.* 114: 712–18, 1957–58.

17. BLOS, P. "The Concept of Acting Out in Relation to the Adolescent Process". *J. Amer. Acad. Child Psychiat.* 2: 118–43, 1963.

19. SHAW, C. R. "Personality Disorders", in Shaw, C. R. and Lucas, A. R., eds., *The Psychiatric Disorders of Childhood,* 2nd ed. Englewood Cliffs, New Jersey, Prentice-Hall, 1970.

22. LAZARUS, A. A.; DAVISON, G. C.; and POLEFKA, D. A. "Classical and Operant Factors in the Treatment of a School Phobia". *J. Abnormal Psychol.* 70: 225–29, 1965.

BARRY GARFINKEL
HARVEY GOLOMBEK

7. Suicide and Depression in Childhood and Adolescence

Suicide in children and adolescents is generally considered a rare occurrence.[3] Hospital records, coroners' reports, and doctors' statements appear to underestimate the true incidence of this psychiatric problem.[38] Frequently, death by suicide is reported as accidental because of pressure exerted by family and society in an attempt to avoid the cultural stigma associated with self-destruction. In addition, the physician may have personal difficulty accepting the possibility that an "accident" could be deliberately self-imposed.[14] Statistics indicating accidents as the leading cause of death in adolescence and childhood appear to include with some degree of certainty death by suicide.[11] In fact, suicide is listed as the world's fifth leading cause of death in the fifteen-to-nineteen-year-old age bracket.[41] In North America alone, it is the second most common cause of death in the fifteen-to-twenty-five-year-old age group.[33] Suicide has been shown to be the second most common cause of death, after accidents, in university-age students.[27] More people die from suicide each year than from breast cancer, hypertension, and asthma combined.[9] Most authors agree that death by suicide in children and adolescents is *not* rare, but because of cultural attitudes is recorded as such only rarely.

Suicide is defined as the deliberate act of self-injury with the intent to kill. Some authors differentiate between those who complete suicide and those whose attempts end in failure, that is, when the suicidal act does not bring about death.[6, 35] Taken as a group, those who succeed in committing suicide differ significantly from those who merely attempt it. In children and adolescents specifically, it is estimated that there are approximately fifty to one hundred times more suicide attempts than completed suicides.[20, 34, 39] Many more girls than boys attempt suicide, yet more boys are successful.[7] No more than 10 per cent of those who make an attempt eventually suicide, while the majority of those who succeed do so on their first attempt.[32] Those who commit suicide appear to be far more socially isolated with less opportunity for others to intervene and stop their destructive actions than those whose suicide attempt does not end in death.[10]

Attempted and completed suicides are further differentiated from suicide gestures, which are acts of self-injury without the intention of dying from the injury. Suicide gestures and threats serve as attempts to communicate distress or to manipulate or punish those in the environment.[35]

"Focal suicides" are associated with self-mutilation and accident-proneness, whereas addictions and alcoholism can be viewed as "chronic suicides", that is, progressive self-destruction.[24, 25] The diabetic adolescent who inadequately controls his disease by refusing to follow his diet and by irregular insulin use may also be an example of the latter group.

Epidemiology

Suicide appears to vary with seasons, with more occurring in the spring and early summer.[28, 29] Children commit suicide most frequently from 15 00 to 24 00 hours, whereas adult suicides more frequently occur between midnight and dawn. Most suicides in children take place at home.[7, 39]

The incidence of suicide varies from country to country, with the over-all suicide incidence in Canada being approximately 11.2 suicides per 100,000 people per year. Hungary, Austria, Germany, Japan, and the Scandinavian countries with the exception of Norway have suicide rates two to three times higher than the rate for Canada. Moslem and Catholic countries appear to have the lowest suicide rates, but it is not clear whether this reflects underreporting due to religious stigma, or whether the structure and stability inherent in a more traditional religious community actually affords immunity to suicide.[20, 22]

Suicides occur more frequently in families experiencing some disruption. Most authors include factors such as homes broken through divorce, separation, abandonment, alcoholism, or death as significantly increasing the incidence of suicide. When a suicide occurs in families that are intact, there is often a high degree of marital discord, physical aggression, and an absence of supportive response to their children's problems.[7, 38] A family history of suicide is found more frequently in those children who commit suicide. School work and peer relationships appear to deteriorate prior to the suicide.

Children and adolescents use overdoses of drugs most frequently in their suicide attempts. Those most widely used are diazepam, barbiturates, aspirin, and anti-depressants.[11, 20] Commonly, the medications have been prescribed for the parents or are household remedies intended for the family's use. Violent methods of destruction, such as jumping from heights or in front of subways, are used less frequently by this age group than by adults.

There appear to be specific ages at which suicide is most likely to occur in childhood and adolescence. Suicide before the age of fourteen is rarely reported, but the incidence increases markedly at this age. The incidence then peaks in the fifteen-to-nineteen-year-old group, with most adolescent suicides occurring within this age group.

Suicide in childhood and adolescence is associated more frequently with a diagnosis of depression than with any other psychiatric diagnosis. Less frequently, particularly in late adolescence, it occurs as part of a psychotic process, as when the teenager uses it as a means of achieving "nirvana" or when he responds to imperative auditory hallucinations demanding that he kill himself or a delusional belief that he can rejoin a dead relative.[4]

In young children suicides occur more frequently as an attempt to alter an intolerable living situation or to punish significant people in the environment. This type of suicide represents an attempt to resolve or escape from a situation that the child believes is beyond his capacity to manage or endure. The young child, who does not understand the finality of death, may view self-destruction as a means of punishing the parents or gaining their love and affection.[19] For him, suicide may be an attempt to teach the parents a lesson and make them feel guilty. Thus, his magical, incomplete comprehension of the permanence of death may lead to his killing himself in a bid to punish the parents, as if he could somehow survive to observe the effect on them.[32]

Psychopathology

The increase in the number of suicides at age fourteen coincides with a developmental process occurring in the early adolescent. During this stage in his progress towards emotional independence (age eleven to fourteen years), the youngster attenuates his attachment to the parents and begins to shift his affections towards peers, cultural heroes, and other significant adults such as coaches, counsellors, and teachers. In relinquishing these family ties he retains as part of his personality only those values and identification he holds in high esteem. To some degree, therefore, the youngster during this phase of development has fewer inner resources to fall back on during stressful times than he had before he began to give up previously held parental values. At the same time, the early adolescent is experiencing an increase in the intensity of all his feelings, so that anger, sadness, and helplessness when they occur are felt with extreme intensity. Frequently adults claim that youngsters at this age tend to "overreact". In fact, it is normal for early adolescents to experience feelings and reactions to events much more intensely than adults.[8]

The early adolescent's personality, rather than maturing in a progressive manner to adulthood, tends to fall back temporarily on previously acquired methods of handling problems. At these times, parents tend to point out, "You're acting like a two-year-old!" This developmental slipping backwards results in the early adolescent's temporarily having fewer and less sophisticated methods of resolving problems. This limits his problem-solving ability, and in stressful situations could lead to his considering suicide as "the only way out". An increase in the suicide rate during this developmental phase, therefore, seems related to more than just a specific psychiatric illness or a reaction to a sad situation. Suicides in this age group thus reflect the youth's view of himself as having fewer inner strengths and fewer internal solutions to difficulties compounded by the increased intensity of feeling during this stage of development.[1]

In later adolescence, suicide follows much the same pattern as in adulthood. The youth may react to a significant loss with profound depression. The loss may be real, as in the death of a parent or the break-up of a romance, or it may be imagined, as when a teenager becomes preoccupied with the thought of not passing a grade, resulting in the imagined loss of status and self-esteem. The adolescent, who previously harboured both positive and negative feelings towards that which he lost, responds by turning against himself his angry, hostile, and blaming feelings. He then becomes increasingly isolated, withdrawn, despondent, full of self-hate and self-blame. If converted into actions, these feelings can result in self-destructive behavior.[15]

Clinical Picture

Almost all children who make suicidal threats, gestures, or acts are reported by their parents, peers, or school to have experienced difficulties prior to the attempt. Children, when depressed, do not show the typical clinical picture of the depressed adult. The adult depressive symptomatology of early-morning awakening, sleep disturbance, diurnal fluctuation in mood, somatic complaints, and specific feelings of self-reproach, guilt, and loss can be seen in late adolescence, but appear only rarely during childhood. Similarly, manic-depressive illness of a depressed type is not commonly seen until late adolescence. If the illness occurs at all before that age, manic symptoms more frequently predominate.[23]

Instead of the typical symptoms of adult depression, one sees one or more *depressive equivalents*. Common depressive equivalents include boredom, restlessness, fatigue, difficulties in concentrating, behavioural problems, and repeated somatic complaints.[26] In two series of one hundred children, each complaining of abdominal pain, only 6 per cent in one study and 8 per cent in the other were found to have organic pathology.[2] These equivalents take the place of an open admission of feeling sad because of a child's tendency to deny or hide his true feelings and to express thoughts and emotions through actions rather than words.[36] Much depressive behaviour has been labelled "acting-out". To say that a child is "acting-out" means that he is expressing his true feelings behaviourally. Common forms of acting-out behaviour in depressed children include running away from home, delinquency, promiscuity, truancy, lateness, bullying younger children, as well as accident proneness. The conclusion, therefore, is that depression in children is not on the surface, but is "masked", or expressed behaviourally.[17]

Suicide is often precipitated by a seemingly trivial event which triggers the self-destructive behaviour. The event produces an impulsive response in the child. It aggravates an ongoing depressive process that previously may have surfaced only intermittently and been expressed episodically and behaviourally. There is often a history of appearing sad, withdrawn, and inhibited. The child demonstrates an extremely poor self-concept, expressing feelings of dissatisfaction, discontent, and rejection. Teachers often comment on abrupt changes in classroom behaviour in a child who formerly had not caused any disturbance. Episodes of marked irritability, low frustration tolerance, and deteriorating academic performance are frequently reported. Observations may show a reversal of behaviour, such as clowning or very active and restless activity instead of the child's usual behavioural pattern. Drug and alcohol abuse are similarly common depressive equivalents in the older child or adolescent.

Clinical Examples

1. Dale was an eleven-year-old boy admitted to the medical wards of a paediatric hospital with a three-year history of persistent, migratory joint pains. There were no associated clinical signs, and despite repeated investigations and consultations no one had been able to establish a diagnosis. It was his failure to improve in response to symptomatic treatment that led to his hospitalization. Following admission, physical, laboratory, and radiological examinations were repeated. When the results were negative, a psychiatric consultation was requested. The request for consultation made it clear that the attending physician and ward staff did not see evidence of a psychiatric illness but that in view of the inability to arrive at a diagnosis they were wondering if they could be overlooking an emotional problem.

   On examination, Dale was a quiet, pleasant, and polite boy who was reserved and lacking in spontaneity. While he did not object to seeing a psychiatrist, he wondered why the consultation had been arranged, since nothing was bothering him. An inquiry into his function in the main areas of his life revealed that his school performance had deteriorated slightly and that his involvements with friends and hobbies had somewhat waned. When asked how he felt about this loss of interest he unexpectedly burst into tears and cried throughout the rest of the interview. He stated that he had no idea why he was so unhappy. He had been feeling sad for years although no one else suspected it, as he had never cried publicly or told anyone, including his parents, how he was feeling.

At this point, Dale's mother entered, according to the prearranged plan to have them seen together. She gave no sign of having noticed that Dale was sobbing, although when asked she did confirm that she had been totally unaware that he was unhappy and that she had not seen him cry in years. Further information revealed that Dale's father had been killed in an industrial accident when Dale was six, that Dale had been thoroughly rejected by his step-father, and that his mother was too depressed and overwhelmed by her own depression and the conflicts in her marriage to recognize, let alone meet, Dale's emotional needs. It seemed clear then that for Dale the deteriorating school performance, the general loss of interest and withdrawal from relationship, and the chronic joint pains represented depressive equivalents.

2. Mark, age sixteen, was seen in consultation along with his parents, who were so frustrated with his behaviour that they were reaching the point where they could no longer tolerate living with him. The second of four children, Mark was lying, stealing, and shirking all responsibilities at home as well as badly underachieving in school. He was in constant conflict with his younger brothers, whom he teased incessantly, while his relationship with his parents shifted from antagonistic confrontation to sullen withdrawal. Any attempt to confront him with his irresponsibility or provocation led to denial, projection of blame, and angry, abusive arguments, which at times deteriorated into physical conflict. His father concluded his presentation of the parents' view of the situation by stating, "I'm exhausted . . . I'm ashamed to admit it, but I've given up . . . My feelings for him are diminishing daily."

On examination, Mark made no attempt to deny his parents' accusations. He agreed that he is frequently belligerent and defensive when confronted, and admitted to being in the wrong 50 to 80 per cent of the time. When asked why he became so defensive when confronted by his parents, he claimed it was because they accused him of being in the wrong 100 per cent of the time. He stated that in any arguments with his brothers the parents never even listened to his side of the story. He felt they were not interested in how he felt, that they did not care about him, that they had written him off. This he said was why he would not talk to them or co-operate with them. By this point, Mark was crying quietly but openly, as he stated that his parents wanted not to help him but to unload him.

In describing Mark, the parents repeatedly stressed the hostile, oppositional aspect of his behaviour (belligerent, un-co-operative, provocative, irresponsible) but at no point showed any evidence of seeing him as unhappy or depressed. When asked specifically—after he had been crying even though actively involved for fifteen minutes—they suggested that since he didn't cry at home, his tears were manipulative rather than an indication of genuine sadness.

After they had left the room, Mark was interviewed alone. While not denying his refusal to co-operate or his anger at his parents for giving up on him and treating him like "scum", Mark remained tearful as he described how alienated he felt from his family. The examiner's impression was that the chronic behaviour disorder represented a depressive equivalent, utilized in Mark's attempt to ward off the feelings of depression, sadness, and rage that had surfaced during the examination. While the depression could be seen at least in part as a response to parental rejection, the predominant symptom of the depression (i.e. the behaviour disorder) had the effect of perpetuating the rejection in a circular manner.

Reported in the child psychiatric literature is the concept of "psychic contagion and suggestion". This refers to the phenomenon of a number of suicides or suicide attempts occurring within a specific environment within a short period of time. It appears that the knowledge of others having committed suicide may point a distraught adolescent in the direction of suicide as a means of resolving his conflicted situation. It is suggested that the mass media may play an important role in suggesting suicide by publicizing and dramatizing the suicidal act and the manner in which it was committed.[16]

Examination and Treatment of a Suicidal Child

Two distinct protocols of assessment are followed in managing the depressed child.

1. *The depressed child*, who may or may not have threatened suicide, is most frequently assessed by the family physician or paediatrician. The physician can offer appropriate management by observing the following guidelines:

a) Serious consideration is given to all of the child's expressions of feelings, both verbal and behavioural.
b) A thorough school, peer, family, and medical history will frequently provide clues to the child's problems. This includes an adequate mental-status assessment and a comparison with the child's previous state of mind as determined from the history. Frequently, this step requires that the physician speak with the parents and teachers.
c) The child is followed in continuous assessment over a period of four to twelve weeks by means of visits at least weekly and more frequently if indicated, during which the physician shows his interest by listening to and counselling the child without giving the impression of being hurried.
d) If the depression fails to remit, a psychiatric consultation should be arranged. The referring physician personally explains to the child the nature of, and reasons for, the psychiatric visit.

2. *Following a suicide attempt* the initial psychiatric assessment is frequently made by the doctor in the hospital emergency department, and should be carried out immediately after any medical problems resulting from the attempt are under control. Pertinent information should be obtained from parents, peers, siblings, teachers, doctors, and psychiatrist in order to arrive at an appropriate treatment plan.

To decide whether or not hospitalization is needed to prevent the child from trying again, one must appraise the seriousness of his intentions. The likelihood of an attempt being repeated can be determined with some degree of certainty by exploring each of the following areas:

a) *Method.* What means did the child select to kill himself? If pills were used did he take all of those available or just a few, and if just a few, why? Did he know the purpose of the pills?
b) *Intent.* Did the child write a suicide note or letter? How detailed were his suicide plans? The content of these notes often describes the true depth of his despair.
c) *Stress.* What was the nature of the precipitating stressful event? How many alternative methods of responding to it were open to the child?
d) *Social Set.* Did the child take steps to prevent anyone from rescuing

him? Was anyone else present in the room or house when the attempt was made? Did anyone know about the suicide attempt either before or immediately after?

e) *History.* Is there a history of previous suicide attempts and gestures; if so, what were they like? Is there a family history of suicide?

f) *Mental Status.* What is the child's present mental status, and how has it changed from the description of him by others before the attempt?

g) *Support.* What kind of support would this child receive from his family, friends, classmates, and teachers if he were sent home?

In-patient admission is recommended when the answers to the above questions leave the examining doctor in doubt about the child's safety. A treatment plan can be initiated while in the hospital and continued after discharge. The admission itself would remove the child from the stressful environment and would defuse the precipitating situation. During the hospitalization, the child's total evaluation could be completed in much more detail over a shorter period of time than on an out-patient basis.

The aim of treatment is to prevent the child from using suicide either as a means of expressing his thoughts and feelings or as a solution to what he understands as his problems. Treatment would therefore depend on developing an honest, frank, and non-judgmental relationship with the child in which the expression of his feelings through play or words would lead to discovering alternate ways of relieving unwanted feelings. This type of relationship would allow the therapist to help the child alter his behaviour through new learning and the provision of a new model for identification. Frequently, parents and members of the child's family will require counselling to improve communication between themselves and the child to help them support his progress towards recovery. In Britain, treatment at times has included anti-depressant medication.[12] There is no convincing evidence, however, that anti-depressants alone are beneficial in children, and if there is serious suicide risk present, the anti-depressant medication could be used to overdose. Electric convulsive therapy is never used for the treatment of depression in children, and seldom with adolescents.[30]

Prevention

Efforts to reduce the incidence of suicide, such as suicide prevention centres, have not shown marked success. However, schools can form a front line of defence in recognizing serious psychiatric problems and the progenitors of suicide and depression in children and adolescents. The teacher is frequently the first person both to recognize the subtle behavioural changes indicative of depression and to initiate action such as professional counselling. Because of their status in the community, teachers may be able to motivate the child and his family to obtain help. Community mental-health services can aid the teacher and school in delineating the situations that require particular attention. Through training, teachers can increase their skills in the area of detection and early intervention.[18]

Chemical compounds, medically prescribed, have become the most frequently used method of self-destruction. This situation is likely to continue. Certain measures have been recommended or implemented to counteract or control this:

1. Limited prescribing of barbiturates;[5]
2. More frequent prescriptions for smaller quantities;
3. Availability of larger pills, more difficult to swallow;[11]
4. Packaging hypnotics individually in aluminum foil to require extra time for thought while unwrapping the pill;[11]
5. Combination of a small amount of emetic with barbiturates as provided in Britain;
6. Use of "less harmful" hypnotics, for example, substitution of benzodiazepines for barbiturates.[5]

Finally the strengthening of poison control centres by staffing them with toxicologists, paediatricians, and psychiatrists in major children's and general hospitals would increase the likelihood of differentiating the true accidental poisoning from undetected suicide attempts.

RECOMMENDED FOR FURTHER READING

1. ANTHONY, E. J. "Two Contrasting Types of Adolescent Depression and Their Treatment". *J. Amer. Psychoanal. Assoc.* 18: 841–59, 1970.
—an excellent psychoanalytic article describing different types of adolescent depression.

5. BARRACLOUGH, B. M. "Are There Safer Hypnotics than Barbiturates?" *Lancet.* 1: 57–60, 1974.
—a good medical article advising physicians about dangers inherent in prescription drugs.

11. CONNELL, H. M. "Attempted Suicide in School Children". *Med. J. Aust.* 1: 686, 1972.
—good description of attempted suicide in children from a medical perspective.

12. CONNELL, P. H. "Suicidal Attempts in Childhood and Adolescence", in Howell, J. G., ed., *Modern Perspectives in Child Psychiatry,* 403–27, New York, Brunner/Mazel, 1971.
—the most comprehensive review of suicide in children.

13. CYTRYN, L., and Mc KNEW, D. H. "Factors Influencing the Changing Clinical Expression of the Depressive Process in Children". *Amer. J. Psychiat.* 131: 879–81, 1974.
—brief but clear description of the depressive process in childhood, discussing the pattern of defences and factors influencing the changing clinical picture with age.

15. FREUD, S. "Mourning and Melancholia", in *The Complete Psychological Works of Sigmund Freud*. Vol. 19, 1917. Standard ed., London, Hogarth, 1915.
—the classical psychoanalytic description of the mechanisms of depression and the aetiology of suicide.

16. GLASER, K. "Attempted Suicide in Children and Adolescents: Psychodynamic Observations". *Amer. J. Psychother.* 19: 220–27, 1965.
—a good clinical understanding of suicide attempts.

17. GLASER, K. "Masked Depression in Children and Adolescents". *Amer. J. Psychother.* 21: 565–74, 1967.
—a good psychodynamic understanding of the behavioural manifestations of depression.

26. MOLL, A. E. "Suicide: Psychopathology". *Can. Med. Assoc. J.* 74: 104–12, 1956.
—an article describing underlying psychiatric causes of suicide.

26. POZNANSKI, E., and ZRULL, J. P. "Childhood Depressions: Clinical Characteristics of Overtly Depressed Children". *Arch. Gen. Psychiat.* 23: 8–15, 1970.
—a descriptive article enumerating the symptoms of depression in children.

31. SHAFFER, D. "Suicide in Childhood and Early Adolescence". *J. Child Psychol. Psychiat.* 15: 275–91, 1974.
—presents the results of a comprehensive survey of all childhood suicides in England and Wales during a period of seven years. Discuss-

es the psychological make-up of these children and such factors as previous suicide attempts, depression, antisocial behaviour, and circumstances leading to the suicides.

32. SHAW, C. R., and SCHELKUN, R. F. "Suicidal Behaviour in Children". *Psychiat.* 28: 157–68, 1965.
—a general review article clearly describing the characteristics of suicidal behaviour.

37. TOOLAN, J. M. "Suicide in Children and Adolescents". *Amer. J. Psychother.* 29: 339–44, 1975.
—a clear discussion of the presenting symptoms, incidence, treatment, and aetiological themes concerned in suicide in children and adolescents.

40. UNWIN, J. R. "Depression in Alienated Youth". *Canad. Psychiat. Assoc. J.* 15: 83–86, 1970.
—discusses psychosocial crises and clinical syndromes among middle-class youth as a result of widespread alienation.

ADDITIONAL READING

2. APLEY, J. *The Child with Abdominal Pains.* 2nd ed. New York, Lippincott, 1975.

3. BAKWIN, H. "Suicide in Children and Adolescents". *J. Pediatr.* 50: 749–69, 1957.

4. BALSER, B. H., and MASTERSON, J. F. "Suicide in Adolescents". *Amer. J. Psychiat.* 116: 400–404, 1959-60.

6. BATCHELOR, I. R. C., and NAPIER, M. B. "Attempted Suicide in Old Age". *Br. Med. J.* 2: 1186–90, 1953.

7. BERGSTRAND, C. G., and OTTO, U. "Suicidal Attempts in Adolescence and Childhood". *Acta Paediatr. Scand.* 51: 17–26, 1962.

8. BLOS, P. *On Adolescence*, p. 170. New York, Free Press, 1962.

9. BROWN, J. H. "Suicide—The Deserted Field". *Can. Psychiat. Assoc. J.* 18: 93–94, 1973.

10. CARSTAIRS, G. M. "Characteristics of the Suicide Prone". *Proc. R. Soc. Med.* 54: 262–68, 1961.

14. DUBLIN, L. I. *Suicide: A Sociological and Statistical Study.* New York, Ronald, 1963.

18. GOLOMBEK, H., and COUCHMAN, R. "Sixty Thousand Children—The Process of Establishing a Mental Health Program in a School

Community". Paper presented to the Ont. Psychiat. Assoc. Meeting, 1974.

19. GOULD, R. E. "Suicide Problems in Children and Adolescents". *Amer. J. Psychother.* 19: 228–46, 1965.

20. JACOBZINER, H. "Attempted Suicides in Adolescents by Poisoning". *Amer. J. Psychother.* 19: 247–52, 1965.

21. JACOBZINER, H. "Attempted Suicides in Children". *J. Pediatr.* 56: 519–25, 1960.

22. LEWIS, A. "Statistical Aspects of Suicide". *Can. Med. Assoc. J.* 74: 99–104, 1956.

23. MALMQUIST, C. P. "Depression in Childhood and Adolescence". *N. Engl. J. Med.* 284: 955–61, 1971.

24. MENNINGER, K. A. *Man Against Himself,* 11. New York, Harcourt, 1938.

27. ROOK, A. "Student Suicides". *Br. Med. J.* 1: 599–603, 1959.

28. SANBORN, D. E., III; CASEY, T. M.; and NISWANDER, G. D. "Monthly Patterns of Suicide and Mental Illness". *Dis. Nerv. Syst.* 30: 551–52, 1969.

29. SANBORN, D. E., et al. "Suicide: Seasonal Patterns and Related Variables". *Dis. Nerv. Syst.* 31: 702–4, 1970.

30. SARGANT, W., and SLATER, E. *An Introduction to Physical Methods of Treatment in Psychiatry*, p. 70. New York, J. Aronson, 1973.

33. Statistics Canada. *Vital Statistics.* Cat. no. 84-202. Ottawa, Information Canada, 1971.

34. STENGEL, E. "Recent Research in Suicide and Attempted Suicide". *Amer. J. Psychiat.* 118: 725–27, 1962.

35. STENGEL, E., and COOK, N. G. *Attempted Suicide*. Maudsley Monograph no. 4. London, Oxford, 1958.

36. TOOLAN, J. M. "Depression in Children and Adolescents". *Amer. J. Orthopsychiat.* 32: 404–15, 1962.

38. TOOLAN, J. M. "Suicide and Suicidal Attempts in Children and Adolescents". *Amer. J. Psychiat.* 118: 719–24, 1961-62.

39. TUCKMAN, J., and CONNON, H. E. "Attempted Suicide in Adolescents". *Amer. J. Psychiat.* 119: 228–32, 1962-63.

41. World Health Organization. *Statistics Annual for 1968.* Geneva, WHO, 1971.

HARVEY R. ALDERTON

8. Psychoses in Childhood and Adolescence

This chapter will classify and describe the various forms of psychosis seen in children and adolescents.

1. Depressive Psychoses

a) ANACLITIC DEPRESSION

The severest form of anaclitic depression occurs if the child is separated from the mothering figure during the second half of the first year, without provision of a substitute. Initial protest is followed by despair. The infant becomes withdrawn, appears sad, loses weight, regresses, and is very prone to infection which may be fatal. In the absence of treatment, survivors show detachment from others and autoerotic behaviour. Treatment is through the provision of a substitute mothering figure.[84]

b) MANIC-DEPRESSIVE PSYCHOSIS

Manic-depressive psychosis is extremely rare in childhood, with only a few unmistakable cases reported before adolescence.[6, 91] Clinical manifestations resemble those in the adult, allowing for the developmental differences. Treatment is similar, including anti-depressive drugs or major tranquillizers in the manic phase. The effect of lithium has not yet been evaluated.

2. Schizophrenic Psychoses

a) CLASSIFICATION

Schizophrenia is a broad diagnostic term encompassing a number of syndromes. These are linked by certain shared characteristics, but each syndrome also has its own particular identifying features.[1] Many authors consider the following syndromes as schizophrenic in nature; others would prefer the use of the less specific term "psychosis" until aetiological or clinical continuity with adult schizophrenia has been more strongly established. The greatest controversy has concerned whether or not early infantile autism should be considered within the group.[77, 79] While options differ on this question, the author feels there is an essential continuity between the syndromes to be described, [8, 14, 42, 7, 21, 89] and for this reason the general term "schizophrenia" will be retained. As in the adult schizophrenias, identical clinical pictures do not necessarily indicate identical aetiology. At the present stage of knowledge, one can identify a number of syndromes, each with its typical clinical picture. Each of these, however, probably represents the outcome of a variety of possible aetiological clusters acting together to produce the clinical picture. A number of different classifications have been proposed, influenced by theoretical persuasion and the particular clinical population studied. At first sight, this results in a confusing array of different terms. However, there is broad agreement that psychosis may first occur within each of the developmental stages outlined in Table 8-1.

The precise clinical picture of the psychotic child will depend upon:

i) the age and developmental level of the child at the point of onset of the psychosis;
ii) the extent and severity of the disruption of normal function by the psychosis;
iii) the nature and extent of ego defences utilized in an attempt to maintain psychological homeostasis.

b) GENERAL CHARACTERISTICS

i) *There is a disturbance in the child's relation to, and his perception of, external reality.* Some authors feel that the core problem is a disturbance in the sense of personal identity, that is, an inability to distinguish what lies within, and what beyond, the orbit of the self.[1, 69] This inability to distinguish "self" from "non-self", also referred to as an uncertainty of ego boundaries, leads to an impaired sense of identity and a deficient awareness of one's separateness from others. As a result, the child has difficulty to a degree that is abnormal for his age in clearly distinguishing internal "private" events, such as thoughts, wishes, feelings, or memories, from external events. This leads to characteristic difficulties

Table 8-1 Schizophrenic Psychoses of Childhood and Adolescence

Age of Onset	*General Characteristics*	*Commonly Occurring Syndromes**
Within the first two years	No clear evidence of prior period of normal personality development Chronic course	Early infantile autism
Age two to five years	Follows apparently normal infancy	Symbiotic psychosis
Latency	Late onset Fluctuating, sub-acute course	Pseudoneurotic schizophrenia or Borderline states
Adolescence		Borderline states or Pseudopsychopathic schizophrenia or Adult-type schizophrenia

* Other diagnostic terms also used to describe these syndromes are listed in the discussion of each syndrome later in the chapter.

in dealing with other people, including a preoccupation with inanimate objects, a disregard for usual object function, and regressive and unusual interests.[17, 19, 51, 71, 80]

Johnny, age three and a half, although apparently quite bright, had never learned to use speech to communicate with others. While he would play contentedly for long periods of time if left alone, he would stiffen and scream if anyone approached him. If someone tried to cuddle him, he would struggle to get away. He was preoccupied with doorknobs, which he would handle and turn endlessly, and spent much time playing with a toy tractor. Instead of "driving it" and making tractor noises like a normal toddler, however, he would repeatedly sniff it, mouth it like an infant, and twirl the wheels on their axles again and again. His symptoms, which had been noted before his second birthday, illustrate serious difficulties in his relationships with people and his dealings with inanimate objects.

Ruth, age four, had seemed normal until her third year of life, at which point she began to experience severe panic reactions whenever her mother left her sight. Even her mother's going into the next room was at times enough to precipitate a panic. Following her mother's return or when a stranger came into the room, she would cling frantically to her mother. Unlike the shyness of the normal child, who may briefly cuddle or cling when a stranger appears on the scene, Ruth would continue to cling endlessly rather than letting go and proceeding to play when the stranger had demonstrated that he did not constitute a threat. Ruth would also experience disproportionate panic if her hair or toenails were cut even by her mother, as if she were losing a vital part of her body on each occasion.

Ricky, age fourteen, who was fascinated with airplanes, suddenly announced he would get a job at the airport. His father remarked that the airport was seventeen miles away, and wondered how he would get to work. Ricky replied that would be easy: he would just get in a plane, fly it home, and land in the middle of his street. Further questioning established that he could see nothing illogical or unrealistic about this proposal.

ii) *Inappropriate emotional responses* may appear as a lack of normal concern or as excessive and apparently illogical anxiety. Sudden mood changes arise apparently from internal sources or from gross misperceptions of external reality.

Bobby, age five, went through a period in which he was convinced that he was a girl. He would become furious at any indication that he was regarded as a boy. At the same time, Bobby was terrified by any sort of mask, which clearly he could not differentiate from a real person.

iii) *Language defects* may include abnormalities in pitch, rhythm, stress, and intonation or neologisms (words made up by the patient, frequently by condensing several other words).[28, 38, 96]

iv) *Motility patterns* may be disturbed, with overactivity or underactivity, bizarre mannerisms, or whirling. The child may alternate overactivity with underactivity. Hand-flapping may accompany anxiety or pleasure. Prolonged rhythmic rocking, head-banging, twirling, jumping up and down, and toe-walking are common. Toys may be used not in the usual way, but may be sniffed or mouthed. Tricycles, instead of being ridden, may be turned on their side so that the wheels can be spun endlessly close to the face of the child. Later some of these activities may turn into more elaborate rituals, such as banging everything three times, kissing dangerous objects, etc.

v) *Disturbances in development* are also characteristic, resulting sometimes in normal or precocious capacity in one or more areas in the face of developmental failure or regression of other functions.

> One child was standing at five months, but at eleven months was already showing bizarre mannerisms. At age two, while showing some echolalia (the repetition of the last words on phrases heard), he was not yet using speech to communicate. At age four, while unable to play with toys in an age-appropriate manner, he mastered jigsaw puzzles that would prove challenging to the average eight-year-old. While he still had no communicative speech, he was able to identify correctly all makes of cars passing by. Another eleven-year-old boy, while able to use speech to communicate in a sing-song and mechanical way, was totally lacking in social skills. While succeeding marginally in school, he was preoccupied with subways and could endlessly reproduce elaborate sketches of various aspects of the subway system of a large metropolitan area.

It is important to note that the clinical features may or may not change significantly as the child becomes older. Some autistic children, for example, remain so, functioning throughout life at a very primitive level. Others gradually become less autistic and begin to display symptoms seen in later-onset psychosis. Children with later-onset psychosis also may undergo a shift in symptoms, with a pseudoneurotic pattern developing pseudopsychopathic features over a period of time. The degree to which ongoing development is blocked (i.e. fixated) and the balance between continuing maturation and behavioural regression will determine the clinical course.

c) PREVALANCE

Treffert[90] reported a prevalence of 3.1 cases per 10,000 children in the state of Wisconsin, of whom one-quarter were classical early infantile autism, 56 per cent were characterized by later onset, while the remaining 19 per cent were probably psychotic but complicated by known organicity. Lotter [58] and Wing et al.[94] found a prevalence of 2.1 cases of classical infantile autism per 10,000 children in a survey of Middlesex County, and a further 2.4 with many of the characteristics of this syndrome.

d) MALE-TO-FEMALE RATIO AND ORDINAL POSITION

Childhood psychosis is more common in boys than girls. Male-to-female ratios for early infantile autism have ranged from 4.25 : 1 to 2.8 : 1.[48, 53, 78, 90] For later-onset psychosis the ratios have varied from 3.4 : 1 to 2.66 : 1.

Findings regarding ordinal position have been contradictory. A tendency for an excess of first-born children to have early infantile autism has been reported,[48, 53] but Treffert found the opposite.[90] Rutter et al.[78] found a higher ratio in first-born children only in two-child families, while Wing et al.[94] reported no particular position.

e) AETIOLOGICAL FACTORS

A variety of interacting influences appear involved in most instances. These include *genetic predisposition*. Most though not all monozygotic twins are concordant for schizophrenia.[46, 85] Estimates of the incidence of schizophrenia in the parents of schizophrenic children range from 10 to 40 per cent,[45, 48, 53, 58, 70, 78] while one study[7] suggests 10 per cent of affected children have two psychotic parents. (Future studies of the adopted children of schizophrenic parents will be particularly valuable in more clearly separating genetic from experimental factors.[7, 37, 53, 92, 95])

Adverse intrauterine and perinatal influences of a nutritional, circulatory, or other nature have been reported in from a third to almost a half of those with infantile autism and a sixth to a quarter with later-onset psychosis.[50, 55, 78, 87, 90, 94]

Minor signs of *brain dysfunction* have been described in as many as one-quarter of the children with infantile autism and in a lesser proportion of those subsequently becoming ill. Gross organic pathology is rare.[3, 18, 43] In such cases it is presumed, but not proven, that there is organic precipitation of psychosis in a genetically predisposed child. A high prevalence of infantile autism has been associated with congenital rubella [15, 22] and epilepsy.[7, 18, 55, 78, 81, 88]

A primary neurophysiological abnormality has been regarded by a number of investigators as being of critical importance.[7, 8, 10, 32, 33,

34 Foetal dysmaturation [7, 35] and disorders of the limbic system[81] or of the reticular formation[74] have been postulated. It has been suggested that the mechanism underlying all the various forms of childhood schizophrenia is the syndrome of *perceptual inconstancy.*[70] Arising from the faulty homeostatic regulation of perceptual input, perceptual inconstancy is related to a specific pathophysiological mechanism which can, at times, be activated by neuropathological conditions. Other hypotheses have included the concept of a *failure of social perception* in autism analogous to the intellectual deficits in the retarded[24] and theories involving the biochemical and neurophysiological substrates of childhood schizophrenia. While an increased incidence of coeliac disease in children with early infantile autism has been used to suggest a possible relationship to disturbed serotonin metabolism,[40] further use of sophisticated biochemical and electroencephalographic techniques is needed to clarify this entire area.[68, 83]

Adverse psychological experiences, especially pathological mother-child relationships[11, 30, 48] and confusing and conflicting family roles and patterns of communication, [12, 57] have also been implicated. Less family pathology has been reported in children with prominent organic features[36, 37] and more in children with later-onset psychosis than in those with infantile autism.[54] Autism has been related to faulty early conditioning, although with little solid evidence to support this relationship.[31] Anthony has studied the children of psychotic parents and described a group where the child's psychosis stems *from*, but antedates, that of the parent.[4] These are children who show a number of somatic factors that Anthony feels are indicative of a genetically determined high-risk for schizophrenia. He contrasts these with two other groups of children. The first group includes children with induced, or parapsychotic, states associated *with* the parental illness, for example, the child who, while exposed to the influence of a paranoid mother, absorbs her delusional belief that everyone is conspiring against her, even though he remains capable of a more realistic assessment of others' motives when no longer continually exposed to his mother's delusional system. The other group includes those children whose disturbance is reactive *to* the parental psychosis. An example might be another child of the paranoid mother described above who, while aware and upset by his mother's delusional system and unpredictable behaviour, developed symptoms in his own right without ever incorporating her delusional view of the world. Anthony stresses the importance of the presence and effectiveness of the non-psychotic parent in minimizing the deleterious effect of the schizophrenic parent on the child.

Other investigators have documented the presence of childhood psychosis in the absence of serious family disturbance and have drawn attention to the effect of the child on the adjustment of other family members.[72, 76] While the emotional environment was held to contribute to either the precipitation or the course of the child's disorder, parental and marital adjustments, while important in determining attitudes to the psychotic child, were not considered a principal cause of the psychosis.[20] The family has also been regarded as significantly influencing the nature of the defences used by the child. This in turn will do much to determine the clinical picture, but familial factors in themselves were not considered sufficient to result in the illness. Developmental phases requiring marked shifts in personality organization and in interpersonal relationships are seen as points of greater vulnerability to breakdown in the predisposed child.[61, 63, 65]

Evidence attempting to relate early infantile autism to the socio-economic status of the parents is contradictory and inconclusive,[53, 66, 75, 90, 94, 95] although severe withdrawal and autism were significantly more frequent in the professional and executive groups.

These apparently conflicting findings on aetiology can be reconciled if a psychobiological viewpoint is maintained and false dichotomies avoided. Childhood psychosis may then be regarded as the outcome of a variety of interacting factors. A purely psychogenic aetiology appears unlikely except perhaps under extraordinarily adverse conditions operating for a prolonged period. No specific psychological experiences have been convincingly associated with the development of psychosis. It is evident, however, that in those neurophysiologically predisposed to schizophrenia (reasons for which might include prenatal and perinatal environmental factors and/or genetic influences), psychotic illness would be more likely if psychological experiences were adverse in certain respects. These would include, for example, environments that increased the difficulties of successful individuation or of establishing object constancy,[5] which did not provide clear differentiation of reality from wish fulfilment[57] or stable identification figures. Family experiences would then be expected to influence the child's symptomatology. The interaction of perinatal, genetic, and experiential factors have been documented in several recent studies,[85] and the concept of schizophrenia as a failure of integration[82]—the outcome of a wide variety of interacting neurophysiological and psychological events—is a useful one. Abnormalities in the child's responses, whether initially physiologically or psychologically determined, influence parental responses to the child,[85] leading in turn to further effects on the developing personality structure.

f) PROGNOSIS

Reports of the outcome of specific syndromes other than infantile autism are sparse, probably because of a lack of diagnostic precision. A number of studies, each containing a proportion of autistic children, confirm the serious outlook for childhood psychosis. Follow-up studies in adolescence and adult life show 33 to 61 per cent of child schizophrenics require continuous in-patient care, while 7 to 14 per cent in three studies and 25 per cent in a fourth function at least well enough to attend a normal class in an ordinary school or to hold a job.[7, 15, 18, 25, 78] The absence of meaningful speech by age five[25] and IQ of less than 60 or inability to be tested at the point of initial diagnosis are poor prognostic signs.[78] With the exception of infantile autism, comments regarding the prognosis for individual syndromes are based on clinical experience rather than on adequate follow-up studies.

g) CLINICAL SYNDROMES

i) *Early Infantile Autism**

This is the earliest form of psychosis, and must be distinguished from symptomatic autism.[26] Mildly autistic behaviour is also seen in deaf, blind, retarded, dysphasic, or severely brain-damaged children. In these cases, the autistic behaviour is more a result of isolation, arising from a combination of reduced sensory input and inadequate social stimulation, and the other characteristic signs of the syndrome are not evident.

Early infantile autism features extreme self-isolation, generally present from infancy.[27, 74] The child, at first, is regarded as very quiet and placid, but it becomes apparent within the first year that he does not

*Other terms used to describe this syndrome include Group I (Mahler);[64] pseudo-defective schizophrenia (Bender);[8] "no-onset type" psychosis (Despert);[23] Group 1 (Anthony);[2] early-onset psychosis.[51]

relate to others. There is failure to develop normal eye contact, and the affectionate relationships with objects such as toys contrast with the lack of interest and involvement with people. Early in the first year the mother may notice the child's lack of response to her and his failure to reach towards her as he is picked up.[62]

A second characteristic sign is the need to preserve the environment of objects unchanged. Even minor alterations prove distressing to the child.

Language may fail to develop or be delayed, and reversal of first and third pronouns is characteristic; that is, if the child has speech, he persists in referring to himself as "he" and to the mother as "I". An inability to use abstract terms and the persistence of immature grammatical structures are frequent. The child's ability to reproduce rhymes and lists of names may be in stark contrast with the lack of communicative speech. Echolalia may be immediate or delayed.[28] These language disorders may derive from perceptual difficulties.[73]

Ritual movements such as hand-flapping, twirling, and toe-walking are often seen. Precocious circumscribed capacities, for example, mechanical or drawing ability, may remain for some children often in marked contrast to the gross failure of development of other functions.

Sometimes normal development in the first eighteen months is followed by withdrawal, loss of language, and a clinical picture indistinguishable from that of children developing symptoms within the first year.

DIFFERENTIAL DIAGNOSIS The two disorders that most need to be distinguished are deafness and mental retardation. In deafness (except when associated in symptomatic autism) the characteristic symptoms of autism are not present, and the child will relate and attempt to communicate. The hearing loss is usually demonstrable, though in doubtful cases cortical audiography is indicated. It must be remembered that some children with early infantile autism also can show hearing deficits.

The mentally retarded child shows a developmental delay in all areas, while in infantile autism motor development is normal or only slightly delayed in contrast with the severe communication and relationship deficits.

In over 50 per cent of cases of early infantile autism, however, the testable IQ is in the mentally retarded range.[78] This does not generally rise in those children who improve clinically,[79] suggesting that mental retardation and infantile autism are both present in many children and that the poor test performance cannot be attributed solely to the disturbed behaviour and social withdrawal. In about one-third of children, despite autistic symptoms no less severe, the IQ is within the average range. The generally higher performance on visuo-spatial than on verbal tasks[77] differs from that pattern found in children with global mental retardation. A tendency towards intellectual deterioration, most evident in those initially estimated to be of normal intelligence, has been reported on follow-up.[42]

Congenital receptive dysphasia is excluded by the presence of echolalia, the pronominal reversals, extreme concreteness, or non-communicative reproduction of rhymes or collections of words. Affective contact remains good, and the child attempts to communicate.

TREATMENT Emphasis is on promoting relationships and communication. Because the child has never learned to relate, intensive efforts are made to lure him into involvement with others and to expose him to peer experiences and social expectations. Some children who respond may then pass into symbiotic relationships with the therapist and other staff. Stereotyped rituals are interrupted and the child is encouraged to interact with others and is socially rewarded for doing so. Kemph et al. have described the phases of psychotherapy with these children,[49] who generally require intensive day[56] or residential treatment[86] directed towards the child's identity difficulties.[16] Wing has provided valuable guidance for parents.[93]

For some children, relationships appear so threatening, or therapeutic attempts to establish them so unrewarding, that behaviour-modification techniques may offer more positive prospects.[59, 60] The child is immediately and consistently rewarded for specified desired behaviour, including speech,[44] using a primary reinforcer, such as food, paired with social reinforcers, such as praise, physical contact, attention, and affection. Starting with very simple behaviours, more complex responses are shaped through a systematic process of reinforcement. By repeated pairing of primary and social reinforcers, it is hoped that the child will ultimately become responsive to the latter alone. There is no doubt that behavioural changes can be obtained, but adequate follow-up studies are not yet available to evaluate this approach.

PROGNOSIS Adequate communicative language by age five years is an important prognostic sign,[24] and in its absence almost no children show even a fair outcome. About half of those children in whom it is present will ultimately make a fair adjustment. Few of these, however, will be well adjusted; of those functioning in the community only 5 per cent seem normal, with the remainder appearing schizoid or showing neurotic symptoms.[14] The inappropriate use of toys and complete lack of speech after age three years have been found of serious significance.[13] An IQ-test level of below 60 when first diagnosed[78] and a late transition from autism to pseudoneurotic phase[42] are unfavourable prognostic signs for later intellectual functioning.

ii) *Symbiotic Psychosis**

In this rare condition the child's relationship with his mother proceeds uneventfully until the normal symbiotic phase, from between twelve and eighteen months to thirty-six months. At this point the child's biological striving towards independence and his increased motor activity, normally given the mother's support and encouragement, lead to a "hatching" from the symbiotic relationship by the process of individuation. In the child with symbiotic psychosis, individuation fails to occur at this stage and the psychosis results. Precipitating factors may include separation of the child from the mother (for example, by hospitalization) or reduced maternal affection and encouragement as with the birth of a sibling or maternal depression.

As the psychosis develops, speech becomes distorted or lost and behaviour regresses. Clinging to others may be seen as an attempt to re-establish interpersonal fusion. Some children frantically test reality by touching, smelling, licking, and feeling as though to define their separateness from their environment. Superficial and unstable identifications with others, for example, in dress or hair style, may represent attempts to maintain a sense of identity. Primary process thinking may become quite evident, stereotyped behaviour is common, and these children usually appear severely disorganized.

DIFFERENTIAL DIAGNOSIS In neurotic regression, which can also occur following separation or the birth of a sibling, the personality remains

*Symbiotic psychosis[61,63] is also referred to as interactional psychosis,[41] disintegrative psychosis,[80] or Group II psychosis.[64]

integrated and psychotic defence mechanisms and confusions of internal and external reality are not apparent. One must also rule out neurotic overattachment, in which there are no signs of psychosis, the behaviour seems purposeful, and the entire clinical picture is understandable from a knowledge of the environmental influences. Progressive cerebral disease (for example, Heller's)[43] is rare; here the child appears sick, and dementia and neurological abnormalties are apparent.

TREATMENT The crucial process of separation-individuation is encouraged. This is done by first promoting a symbiotic relationship with a therapeutic adult and then encouraging independence and separation at a pace the child can tolerate without disruptive anxiety or the need for pathological defences.[62] The child is helped to reality-test within the security of the therapeutic relationship, with the anxiety level kept down by the provision of structure, predictability, safe limits, clear reality communications, and supportive relationships with others.[62] When anxiety is marked, the phenothiazines may contribute to over-all treatment planning.

PROGNOSIS The prognosis for symbiotic psychosis is usually regarded as very poor.[26, 78] Some children remain secondarily autistic, others continue to function at a severely regressed level, while some show a gradual improvement with residual deficits.[63]

iii) *Pseudoneurotic Schizophrenia**

This syndrome is typically seen in latency.[8] Ego functions are sufficiently developed for a variety of neurotic defence mechanisms to be apparent. These include denial, repression, dissociation, reaction formation, displacement, and intellectualization. Repetitive questioning and bizarre rituals and mannerisms are often seen. Great difficulty distinguishing between fantasy and reality may be evident, with terrifying nightmares and marked identity confusion. Omnipotent feelings and extremely controlling behaviour may be apparent. Relationships

*Pseudoneurotic Schizophrenia has also been referred to as Group III (Mahler);[64] as schizophreniform psychosis (Group for the Advancement of Psychiatry classification);[41] as the "normal-neurotic" group (Brown and Reiser);[14] as Group II (Anthony).[2]

are superficial and withdrawal and dependency are usual. Typically the onset is sub-acute or chronic, with failing school performance and increasing ritualistic preoccupations. Obsessive concern with death, disaster, and events such as earthquakes and volcanoes may be marked. These represent threatening internal forces and are dealt with by attempts at intellectual mastery.[64]

Drawings may reveal these concerns and/or the defences against them. Compulsive accumulation of information on unusual topics may occupy much of the child's time. Sometimes an acute onset occurs, with diffuse anxiety or psychosomatic complaints, phobias, insomnia, withdrawal, and disorganization. A thought disorder may become clearly evident, and delusions and hallucinations may occur, although they are not necessary for the diagnosis. Affective inappropriateness and episodes of marked regressive behaviour may be seen.

DIFFERENTIAL DIAGNOSIS Differential diagnosis is chiefly from severe neurotic states, especially obsessive-compulsive neurosis. These neurotic states are excluded by evidence in pseudoneurotic schizophrenia of identity confusion and confusion of internal and external experience, which may sometimes be recognized easily or at others may be evident only through the use of drawings and other projective techniques. Affective inappropriateness and marked regressive behaviour also exclude psychoneurosis. The child's description of his thought content is characteristically vague, illogical, and hard to follow.

TREATMENT A relatively satisfactory adjustment may be maintained except at times of external stress. This may result from family disequilibrium, rapid changes in the child's life situation such as a move to a new school or neighbourhood, and feared or actual relationship loss. Emphasis is on reducing stress to a tolerable level and encouraging social relationships and involvement. If decompensation is marked, brief admission may be necessary with a return to the family at the earliest opportunity. Concurrent work with parents in family therapy may be indicated to clarify communications within the family and to help members derive adaptive ways of dealing with and resolving conflict and disturbing effect.

Medication may be helpful to reduce the disorganizing effects of anxiety or to control severely impulsive behaviour. Because of the relative instability of the neurotic defences, psychotherapy when indicated is generally of a supportive nature.

PROGNOSIS The prognosis frequently appears good in those children whose decompensation is clearly referrable to stress and whose prior adjustment was relatively stable. Continued satisfactory functioning may be maintained during adolescence.[9]

iv) *Borderline States*

Regardless of the presenting symptoms, the borderline states have been ascribed to a specific developmental arrest caused by the inability of the borderline child's mother to tolerate the child's attempts to hatch from the normal symbiotic stage. As a result, any move in the direction of normal independence or separation brings with it the massive threat of abandonment, which threatens to overwhelm the child.[65] Rapid fluctuations in the level of ego functioning are characteristic. At times, adjustment may seem relatively intact, but neurotic symptoms or psychotic defences and primary process thinking may abruptly appear, only to revert with equal suddenness to higher functioning.[29] These regressive shifts occur particularly in response to real or feared loss of relationships, without which the precarious ego integration cannot be maintained, or under the impact of threatening inner experiences. Some children show omnipotent delusions or project their anger on to the environment, which is then experienced as dangerous and about to destroy them. A preoccupation with space, monsters, and world catastrophes is frequently apparent, at times reaching delusional proportions. Drawings are a valuable diagnostic aid in these children and in assessing progress. A clear thought disorder may be present and delusions and hallucinations may appear although much less commonly than in adult schizophrenia. Children have been reported to progress from an infantile autistic state to one with pseudoneurotic or borderline characteristics.

Children showing this syndrome are generally neither as well as they appear when at their best (because of their propensity for disorganization under minor stress) nor as ill as they seem when most regressed (in view of their capacity to reintegrate to their former level).

DIFFERENTIAL DIAGNOSIS The rapid and often quickly reversible shifts in ego functioning in response to internal or external stimuli are quite characteristic and, when observed, pathognomonic. Less severely disturbed youngsters may require intensive in-patient observation to establish the diagnosis.

TREATMENT A search is made for the factors producing the regressive shifts. Such children, because they cannot maintain a stable level of functioning, are generally more vulnerable than those showing a chronic pseudoneurotic clinical picture. Individual psychotherapy, while placing severe demands and requiring great skill on the part of the therapist, is often indicated and frequently needs to be prolonged because of the fragility of the defences.[29, 65] Concurrent medication with one of the phenothiazines may significantly reduce regression and enhance the capacity to tolerate psychotherapeutic involvement. Some of these youngsters respond well to residential treatment in a highly predictable, structured setting.

PROGNOSIS Some cases with intensive treatment respond well and appear to sustain the good outcome for years after their regular psychotherapy has been discontinued. Following the period of intensive treatment, it often appears useful in times of crisis for the patient to have access briefly to his therapist, who serves as a "refuelling" station, thus helping him reorganize the defences temporarily overwhelmed by the crisis.

v) *Pseudo-psychopathic Schizophrenia*

Characteristically seen in adolescence, this syndrome may originate at that time or it may develop from an earlier but different syndrome. A very careful case history is therefore extremely important. Children with similar difficulties in latency may initially be thought to have a personality disorder, with the diagnosis only becoming clear after prolonged observation.

The clinical picture is characterized by antisocial acting-out, sometimes of a very serious nature with relatively little anxiety, concern, or guilt. There is an absence of the dominant neurotic mechanisms seen in pseudoneurotic schizophrenia. Markedly impulsive behaviour, little empathy for others, poor social judgment, and clear paranoid ideation may be present. Delusions and hallucinations may occur but may be concealed. A thought disorder may not be evident. Bender has commented on the improvement seen in some schizophrenic children in early adolescence, although often not sustained throughout this period.

DIFFERENTIAL DIAGNOSIS This is chiefly from reactive disorders and personality disorders of adolescence. Projective psychological tests that include drawings may be of great help in revealing identity confusion and body-image distortions in those subjects in whom delusions, hallucinations, or thought disorder are not apparent. The diagnosis of schizophrenia is especially difficult in adolescence. Emphasis should be placed on the previous history for evidence of earlier psychotic difficulties, and on the current situation. The development of antisocial behaviour during latency or adolescence in the absence of evident environmental cause should always raise the possibility of schizophrenia. This is particularly so if prior evidence of personality disorder is not obtained. When resulting chiefly from a disturbed interpersonal environment, children with personality disorders manifest difficulties from the pre-school or early latency periods.

TREATMENT Emphasis is on reducing the adolescent's paranoid interpretation of his environment by establishing feelings of trust and security within the therapeutic relationship. Depending on the nature of the acting-out, this may initially require residential treatment or intensive individual psychotherapy several times a week. Once trust can be secured, it becomes possible to help the youngster discover what it is he does that leads to hostility and rejection from his environment, and to assist him in finding more adaptive ways of dealing with stress and experiential difficulties. These youngsters are often very hard to reach because of their suspiciousness and ability to disguise symptoms.

PROGNOSIS Outlook appears poor but definitive follow-up studies are lacking. Florid breakdown may be followed by withdrawal, panneurotic, psychosomatic, or catatonic symptomatology.[9]

vi) *Adult-Like Schizophrenia*

In adolescence, and occasionally in latency, a clinical picture resembling adult schizophrenia has been reported.[52] Symptoms include a thought disorder, affective blunting, mood disturbance, especially early perplexity, and manneristic behaviour. Hallucinations, most commonly auditory but sometimes accompanied by the visual and somatic variety, and delusions are also described.

h) CONCLUSIONS

In conclusion, it should be noted that, for those psychotic children and adolescents capable of relating, the availability on a very long term basis of a therapist who will provide support, understanding, and commitment may be crucial. Many show a lifelong vulnerability necessitating therapeutic intervention at times of stress or when rapid need for fresh adaptive changes cannot be met. No evidence currently exists to support the use of megavitamins in child psychosis.[39]

RECOMMENDED FOR FURTHER READING

1. ALDERTON, H. R. "A Review of Schizophrenia in Childhood". *Can. Psychiat. Assoc. J.* 11: 276–85, 1966.
—an overview of the subject, relating constitutional to experiential factors, and the clinical picture to developmental level.

2. ANTHONY, E. J. "A Clinical Evaluation of Children with Psychotic Parents". *Amer. J. Psychiat.* 126: 177–84, 1969.
—relates the type of disturbance found in children of psychotic parents to the type of relationship between the sick parent and the child.

6. ANTHONY, E. J., and SCOTT, P. "Manic-Depressive Psychosis in Childhood". *J. Child Psychol. Psychiat.* 1:53–72, 1960.
—a good summary article on the subject.

10. BERGMAN, P., and ESCALONA, S. K. "Unusual Sensitivities in Very Young Children". *Psychoanal. Stud. Child.* 3–4: 333–52, 1949.
—a classical paper, illustrating one type of predisposition to psychosis.

27. EISENBERG, L., and KANNER, L. "Early Infantile Autism, 1943–1955." *Amer. J. Orthopsychiat.* 26: 556–66, 1956.
—a useful review of the syndrome.

34. FISH, B., SHAPIRO, T.; HALPERN, F.; and WILE, R. "The Prediction of Schizophrenia in Infancy. 3: A Ten-Year Follow-up Report of Neurological and Psychological Development". *Amer. J. Psychiat.* 121: 768–75, 1964–65.
—predicts vunerability to schizophrenia from uneven early development.

49. KEMPH, J. P.; HARRISON, S. I.; and FINCH, S. M. "Promoting the Development of Ego Functions in the Middle Phase of Treatment of Psychotic

Children". *J. Amer. Acad. Child Psychiat.* 4: 401–12, 1965.
—describes the phases of psychotherapy with psychotic children.

60. LOVAAS, O.I.; FREITAS. L.; NELSON, K.; and WHALEN, C. "The Establishment of Imitation and Its Use for the Development of Complex Behaviour in Schizophrenic Children". *Behav. Res. Ther.* 5: 171–81, 1967.
—a description of a current behaviour therapy approach.

61. MAHLER, M. S. "On Child Psychosis and Schizophrenia: Autistic and Symbiotic Infantile Psychosis". *Psychoanal. Stud. Child.* 7: 286–305, 1952.
—a presentation of a psychoanalytic viewpoint on childhood psychosis.

65. MASTERSON, J. F. *Treatment of the Borderline Adolescent: A Developmental Approach.* New York, Wiley-Interscience, Division of John Wiley and Sons, 1972.
—the most definitive statement regarding the clinical management of the borderline adolescent.

71. ORNITZ, E. M.; and RITVO, E. R. "Perceptual Inconstancy in Early Infantile Autism". *Arch. Gen. Psychiat.* 18: 76–98, 1968.
—an important recent view of a possible neurophysiological basis for childhood schizophrenia and autism.

92. WENDER, P. H. "The Role of Genetics in the Etiology of Schizophrenias". *Amer. J. Orthopsychiat.* 39: 447–58, 1969.
—a description of an important approach which makes it possible to separate genetic from experiential factors.

ADDITIONAL REFERENCES

3. ANTHONY, E. J. "An Experimental Approach to the Psychopathology of Childhood: Autism". *Brit. J. Med. Psychol.* 31: 211–25, 1958.

4. ANTHONY, E. J. "Low-Grade Psychosis in Childhood", in Richards, B. W., ed., *Proceedings of London Conference on Scientific Study of Mental Deficiency.* Vol. 2. London, May and Baker, 1962.

5. ANTHONY, E. J. "The Significance of Jean Piaget for Child Psychiatry". *Brit. J. Med. Psychol.* 29: 20–34, 1956.

7. BENDER, L. "Childhood Schizophrenia". *Psychiat. Quart:* 27: 663–81, 1953.

8. BENDER, L. "Schizophrenia in Childhood—Its Recognition, Description, and Treatment." *Amer. J. Orthopsychiat.* 26: 499–506, 1956.

9. BENDER, L. "The Concept of Pseudopsychopathic Schizophrenia in Adolescents". *Amer. J. Orthopsychiat.* 29: 491–509, 1959.

11. BETTLEHEIM, B. *The Empty Fortress: Infantile Autism and the Birth of Self.* New York, The Free Press, 1967.

12. BOATMAN, M. J., and SZUREK, S. A. "A Clinical Study of Childhood Schizophrenia", in Jackson, D., ed., *The Etiology of Schizophrenia,* 389–440. New York, Basic Books, 1960.

13. BROWN, J. L. "Prognosis from Presenting Symptoms of Preschool Children with Atypical Development". *Amer. J. Orthopsychiat.* 30: 382–90, 1960.

14. BROWN, J. L., and REISER, D. E. "Follow-up Study of Preschool Children of Atypical Development (Infantile Psychosis): Later Personality Patterns in Adaptation to Maturational Stress". *Amer. J. Orthopsychiat.* 33: 336–38, 1963.

15. CHESS, S. "Autism in Children with Congenital Rubella". *J. Autism Child. Schiz.* 1: 33–47, 1971.

16. COHEN, R. S. "Some Childhood Identity Disturbances: Educational Implementation of a Psychiatric Treatment Plan". *J. Amer. Acad. Child. Psychiat.* 3: 488–99, 1964.

17. CREAK, E. M. "The Schizophrenic Syndrome in Childhood—Progress Report of a Working Party". *Brit. Med. J.* 2: 889–90, 1961.

18. CREAK, E. M. "Childhood Psychosis: A Review of 100 Cases". *Brit. J. Psychiat.* 109: 84–89, 1963.

19. CREAK, E. M. "The Schizophrenic Syndrome in Childhood—Further Progress Report of a Working Party". *Develop. Med. Child. Neurol.* 6: 530–35, 1964.

20. CREAK, M., and INI, S. "Families of Psychotic Children". *J. Child. Psychol. Psychiat.* 1: 156–75, 1960.

21. DARR, G. C., and WORDEN, F. G. "Case Report Twenty-Eight Years After an Infantile Autistic Disorder". *Amer. J. Orthopsychiat.* 21: 559–70, 1951.

22. DESMOND, M. M.; WILSON, G. S.; VERNIAUD, W. M.; MELNICK, J. L.; and RAWLS,

W. E. "The Early Growth and Development of Infants with Congenital Rubella". *Advances in Teratology,* 4: 39–63, 1970.

23. DESPERT, J. L. "Schizophrenia in Children". *Psychiat. Quart.* 12: 366–71, 1938.

24. EISENBERG, L. "The Autistic Child in Adolescence". *Amer. J. Psychiat.* 112: 607–12, 1955–56.

25. EISENBERG, L. "The Course of Childhood Schizophrenia". *Arch. Neurol. Psychiat.* 78: 69–83, 1957.

26. EISENBERG, L. "The Classification of Childhood Psychosis Reconsidered". *J. Autism Child. Schiz.* 2: 338–42, 1972.

28. EKSTEIN, R. "On the Acquisition of Speech in the Autistic Child". *Reiss-Davis Bull.* 1: 63–79, 1964.

29. EKSTEIN, R. *Children of Time and Space, Action and Impulse,* pt. 2: 89–122. New York, Appleton-Century-Crofts, 1966.

30. ERIKSON, E. *Childhood and Society*. 2nd ed., pp. 195–208. New York, W. W. Norton, 1963.

31. FERSTER, C. B. "Positive Reinforcement and Behavioural Deficits of Autistic Children". *Child. Devel.* 32: 437–56, 1961.

32. FISH, B. "Longitudinal Observations of Biological Deviations in a Schizophrenic Infant". *Amer. J. Psychiat.* 116: 25–31, 1959–60.

33. FISH, B., and ALPERT, M. "Patterns of Neurological Development in Infants Born to Schizophrenic Mothers". *Rec. Adv. Biol. Psychiat.* 5: 24–37, 1962–3.

35. FREEDMAN, A. M. "Maturation and Its Relation to the Dynamics of Childhood Schizophrenia". *Amer. J. Orthopsychiat.* 24: 487–91, 1954.

36. GOLDFARB, W. *Childhood Schizophrenia.* Cambridge, Mass., Harvard University Press, 1961.

37. GOLDFARB, W. "An Investigation of Childhood Schizophrenia: A Retrospective View." *Arch. Gen. Psychiat.* 11: 620–34, 1964.

38. GOLDFARB, W.; BRAUNSTEIN, P.; and LORGE, I. "A Study of Speech Patterns in a Group of Schizophrenic Children". *Amer. J. Orthopsychiat.* 26: 544–55, 1956.

39. GREENBAUM, G. H. C. "An Evaluation of Niacinamide in the Treatment of Childhood Schizophrenia". *Amer. J. Psychiat.* 127: 89–92, 1970–71.

40 GRAFF, H., and HANDFORD, A. "Celiac Syndrome in the Case Histories of Five Schizophrenics". *Psychiat. Quart.* 35: 306–13, 1961.

41. Group for the Advancement of Psychiatry. *Psychopathological Disorders in Childhood: Theoretical Considerations and a Proposed Classification.* Vol. 6, Report no. 62. New York, Group for the Advancement of Psychiatry, 1966.

42. HAVELKOVA, M. "Follow-up Study of Seventy-One Children Diagnosed as Psychotic in Preschool Age". *Amer. J. Orthopsychiat.* 38: 846–57, 1968.

43. HELLER, T. "Ueber Dementia Infantilis" *Ztschr. Kinderforsch.* 37: 661–67, 1930. Reprinted in Howells, J., ed., *Modern Perspectives in International Child Psychiatry,* 610–16. Edinburgh, Oliver and Boyd, 1969.

44. HEWETT, F. M. "Teaching Speech to an Autistic Child Through Operant Conditioning". *Amer. J. Orthopsychiat.* 35: 927–36, 1965.

45. KALLMAN, F. J., and ROTH, B. "Genetic Aspects of Preadolescent Schizophrenia". *Amer. J. Psychiat.* 112: 599–606, 1955–56.

46. KAMP, L. N. "Autistic Syndrome in One of a Pair of Monozygotic Twins". *Psychiat. Neurol. Neurochir.* 67: 143–47, 1964.

47. KANNER, L. "Autistic Disturbances of Affective Contact". *Nerv. Child.* 2: 217–50, 1942–43.

48. KANNER, L. "Genetics and the Inheritance of Integrated Neurological Psychiatric Patterns". *Prac. Assoç. Res. Nerv. Ment. Dis.* 33: 378–85, 1953.

50. KNOBLOCH, H., and GRANT, D. K. "Etiological Factors in 'Early Infantile Autism' and 'Childhood Schizophrenia' ". *Amer. J. Dis. Childhood.* 102: 535–36, 1961.

51. KOLVIN, I. "Studies in Childhood Psychoses. 1: Diagnostic Criteria and Classification". *Brit. J. Psychiat.* 118: 381–84, 1971.

52. KOLVIN, I.; OUNSTED, C.; HUMPHREY, M.; and McNAY, A. "Studies in Childhood Psychoses. Phenomenology of Childhood Psychoses". *Brit. J. Psychiat.* 118: 385–95, 1971.

53. KOLVIN, I.; OUNSTED, C.; RICHARDSON, L. M.; and GARSIDE, R. F. "Studies in Childhood Psychoses. 3: The Family and Social Background in Childhood Psychoses". *Brit. J. Psychiat.* 118: 396–402, 1971.

54. KOLVIN, I.; GARSIDE, R. F.; and KIDD, J. S. "Studies in Childhood Psychoses. 4: Parental Personality and Attitude and Childhood Psychoses". *Brit. J. Psychiat.* 118: 403–6, 1971.

55. KOLVIN, I.; OUNSTED, C.; and ROTH, M. "Studies in Childhood Psychoses. 5: Cerebral Dysfunctions and Childhood Psychoses". *Brit. J. Psychiat.* 118: 407–14, 1971.

56. LA VIETES, R. L.; HULSE, W. C.; and BLAU, A. "A Psychiatric Day Treatment Centre and School for Young Children and Their Parents". *Amer. J. Orthopsychiat.* 30: 468–82, 1960.

57. LIDZ, T., and FLECK, S. "Family Studies and a Theory of Schizophrenia", in Lidz, T.; Fleck, S.; and Cornelison, A. R., eds., *Schizophrenia and the Family,* pp. 362–76. New York, IUP, 1965.

58. LOTTER, V. "Epidemiology of Autistic Conditions in Young Children: I. Prevalence". *Soc. Psychiat.* 1: 124–37, 1966.

59. LOVAAS, O. I.; FREITAG, G.; KINDER, M.I.; RUBENSTEIN, B.D.; SCHAEFFER, B.; and SIMMONS, J. Q. "Establishment of Social Reinforcers in Two Schizophrenic Children on the Basis of Food". *J. Exp. Child. Psychol.* 4: 109–25, 1966.

62. MAHLER, M. S., "On Sadness and Grief in Infancy and Childhood: Loss and Restoration of the Symbiotic Love Object". *Psychoanal. Stud. Child.* 16: 332–51, 1961.

63. MAHLER, M. S., and GOSLINER, B. J. "On Symbiotic Child Psychosis: Genetic, Dynamic, and Restitutive Aspects". *Psychoanal. Stud. Child.* 10: 195–212, 1955.

64. MAHLER, M. S.; ROSS, J. R.; and De FRIES, Z. "Clinical Studies in Benign and Malignant Cases of Childhood Psychosis". *Amer. J. Orthopsychiat.* 19: 295–305, 1948.

66. McDERMOTT, J. F.; HARRISON, S. I.; SCHRAGER, J.; LINDY, J.; and KILLINS, E. "Social Class and Mental Illness in Children: The Question of Childhood Psychosis". *Amer. J. Orthopsychiat.* 37: 548–57, 1967.

67. MEDNICK, S., and SCHULSINGER, F. "Some Premorbid Characteristics Related to Breakdown in Children with Schizophrenic Mothers",

in Rosenthal, D. and Kety, S., eds., *The Transmission of Schizophrenia.* Oxford, Pergamon Press, 1968.

68. NARASIMACHARI, N., and HIMWICH, H. E. "Biochemical Studies in Early Infantile Autism". Paper Presented at the Conference on Psychiatric Problems of Childhood, New York City, Jan. 31–Feb. 2, 1974. In Press.

69. *Neurology and Psychiatry in Childhood.* p. 468. Proceedings of the Association for Research in Nervous and Mental Disease. Baltimore, Williams and Wilkins, 1956.

70. O'GORMAN, G. "Childhood Schizophrenia", in O'Gorman, G., ed., *The Nature of Childhood Autism.* 2nd ed., 15–23. London, Butterworth, 1970.

72. PECK, H. B.; RABINOVITCH, R. D.; and CRAMER, J. B. "A Treatment Program for Parents of Schizophrenic Children". *Amer. J. Orthopsychiat.* 19: 592–98, 1949.

73. PRONOVOST, W.; WAKESTEIN, M.P.; and WAKESTEIN, D. J. "A Longitudinal Study of the Speech Behaviour and Language Comprehension of Fourteen Children Diagnosed Atypical or Autistic". *Except. Child.* 33: 19–26, 1966–67.

74. RIMLAND, B. *Infantile Autism.* New York, Appleton-Century-Crofts, 1964.

75. RITVO, E. R.; CANTWELL, D.; JOHNSON, E.; CLEMENTS, M.; BENBROOK, F.; SLAGLE, S.; KELLY, P.; and RITZ, M. "Social Class Factors in Autism". *J. Autism Child. Schiz.* 1: 297–310, 1971.

76. RUTTER, M. "The Influence of Organic and Emotional Factors on the Origins, Nature, and Outcome of Childhood Psychosis". *Develop. Med. Child. Neurol.* 7: 518–28, 1965.

77. RUTTER, M. "Behavioural and Cognitive Characteristics of a Series of Psychotic Children" in Wing, J.K., ed., *Early Childhood Autism: Clinical, Educational, and Social Aspects.* London, Pergamon Press, 1976.

78. RUTTER, M.; GREENFELD, D.; and LOCKYER, L. "A Five to Fifteen Year Follow-up Study of Infantile Psychosis". *Brit. J. Psychiat.* 113: 1169–99, 1967.

79. RUTTER, M. "Concepts of Autism: A Review of Research". *J. Child. Psychol. Psychiat.* 9: 1–25, 1968.

80. RUTTER, M. "Childhood Schizophrenia Reconsidered". *J. Autism Child. Schiz.* 2: 315–37, 1972.

81. SCHAIN, R. J., and YANNET, H. "Infantile Autism: An Analysis of Fifty Cases and a Consideration of Certain Neurophysiologic Concepts". *J. Pediat.* 57: 560–67, 1960.

82. SINGER, R. D. "Organisation as a Unifying Concept in Schizophrenia". *Arch. Gen. Psychiat.* 2: 61–74, 1960.

83. SMALL, J. G. "Sensory Evoked Responses of Autistic Children", in *Infantile Autism,* 224–39. Churchill, D.W.; Alpern, G. D.; and DeMyer, M. K., eds. Illinois, Charles C. Thomas, 1971.

84. SPITZ, R. A. "Anaclitic Depression: An Inquiry into the Genesis of Psychiatric Conditions in Early Childhood, II" *Psychoanalyt. Stud. Child* 2: 313–42, 1946.

85. STABENAU, J. R., and POLLIN, W. "Early Characteristics of Monozygotic Twins Discordant for Schizophrenia". *Arch. Gen. Psychiat.* 17: 723–34, 1967.

86. SZUREK, S.A.; BERLIN, I. N.; and BOATMAN, M. J. *Inpatient Care for the Psychotic Child.* New York, Science and Behav. Books, 1971.

87. TAFT, L. T.; and GOLDFARB, W. "Prenatal and Perinatal Factors in Childhood Schizophrenia". *Develop. Med. Child. Neurol.* 6: 32–43, 1964.

88. THOM, D. A. "Convulsions of Early Life and Their Relation to the Chronic Convulsive Disorders and Mental Defect". *Amer. J. Psychiat.* 98: 574–80, 1941–42.

89. TOLOR, A., and RAFFERTY, W. "Incidence of Symptoms of Early Infantile Autism in Subsequently Hospitalized Psychiatric Patients". *Dis. Nerv. Syst.* 24: 423–29, 1963.

90. TREFFERT, D. A. "Epidemiology of Infantile Autism". *Arch. Gen. Psychiat.* 22: 431–38, 1970.

91. VARSAMIS, J., and MACDONALD, S. M. "Manic-Depressive Disease in Childhood". *Canad. Psychiat. Ass. J.* 17: 279–81, 1972.

93. WING, L. *Austistic Children.* New York, Brunner/Mazel, Inc., 1972.

94. WING, J. K.; O'CONNOR, N.; and LOTTER, V. Autistic Conditions in Early Childhood: A Survey in Middlesex". *Brit. Med. J.* 3: 389–92, 1967.

95. WOLFF, S., and CHESS, S. "A Behavioural Study of Schizophrenic Children". *Acta. Psychiat. Scand.* 40: 438–66, 1964.

96. WOLFF, S., and CHESS, S. "An Analysis of the Language of Fourteen Schizophrenic Children". *J. Child. Psychol. Psychiat.* 6: 29–41, 1965.

ROBERT SIMMONS

9. Psychophysiological Disorders in Childhood and Adolescence

A psychophysiological disorder is present when a child, exposed to a stressful or upsetting situation, responds simultaneously along two dimensions:

1. At the *psychological* level, he reacts subjectively, feeling upset, tense, anxious, or angry.
2. At the *physiological* level, the stress activates the autonomic nervous system, causing an alteration of functioning (e.g. spasm, oversecretion, overbreathing) which, if it persists, may lead to changes in structure (e.g. ulceration, obesity).

The child may or may not be fully aware of the psychological component of his reaction. Some children recognize that when upset their abdominal pains, headaches, or other somatic symptoms occur or become worse. In others, the activation of the autonomic nervous system takes place without conscious recognition, so that at times of stress the child experiences the symptoms resulting from disordered function (e.g. the spasm or pain) with little awareness of their connection with emotional events.

Under normal circumstances, transitory physiological responses frequently accompany emotional states (e.g. blushing). Why in some cases these reactions result in organic pathology is not clear, but a number of factors appear to contribute to the pathogenesis:

1. *Genetic Endowment*. In both diabetes mellitus and asthma there are family histories with strong genetic loadings. This probably is true of

other conditions, although the genetics of each has not been completely defined.

2. *Autonomic System*. Evidence suggests that predominance of a sympathetic or parasympathetic response pattern influences the production of a disorder. For years, autonomic regulation was considered beyond voluntary control, but recent investigations have shown that voluntary control can be achieved through learning and experience.[1] Some people are better able to achieve this control than others. Far Eastern cultures have made use of this factor in Yoga and Transcendental Meditation. Biofeedback mechanisms are being extensively and most promisingly investigated for their effects on heart rate and blood pressure.

3. *Psychoendocrine mechanisms*. Linkages between brain cells and the endocrine system have been elaborated, particularly those between the hypothalamus and the release of tropic hormones. The influence of psychological factors on hormone secretion and resulting fluctuations in menstrual cycles and growth has been documented.

4. *Psychosocial factors* in the child, the family and the social milieu may encourage the expression of emotions via somatic pathways rather than through behaviour or verbalization. For example, a family that generates intense tension and hostility but reacts explosively to overt expressions of rage predisposes to a child's learning to internalize—and possible discharge via somatic pathways—his angry feelings.

Psychophysiological disorders should be distinguished diagnostically from:

1. *Conversion Reactions*. Here anxiety generated by unconscious conflict is converted into a somatic symptom that has no associated structural change (i.e. pathology). The symptom reduces the consciously experienced anxiety (for a further discussion of conversion reactions, see Chapter 5). Physical disease can coexist with a conversion reaction, but is not caused by the underlying conflicts.

2. *Hypochondriasis*. The hypochondriacal child has an exaggerated concern about a real or imagined disturbance in his body function. This is often a symptom of psychoneurosis (especially depression) but occasionally is related to an underlying psychosis.

3. *Self-Inflicted Disorders*. Here the child creates the symptom for psychological reasons (e.g. diarrhoea caused by excessive use of laxatives) often in an attempt to gain attention or help.

4. *Malingering*. The malingering child knowingly pretends to be ill,

usually to avoid an unpleasant situation. Should such avoidance of difficult or unpleasant situations become a pattern, an underlying psychoneurosis or behaviour disorder is indicated. Professionals, as well as parents, often resent being manipulated. The term "malingering", with its pejorative overtones, may reflect this not always recognized resentment. One must carefully avoid letting such personal reactions block the recognition, diagnosis, and appropriate management of the underlying condition.

Psychophysiological disorders can develop in any organ system. The developmental stage of the child influences the psychophysiological manifestation. The infant, for example, handles stress by a gross physiological reaction, because of its lack of experience and psychological development. The extreme example of such a global reaction is to be seen in the marasmic infant (see Chapter 5). Colic in some babies may be a more moderate response to a less severe stress.

Psychophysiological disorders can be classified as falling into one of two categories depending on whether or not structural change has occurred. The first group consists of those disorders in which there is a disturbance of function without an associated change of structure (e.g. the child who has pylorospasm and hypersecretion). The second group includes conditions in which, as a result of prolonged disturbance in function, structural change has occurred (e.g. the child with peptic ulcer).

Common Psychophysiological Disorders of Children and Adolescents

BREATH-HOLDING SPELLS

Breath-holding is a common disorder before age four. Boys and girls are affected with equal frequency. The spells are characterized by a holding of the breath in response to some adverse circumstance. In severe cases, the child goes on to apnoea, cyanosis, and unconsciousness before recovering. In all instances, it is benign and self-limiting.

Two sets of factors seem to contribute to a pattern of breath-holding in response to stress. The occurrence of spells during the newborn period before the child attains any significant awareness of the environment suggests the influence of a constitutional factor. This contention is supported by the frequency with which a family history of breath-holding is obtained. It has been noted, however, that many attacks are precipitated by severe crying due to frustration and anger.

Some children appear to react to any unpleasant situation by breath-holding. For such children, over and above the involuntary and constitutional component, the breath-holding serves as a conscious attempt to control and manipulate the environment.

In management, the parents need reassurance that the episodes are benign and that ignoring them often handles the immediate situation. Parents may need assistance in helping their youngster develop greater frustration tolerance and more appropriate ways of handling unpleasant situations.

HYPERVENTILATION SYNDROME AND SIGHING RESPIRATIONS

This situation presents most frequently to the primary physician or to a hospital emergency department. Approximately 5 per cent of all children for whom a psychiatric diagnosis was given in the emergency department of a large paediatric hospital (Hospital for Sick Children, Toronto, 1974) presented with hyperventilation. The affected child, often described as nervous or highly strung, is characteristically overbreathing, his face flushed rather than cyanotic. If the overbreathing has been prolonged, the child may complain of tingling in the fingers and toes or even demonstrate tetany secondary to hypocalcaemia produced by the respiratory alkalosis. One must carefully distinguish this syndrome from dyspnoea of cardiac or pulmonary disease, from overbreathing caused by ketoacidosis in the diabetic child and from salicylate poisoning. A wide variety of emotional states from joy through fear may trigger the autonomic response, but actual pathways and triggering sites have not yet been defined.

Treatment

Treatment consists of having the patient hold his breath or breathe and rebreathe the same air from a paper bag. As the rebreathing continues, the concentration of carbon dioxide within the bag increases. The carbon dioxide, when inspired, corrects the respiratory alkalosis and activates the Hering-Breuer reflex which effectively limits the respiratory excursion. This treatment, with reassurance in a confident, tranquil atmosphere, is usually sufficient to abort the attack. Only occasionally are antianxiety drugs necessary. If the attacks are recurrent, further investigation to identify the sources of tension and to differentiate the symptom from a conversion reaction is indicated.

Table 9-1

	Control	A	B	C	D
Scale 0–4	N=82	N=64	N=87	N=107	N=57
Severity of clinical components	0	1	2	3	4
Severity of airway resistance between attacks	0	0	0	2	4
Allergic components	1/2	1	1 1/2	3	4
Psychosocial component	0	0	0	1	4

BRONCHIAL ASTHMA

This condition is characterized by dyspnoea featuring recurrent wheezing with laboured and prolonged expiration due to narrowing of the smaller bronchi and bronchioles.

Psychophysiology

In order to develop asthma, the child must be allergic, but a number of factors acting alone or in combination may trigger a particular attack. These may include the exposure to allergens to which the child is sensitive, exercise creating overbreathing, or anxiety from environmental stress or neurotic conflicts. The anxiety acts directly by affecting bronchiole secretion and constriction or by indirectly inducing hyperventilation. In addition, anxiety generated in the child and parents by the attack itself may potentiate the above factors, increasing the severity of the attack and possibly pushing the child into status asthmaticus.

McNicol et al.[12] studied 315 asthmatic children aged seven to fourteen, comparing them to a control group of 82 children. The asthmatic children were divided into four groups according to the frequency and persistence of asthma to fourteen years of age. The findings appear in Table 9-1.

The chronic asthmatic group (D) shows the greatest severity in all components.

Management

1. Treatment of the acute attack by medical means, regardless of the triggering mechanism.
2. Weighing of both allergic and psychological factors contributing to the production of attacks. If neurotic conflicts or family difficulties

seem prominent, intervention towards defining and resolving these is indicated.

Any family with an asthmatic child needs counselling regarding the emotional factors associated with the disease. Minimizing the emotional component along with appropriate treatment of the allergic factor can help reduce the frequency and severity of attacks. In the most severe cases where the family's anxiety has reached such a pathological degree that they cannot manage the child's attacks, "parentectomy" (that is, placing the child in a residential treatment centre for asthmatic children) may have to be considered.

Removal of a pet to which the child is allergic or the curtailment of the child's activities requires an appreciation of the psychological impact this decision may have on the child. While the decision may still have to be made on medical grounds, the way the child's feelings about it are handled can be significant in the control of attacks.

> Six-year-old John, an only child, had a history of bronchitis, beginning at age one year and progressing to clinical asthma by age four. Allergy testing showed him to be mildly sensitive to house dust and tobacco smoke. Many of his attacks were precipitated by infection, usually of viral origin. The parents were in their early forties. With each attack, his mother would panic and John's wheezing would become worse in spite of medication. He would be rushed to the hospital, where he would be admitted because he was so ill, only to clear with minimal treatment within twenty-four hours. The situation was becoming worse with multiple hospital admissions, a great deal of time absent from school and the parents becoming more upset and feeling increasingly inadequate.
>
> Discussion with the parents revealed how anxious they were about this child who meant so much to them. The physician also learned that the father resented having to give up smoking because of the child. He did not criticize them by telling them that they were overprotective, as this would have increased their feelings of inadequacy. The father was helped to recognize some of his feelings and was shown how he could continue smoking in a way that would not affect John, who was only mildly sensitive to tobacco smoke.
>
> In discussion with the physician, much of the family

stress in response to the illness was relieved. John continued to have asthmatic attacks with every severe cold, but these became less distressing to all members of the family, to the point where they usually could be handled at home without hospitalization and with less time off school.

ABDOMINAL PAIN

Some forms of abdominal pain result when tension creates cramping of the abdominal muscles or dysfunction of the gastrointestinal tract. This occurs commonly between seven and twelve years of age, equally in boys and girls. This may also be the origin of some forms of infant colic in children who experience a great deal of tension from the environment. Children with school phobia (or school refusal) often present with chronic abdominal pain (For a discussion of school phobia, see Chapter 6.) Physical and radiological examination are typically negative.

> An eight-year-old girl complained of intermittent abdominal pain for six months. Appetite and bowel function were normal. Physical and radiological investigation revealed nothing. This girl had been an only child up until six months previously, when a younger brother had been born. According to the parents, their daughter was pleased by the new baby and showed no jealousy.
>
> When the physician asked the girl how she felt about her younger brother, it became apparent that although she felt quite jealous she was afraid to express this for fear of upsetting her parents. When they were made aware of her feelings and could allow her to express them more openly, the abdominal pain disappeared.

Management

1. A thorough physical examination, to reassure all concerned that there is no evidence of serious organic pathology.
2. Identification of the major source of stress which may be: (a) a developmental crisis (see Chapter 5); (b) a change within the family; (c) family discord and/or breakdown (see Chapter 20). Adequate handling of the major sources of stress will help to relieve the symptom.
3. If the pain is masking a school refusal, the child should be sent back to school, the reasons for the school refusal explored and dealt with.

PEPTIC ULCER

There has been some controversy over the incidence of ulcers in children and adolescents. A survey of twenty-nine paediatric centres in North America revealed approximately two new cases per hospital per year.[18] A Swedish study of 417, 251 children and adolescents seen in a paediatric department from 1953 to 1962 revealed 184 patients with peptic ulcers, an incidence of 4.4 per 10,000 patients.[17]

Diagnosis

The symptoms are usually atypical, less clearly related to food intake, early morning discomfort, anorexia, and headaches than in the adult. The diagnosis is not infrequently made only secondary to complications (e.g. haemorrhage).

Psychophysiology

In a study of 337 children with ulcers, 324 had significant emotional problems. In adults, Wolf has shown that the gastric mucosa does respond to emotional states. Ulcer patients are known to be hypersecretors of hydrochloric acid, and Weiner et al. demonstrated that those likely to develop an ulcer under stress can be predicted through serum pepsinogen levels.

Psychologically, children with ulcers are characterized by marked conflict around their dependency needs. As a result, they remain immature and have difficulties functioning assertively and independently.

Treatment

1. Medical management of the ulcer.
2. Help the child (via parent counselling and/or psychotherapy of the child) to become a more competent and independent person.

FUNCTIONAL CONSTIPATION

Psychophysiology

The child involved is typically obstinate, highly ambivalent, and passive-aggressive or compulsive. His parents are chronically preoccupied with the presence or absence of his daily bowel movement, regularly cajoling its appearance with laxatives and enemas. The child increasingly resists the pressure to comply with his parents' wishes. The resulting power struggle leads to the child withholding faeces. As the faecal mass becomes larger and harder, pain on attempted defecation encourages further withholding. Overflow incontinence may lead to diarrhoea and soiling of the underclothing (encopresis). In persistent cases, a functional megacolon may be produced. The older the child and the more severe the psychopathology of parents and child, the poorer the prognosis.

Treatment

1. Medical: assist the child towards normal bowel function and bowel re-education, using stool-softening agents if necessary.
2. Help achieve a general de-emphasis of elimination through counselling or psychotherapy.

ULCERATIVE COLITIS

Incidence

Ulcerative colitis occurs in all age groups with the incidence increasing towards puberty. It presents with equal frequency in males and females.

Diagnosis

Ulcerative colitis is diagnosed from a history of diarrhoea and rectal bleeding associated with crampy abdominal pain. It is confirmed by radiological studies and sigmoidoscopy. In the early phase, a barium enema may be negative but as the illness progresses, a distorted mucosal pattern followed by ulcers appearing as shaggy barium-filled niches is typical. On sigmoidoscopy in early stages one finds hyperaemic mucosa that bleeds easily. Only later are ragged ulcers and pseudopolyps seen.

The psychological impact of these investigations on the child, particularly sigmoidoscopy, needs to be taken into account. What may seem a routine procedure to medical and technical staff can prove extremely uncomfortable, embarrassing, and upsetting to the child or adolescent involved. If the child is adequately informed about what to expect during the procedure and given an opportunity to discuss his concerns, what might otherwise be interpreted as an attack is usually well tolerated.

Psychophysiology

The colon is affected by emotions via the cerebral cortex by way of the hypothalamus and the autonomic-parasympathetic nervous system.

The emotional factors influencing the onset and exacerbations are not specific to this disease. Whether or not there are predisposing biological influences also remains unclear. Currently the most promising approach to explaining the aetiology is an autoimmune one. Prognosis is considered by some as related to the degree of psychological disturbance.[16]

Management and Prognosis

1. Medical: Use of steroids (including steroid enemas), asulfadines and transfusions if necessary. In rare cases immuno-suppressive therapy with azothiozine (immuran) is indicated.
2. Supportive psychological care for the child and parents, to minimize the distress of the disease and to increase their ability to deal with its psychological impact and stress generally. Children of those families who can acknowledge and tolerate treatment for psychological stresses may benefit greatly from intensive psychotherapy.
3. Surgical: For continued exacerbations uncontrolled by medical and psychological treatment, removal of the diseased bowel may be necessary. The risk of neoplastic change has led to removal of chronically diseased bowel.

ANOREXIA NERVOSA

A number of adolescents show transient anorexia; but the more serious syndrome of anorexia nervosa is a self-imposed dietary restriction that results in severe weight loss with all the symptoms of malnutrition. The weight loss is significant, at times reaching 20-35 per cent of body weight. It begins typically during adolescence, with the incidence of onset reaching a peak around seventeen to eighteen years of age. Girls are affected nine times as commonly as boys.

Ammenorrhea occurs in girls usually at the time of dietary restriction and before significant weight loss has been established. In spite of the inadequate calorie intake, these individuals are full of energy and perform many physical feats which contrast strikingly with their physical condition. Prognosis for the acute episode is good, although the occasional patient dies. About 50 per cent of patients show some degree of obesity in later years.

Psychophysiology

The patient starves herself for psychological reasons. The psychic stimulus may be mediated through the appetite centre in the hypothalamus. If the anorexia persists, this centre becomes sufficiently suppressed to resist stimulation even when the patient wishes to eat again. The neurophysiological apparatus is theoretical and not clearly understood. However, these patients still have hunger pains and are aware of them but are not prepared to recognize them. The psychological problems are non-specific, ranging from mild adjustment problems with a fear of obesity through obsessions with food (food fads) to delusions about food in a schizophrenic (fear of being poisoned). Psychological concerns are usually related to the ongoing problems of adolescent development, including:

1. Conflict around independent strivings, in which eating becomes a battle ground between patient and family.
2. Conflict around sexual impulses, as a result of which the patient attempts to deny her developing sexuality, e.g. breast development.
3. A distortion of body image.

A family preoccupation with food and feeding may have a great deal to do with food refusal being used by the patient as a symptom and a weapon.

Management

1. Medical. Medical management begins with a thorough physical examination and elimination of other causes for weight loss. A dietary regime sufficient to maintain health and restore weight must be instituted, avoiding as much as possible struggles with the patient around food. One should try to contract with the patient (not the parents) to assume responsibility for attaining an agreed-upon level of weight. Should this not prove successful, the degree of malnutrition may necessitate hospitalization. One means of encouraging weight gain while in hospital is through the use of a behaviour-modification program. The patient is initially restricted to minimal activity but, dependent upon weight gain, can earn additional privileges. This usually motivates patients to eat and retain food in spite of the lack of appetite, but in cases which fail to respond, D-tube or intravenous feeding may be life-saving. In hospital, these patients may present serious management problems because of their ability to entangle ward staff in the same demoralizing struggle that they have engaged in with their parents.
2. Specific treatment for the psychological problems. With the less severely psychologically disturbed patient, firm reassurance and

clear expectations are usually enough. For the more deeply disturbed patient who is unable to respond to simple support and an appeal to reason, psychotherapy of the child and parents is indicated. Phenothiazines may prove helpful for the anorexic patient who is basically schizophrenic.

Claire was a fourteen-year-old girl, oldest in a sibline of three, who began on a diet when she became concerned that she was becoming fat. Her mother was moderately overweight and the relationship between the parents was distant. At first her parents were not alarmed by her dieting. As her diet became more restricted and her exercising increased each day, her weight began to drop more precipitously. When she became amenorrhoeic her parents grew concerned. They tried to beg, bribe, and threaten her to eat, but when all their efforts failed first they and then her siblings became increasingly frustrated. This reached the point where the entire family was becoming increasingly preoccupied with her eating habits.

The parents described Claire prior to her illness as an extremely conforming girl who was an excellent student. Her friendships were few and superficial, and the emotional bond between mother and daughter was extremely intense. Claire seemed to be struggling to emancipate herself from this overly close relationship and to develop her own separate identity.

As Claire had lost 10 kg, she was placed in hospital with privileges and activities restricted. Although she had no appetite, goals were set for her to gain weight and within two weeks she was gaining adequately. Initially, her psychiatrist confined himself to encouraging and supporting her. After 4 kg had been gained, family therapy was instituted in an attempt to bring mother and father closer together and to allow Claire to develop interests outside the family. After ten weekly sessions, Claire had improved enough to be discharged from hospital. She was more involved in school and beginning to show an interest in boys. The parents were working together to consolidate their marriage, instead of remaining preoccupied with their daughter. As the focus of the therapy shifted to the marital relationship, direct treatment of Claire stopped. Follow-up two years later found her to be functioning well.

OBESITY

Obesity does not present a problem until the child enters school, when being overweight results in his missing out on many athletic activities and being vulnerable to teasing. The consequences are even greater in adolescence, when concern with physical attractiveness and social acceptance are particularly acute.

Psychophysiology

The psychophysiology of obesity is only partially understood. Among the dynamic factors thought to contribute to the aetiology are:

1. Family eating habits. These include a family preoccupation with food and eating.
2. Genetic loading in the patient where other family members are also obese.
3. The soothing effect of having something (e.g. thumb, cigarette, gum, etc.) in one's mouth. For the obese patient, food serves as a pacifier in times of tension or distress, just as acting-out does for the child with a neurotic behaviour disorder. (See Chapter 6.)
4. Some children who feel deprived or depressed may try to substitute food for emotional needs that they can't satisfy otherwise.

Management

1. Try to help both child and family appreciate and deal with the underlying problem. The child's image of himself is important. Unless he can acknowledge the extent of the problem and determine to do something about it, attempts at medical treatment (e.g. dieting) will prove an exercise in frustration.

   Successful weight reduction demands considerable self-control, but obese children typically have difficulty establishing and maintaining control over their impulses (including hunger), their behaviour, and their relationships.
2. Medical. A long-term approach towards changing both the child and family's eating habits, with gradual weight reduction through diet restriction and increased exercise, is recommended.
3. Self-help groups provide the needed support for a food addict as Alcoholics Anonymous does for the alcoholic.

DIABETES MELLITUS

For some time diabetic control has been known to be influenced by emotional factors. Some diabetic children with behaviour disorders cheat on their diets, take insulin overdoses, refuse their insulin, or fast in order to precipitate a reaction. This behaviour provokes anxiety in the family thus manipulated by these episodes. In some cases, such behaviour may serve as a depressive equivalent or "chronic suicide" (see Chapter 7). Other children, in response to emotional states may show biochemical alterations leading to difficulties in achieving diabetic control. This represents a true psychophysiological reaction. Preliminary investigation of children who frequently experience life-threatening ketoacidosis has shown that psychological or family stresses precipitate these bouts. In the experience of Minuchin et al.,[16] of the Philadelphia Children's Hospital, and the author, at the Hospital for Sick Children, Toronto, this occurs more frequently in girls, usually just before puberty or in early adolescence.

Psychophysiology

A suggested explanation is that anxiety stimulates the sympathetic nervous system causing the release of catecholamines. The catecholamines facilitate lipolysis in fat tissues releasing free fatty acids. These the liver metabolizes in a manner similar to that used to break down ketones, causing an overloading of the system resulting in ketosis. Why this pathway is chosen seems somewhat related to the constitutional state of the individual. Such children generally avoid open expression of emotional concerns.

Management

Minuchin et al. have used family therapy to decrease stress within the child and family, thus achieving an increase in diabetic control. Some such situations, however, are highly resistant to therapeutic intervention, since family break-up and intractable rejection seem at the root of the problem. In such cases, removal of the child, usually a teenager, from the rejecting family and placement in a group home with supportive counselling can help achieve better diabetic control.

RECOMMENDED FOR FURTHER READING

2. BARBERO, G. J. "Ulcerative Colitis", in Vaughan, V. C.; McKay, R. J.; and Nelson, W. E., eds., *Nelson Textbook of Pediatrics.* 10th ed. Philadelphia, W. B. Saunders, 1975.
—a good description of the medical picture in ulcerative colitis.

4. BRUCH, H. *Eating Disorders.* New York, Basic Books, 1973.
—the most comprehensive book on the subject.

8. LIEBMAN, R.; MINUCHIN, S.; and BAKER, L. "An Integrated Treatment Program for Anorexia Nervosa". *Amer. J. Psych.* 131: 432–36, 1974.
—presents the case for a family approach to management.

9. LIEBMAN, R.; MINUCHIN, S.; and BAKER, L. "The Use of Structural Family Therapy in the Treatment of Intractable Asthma". *Amer. J. Psychiat.* 131: 535–40, 1974.
—discusses characteristics of family organization and functioning associated with psychosomatic illness (e.g. chronic relapsing asthma) and reports the goals, process, and technique of a successful therapeutic approach to changing these.

10. LIVINGSTON, S. "Breath-Holding Spells in Children: Differentiation from Epileptic Attacks". *J. A. M. A.* 212: 2231–35, 1970.
—differentiates breath-holding from seizure disorders and discusses management of spells.

12. McNICHOL, K. N.; WILLIAMS, H. E.; ALLAN, J.; and Mc ANDREW, I. "Spectrum of Asthma in Children: 1. Clinical and Psychological Components; 2. Allergic Components; 3. Psychological and Social Components". *Brit. Med. J.* 4: 7–20, 1973.
—the most comprehensive study available today looking at all factors contributing to asthma.

15. MILLER, N. E. "Learning of Visceral and Glandular Responses". *Science* 163: 434–45, 1969.
—preliminary report that the autonomic nervous system is influenced by experience.

16. MINUCHIN, S.; BAKER, L.; ROSMAN, B. L.; LIEBMAN, R.; MILMAN, L.; and TODD, T. C. "A Conceptual Mode of Psychosomatic Illness in Children: Family Organization and Family Therapy". *Arch. Gen. Psychiat.* 32: 1031–38, 1975.
—provides a useful family model in approaching psychophysiological disorders.

17. MOLDOFSKY, H., and GARFINKEL, P. E. "Problems of Treatment of Anorexia Nervosa". *Canad. Psychiat. Assoc. J.* 19: 169–75, 1974.
—a good discussion of problems in clinical management.

18. O'CONNOR, J. F.; DANIELS, G.; KARUSH, A.; FLOOD, G.; and STERN, L. O. "Prognostic Implications of Psychiatric Diagnosis in Ulcerative Colitis". *Psychosomat. Med.* 28: 375–81, 1966.
—an adult study, examining the relation of psychiatric disorder to the course of ulcerative colitis.

19. POS, R. "Psychological Assessment of Factors Affecting Pain". *Canad. Med. Assoc. J.* 111: 1213–15, 1974.
—assessment of patients with chronic pain should focus on both the organic factors and the psychological process contributing to the pain. The traditional tendency to see organic and psychogenic pain as distinct entities leads to physician confusion and interferes with patient care.

21. REINHART, J. B.; KENNA, M. D.; and SUCCOP, R. A. "Anorexia Nervosa in Children: Outpatient Management". *J. Amer. Acad. Child Psychiat.* 11: 114–31, 1972.
—describes a method of managing children with anorexia nervosa and their families, stressing particularly the importance of the psychological conflict. Helpful case reports.

23. SPERLING, M. "Asthma in Children: An Evaluation of Concepts and Therapies". *J. Amer. Acad. Child Psychiat.* 7: 44–58, 1968.
—strongly psychoanalytical in its approach: points out the chief contributing psychological patterns.

24. TOLSTRUP, K. "The Treatment of Anorexia Nervosa in Childhood and Adolescence". *J. Child Psychol. Psychiat.* 16: 75–78, 1975.
—brief review of various approaches to treatment and a brief evaluation of results obtained.

25. TUDOR, R. "Peptic Ulcer in Childhood", in Sleisenger, M. H., and Fordtran, J. S., eds., *Gastrointestinal Disease*. Philadelphia, W. B. Saunders, 1973.
—very comprehensive article dealing with medical aspects of peptic ulcer.

ADDITIONAL READING

1. APLEY, J. "The Child with Recurrent Abdominal Pain". *Pediat. Clin. N. Amer.* 14,1: 63–72, 1967.

3. BRUCH, H. "Obesity in Adolescence", in Howells, J. G., ed., *Modern Perspectives in Psychiatry*. Vol. 4: 254–73, Brunner/Mazel, New York, 1971.

5. HOLLAND, B. C., and WARD, R. S. "Homeostasis and Psychosomatic Medicine", in Arieti, S., ed., *American Handbook of Psychiatry*. Vol. 3: 344–62. New York, Basic Books, 1966.

6. KARLSTROM, F. "Peptic Ulcer in Children in Sweden During the Years 1953–1962". *Ann. Paediat* (Basel). 202: p. 218, 1964.

7. KHAN, A. U. "Present Status of Psychosomatic Aspects of Asthma". *Psychosomat.* 14: 195–200, 1973.

11. MASON, J. W. "Organization of the Multiple Endocrine Responses to Avoidance in the Monkey". *Psychosomat. Med.* 30: 774–90, 1968.

13. MERCER, R. D. "Constipation". *Pediat. Clin. N. Amer.* 14: 175–84, 1967.

14. MILLAR, T. P. "Peptic Ulcers in Children", in Howells, J. G., ed., *Modern Perspectives in International Child Psychiatry*. Vol. 3: 471–93. Modern Perspectives in Psychiatry, Edinburgh, Oliver and Boyd, 1969.

20. PRUGH, D. G., and JORDON, K. "The Management of Ulcerative Colitis in Childhood" in Howells, J. G., ed., *Modern Perspectives in International Child Psychiatry*. Modern Perspectives in Psychiatry. Edinburgh, Oliver and Boyd, Vol. 3: 494–530, 1969.

22. SINGLETON, E. B., and FAYKUS, M. H. "Incidence of Peptic Ulcer as Determined by Radiologic Examination in the Pediatric Age Group" *J. Pediat.* 65: 858–62, 1964.

26. WAHL, C. W. "Commonly Neglected Psychosomatic Syndromes—Hyperventilation Syndrome", in Arieti, S., ed., *American Handbook of Psychiatry*. Vol. 3: 158–65. New York, Basic Books, 1966.

27. WOLF, S. G. and WOLFE, H. G. *Human Gastric Function*. New York, Oxford Univ. Press, 1947.

MILADA HAVELKOVA

10. Organic Brain Syndromes in Childhood and Adolescence

The patterns of behaviour found in organic brain syndromes occur not only in children in whom organic damage is demonstrable but also in children in whom no organic abnormality can be detected by present techniques. Without doubt these patterns of behaviour result from a group of conditions of widely differing aetiology. The behaviour pattern common to all organic brain syndromes is a disorganization of brain function evident in the child's earlier development and in his present physical, emotional, intellectual, and social functioning.

Depending upon the presence or absence of definite signs of organic disease, one can divide the syndromes into two main groups.

GROUP 1: *The Brain Damage Syndrome* In these children there is definite evidence of abnormal functioning of the central nervous system, either in the history (e.g. convulsions) or in the present examination (e.g. cerebral palsy). The behavioural problems of these children are likely to be associated with the child's cerebral pathology. The exact symptoms will vary with the location and extent of the disease, with the age of the child, with his innate personality (aggressive-passive), with his intellectual ability, and with the way the family interacts with the child.

GROUP 2: *The Brain Dysfunction Syndrome* Although clinically this syndrome may appear almost identical to the Brain Damage Syndrome, there is no evidence in the historical data or in the physical examination that would justify the diagnosis of definite organic cerebral disease. In these cases, it is presumed that the behaviour arises from an organic origin which is not detectable by our present diagnostic tools and techniques. It is possible that in many of these children the origin of the behaviour lies in abnormalities of biochemical function and not with structural damage to the central nervous system. In a number of children the origin may be constitutional or hereditary since there is frequently a history of similar patterns of behaviour in close relatives. The importance of the concept of brain dysfunction is that the behaviour is considered to be due to factors within the child and not primarily the result of environmental or external relationships. Thus problems arise from an innate inability of the child to deal with his environment as the normal child does.

Symptomatology

The signs and symptoms seen in these children may be classified under the following headings:

1. *Primary signs and symptoms.* These are the direct result of disorganized brain function.
2. *Secondary signs and symptoms.* These are the defensive reactions to the excessive and diffuse anxiety which is a primary symptom in most cases.
3. *Tertiary signs and symptoms.* These result from the ongoing interaction between the child and his environment, originally his family and later society.

The diagnosis of an organic brain syndrome can only be made if a large number of *primary symptoms* are present. The secondary and tertiary symptoms, while often the reason for the consultation, are not pathognomonic of the organic brain syndrome. On the other hand, they are often target symptoms for treatment after the diagnosis has been made.

THE SECONDARY SIGNS AND SYMPTOMS

These represent the defences of the child against the excessive anxiety which is present as a primary symptom in the majority of cases. The nature of the secondary symptoms will depend upon the child's age, on his intellect and personality, and on the way his family deals with his anxiety. The amount of anxiety the child is experiencing, his innate ability to cope with anxiety, and the example set by his parents and siblings as they deal with their anxieties will all influence the degree to which a particular defence is used. In many children, the defensive

Table 10-1 Primary Signs and Symptoms of Brain Dysfunction

Major areas of disturbance resulting directly from disorganized brain function	*Signs and symptoms resulting from the disturbance in brain function*
1. Disorders of *development*	Uneven development of intellect Uneven physical development Uneven emotional development
2. Disorders of *learning*	Pre-schooler: does not learn from experience School-age child: likely to have specific learning deficits
3. Disorders of *thinking*	Poor organization of thoughts Lack of goal-directedness Poor judgment of cause-and-effect Poor concept formation Poor generalization Delayed abstractions
4. Disorders of *memory*	The child often has problems of retaining what he has learned either through auditory channels or visual channels
5. Disorders of *attention*	Short attention span Problems in concentration Problems of perseveration
6. Disorders of *activity level*	Hyperactivity Hypoactivity (less often)
7. Disorders of *feeling*	*Excessive generalized anxiety* Lack of normal anxiety (rarely) Impulsivity Low frustration tolerance Emotional lability

reaction may interfere with the child's functioning and aggravate the problems created by his primary defect. There are many patterns of secondary symptoms, but withdrawals, phobias, obsessions and compulsions, somatizations of the anxiety, and depressions are most frequently seen.

In a few children who are probably constitutionally predisposed to psychosis, the anxiety may be so great that the defences collapse and a clinical picture akin to a childhood psychosis may appear. This may be evident only during periods of excessive stress or may be present most of the time. In such children, the clinical picture will show a mixture of the signs and symptoms of an organic brain syndrome and those of a childhood psychosis.

THE TERTIARY SIGNS AND SYMPTOMS

These include the child's reactions, emotional and social, to his family's acceptance or non-acceptance of him, to stress within the family, and to stresses at school, in the neighbourhood, and in the broad community. The organic child, difficult, poorly adaptable, immature, and self-centred, easily becomes the scapegoat for a troubled family and may become a battered child if his parents, sufficiently deprived and immature, interpret his difficult behaviour as directed against them. Practically all parents of handicapped or difficult children harbour some rejection and guilt and often a mixture of both. From observation in the office and from parents' reports, one may have difficulty deciding which of these is more prevalent in a given case. The following are common patterns of behaviour seen as tertiary symptoms:

1. *Negativism* may be the reaction to excessive parental pressures.
2. *Excessive dependency* may be the reaction to overprotective, over-directing parents.
3. *Controlling behaviour* may be the reaction to overprotective and indulgent parents who are unable to stand up to the pressures of the child.
4. *Aggressive, hostile behaviour* may be the reaction to parents' overt or covert rejection.
5. *Poor peer relationships* may result from the child's envy of other children who appear to have a much easier and more comfortable life.

Many children with an organic brain syndrome may be rigid, self-centred, negativistic, and controlling due to a handicap that is often invisible to the family and others. One must remember that poor social adaptability may be present to some degree even in what might be considered an optimal environment. If the organic syndrome remains unrecognized, the conflict between the child and his parents may intensify, spread into school, and involve teachers and peer groups. In some cases this leads to antisocial and delinquent behaviour in the adolescent years.

DIAGNOSIS

The diagnostic process requires experience, since the presenting picture may vary considerably and since the syndrome may be caused by abnormalities of function at any level of the central nervous system, including the highest structures, which are often mute on neurological examination. An adequate history, neurological examination, and, when indicated, special investigations should be used to confirm or rule out the presence of an organic brain syndrome. A formal neurological assessment, especially of the child presenting with a behaviour disorder and/or hyperactivity, may be impossible, and clear evidence of organicity may be meagre.

The following historical data may suggest a diagnosis of an organic brain syndrome:

1. A history of *lifelong difficulties* in motor, emotional, intellectual, and social development.
2. a) *Lack of oxygen in the perinatal period,* with evidence of foetal or neonatal distress. This may result from complications of the pregnancy and delivery.
   b) *Toxic influences* including drugs taken by the mother during pregnancy, severe toxemia of pregnancy, or maternal thyrotoxicosis.
   c) *Blood incompatability* leading to erythroblastosis due to Rh, ABO, or other factors.
   d) *Infections* (especially viral) of the mother during pregnancy, or severe infections of the child in early life. The effect may be through a specific attack upon the nervous system (e.g. meningitis, encephalitis) or may result from any acute febrile illness with sustained high fever, especially when accompanied by dehydration (e.g. severe gastroenteritis).
   e) *Trauma,* including perinatal injuries or subsequent severe head injuries with associated concussion.
   f) *Seizures.*
3. The type of examination carried out on the child will vary, depending upon the age of the child and the degree of co-operation obtained. Instead of attempting a full neurological assessment of the difficult child, one provides a relaxed atmosphere with play materials available and examines the child more through observation than by formal testing. On observing a suspected abnormality, one then selectively tests the related aspects of the child's neurological function through, for example, a reflex or a test of perception, in order to confirm or exclude the suspected difficulty. Toys and games may aid in assessing the child's size, shape, and colour concepts. The child

may be asked to identify pictures and solve puzzles appropriate to his age. Provided the child is motivated and co-operating, his drawings—and later his speech, reading, printing, writing, and computing—may offer a general indication of his developmental level and his perceptual and motor functioning. The child's play and work, both spontaneous and in response to direction, may help assess his developmental level, his attitudes and approaches to play materials and assigned tasks, his goal-directedness, and the quality of his ideas, imagination, and spontaneity as compared to other children of his age.

At the completion of the examination, one may have found a number of soft neurological signs with an occasional hard neurological sign.* It must be remembered that several soft neurological signs can be present in what are essentially normal children. Very often one cannot be certain whether or not the findings indicate organic disease and consultation with a neurologist may be indicated. Depending upon the philosophy of the neurologist, the report may suggest possible organic symptoms and a suggestive history. The findings of this nature tend towards the confirmation of the diagnosis of an organic brain syndrome.

4. In arriving at a diagnosis, one must also consider and exclude a number of conditions which, while of psychogenic origin, may mimic the clinical picture of an organic brain syndrome. These would include:
   a) The normal child who, in response to rigid and excessive parental expectations, may show many of the tertiary signs and symptoms of brain dysfunction.
   b) The child who is chronically and acutely anxious. In addition to showing many of the tertiary signs and symptoms, he may show impairments of memory and attention, along with associated deficits in learning because of the chronic interference of intolerable anxiety.
   c) The child who is mentally retarded may present an almost iden-

Soft neurological signs include transient esotropia, unsteadiness of the outstretched hands, hyperreflexia, ambiguous plantar responses, awkwardness, and minor degrees of incoordination, poor balancing, and hopping, etc. *Hard neurological signs* indicate unequivocal findings of abnormalities such as a definite extensor or plantar, a consistent esotropia, a definite intention tremor, etc.

tical clinical picture. A careful developmental history and demonstration of the intellectual deficit through psychological testing usually make possible an accurate diagnosis.

d) The child of parents who are depressed and withdrawn may appear hyperactive when, in effect, one is seeing a high level of attention-seeking behaviour which represents the child's response to his parents' unresponsiveness.

e) The child who is responding to a chaotic family situation may show any of the tertiary signs and symptoms of brain dysfunction along with disorders of development, learning, attention, activity level, and feeling.

5. In doubtful cases the physician may extend his assessment by seeking consultation from specialists in a variety of related fields. Depending on the clinical picture, one or more of the following might prove helpful in arriving at a diagnosis:

   a) *The teacher,* who can provide information about the child's ability, learning patterns and functioning on a day-to-day basis over an extended period of time. This allows a comparison of the child's intellectual, emotional, social, and motor functioning with that of other normal children.

   b) *The child psychologist,* who can assess developmental, motor, and perceptual functioning, and who can delineate and measure various defects as well as offer a second opinion.

   c) *The speech pathologist,* who can evaluate and quantify disorders of speech or language, in addition to providing a second opinion.

   d) *The otolaryngologist,* who can exclude peripheral defects in auditory perception and arrange for audiometry if indicated.

   e) *The ophthalmologist,* who can exclude peripheral defects in visual perception.

   f) *The neurologist,* who through his clinical examinations and through electroencephalography* may do much to clarify a confusing clinical picture.

*Such children often have EEGs described as borderline or marginal, with poor organization of wave forms, a relative increase in the number of slow waves, slight asymmetry between the two hemispheres, and increased sensitivity to hyperventilation. They often show a pattern that would be normal at a younger age. Such a pattern may represent either immaturity or actual pathology of cerebral function.

g) *The paediatrician,* who, if not already consulted, may help clarify a confusing diagnostic picture by excluding other conditions in the differential diagnosis.
h) *The occupational therapist,* who can assess motor and perceptual functioning, comparing them to the norm for any given age.
i) *The public-health nurse,* who through home visits and as a result of her contact with school and health agencies with whom the family have had contact in the past, may be able to do much to clarify the level of the family's functioning both within the home and within society.

Symptomatology

The following syndromes can be differentiated and related to age:

1. *In infancy.* The clinical picture commonly seen in this age group is that of the hypertonic, colicky infant.
2. *In the pre-school years.*
   a) The restless, hyperkinetic child's behaviour is dominated by motor unrest and excessive and poorly controlled motor activity resulting from inadequate suppression by the higher centres of the central nervous system. These children are hyperactive, emotionally labile and irritable. Their behaviour does not settle in a different environment, such as nursery school.
   b) The clumsy child may not be hyperactive but is awkward in both gross and fine motor skills and poor in games and sports. These problems often make these children reluctant to play with others, and interfere with their social adjustment.
   c) The child may be delayed in learning to speak both single words and sentences. These children may have adequate perception and comprehension of speech, and the problem is primarily in the expressive area. They usually develop reasonable language skills as they grow older, often after a period of infantile speech or lalling.
3. *In the school-age child.*
   a) Specific learning disorders and/or associated behaviour problems may dominate the picture. Such children may demonstrate agnosia, speech and language defects, defects in visual or auditory perception, perceptuo-motor problems, mixed laterality (e.g. right-handed child with left eye dominant), etc. These children may or may not have associated hyperkinesis, short attention

span, and lack of concentration. If so, they function poorly in groups and disturb the class. Teachers unaware of the reason for their difficulty often believe that they could learn if they wanted to and ascribe their failure to laziness or lack of motivation.

b) From the age of nine to adolescence, secondary and tertiary symptoms frequently predominate and the child falls further behind academically. He may increasingly seek to avoid school (via truancy, hysterical symptoms often presented as vague somatic complaints) or may gradually drift into antisocial behaviour and delinquency, ultimately dropping out of school.

There may be a relationship between the patterns noted in the organic syndrome and the actual organic disease. For example, epileptic seizures in a child may evoke anxiety, guilt, overprotection, or rejection on the part of the parents. These in turn may lead to excessive restrictions, which make the child feel inadequate, different, or unloved. The child may react by becoming depressed or by warding off feelings of depression by aggressive, acting-out behaviour.

COMMON ERRORS IN DIAGNOSIS

1. The hyperactive child, when seen alone and given undivided attention, may seem quite normal over a short contact. Often these children are not hyperkinetic in a one-to-one relationship or when involved in a specific task. In a group situation or one which is less involving, however, the hyperkinetic behaviour becomes evident. A school history or other independent assessment should be obtained before deciding that the child is normal and that the real problem lies with the environment. Exposing the child to some frustration during the assessment may help to avoid this error.
2. Very often the relationship between parent and child is poor at the time when the child is brought for assessment. In such cases, it is obvious that the relationship plays a part in the behavioural problems of the child. However, these problems are the result, not the cause, of the child's primary difficulty. Too often the underlying organic syndrome is missed and the parents are criticized and held responsible for the resulting behavioural problems.
3. The child's intellectual functioning may be extremely variable. One must remember that children with organic syndromes may have widely differing levels of function in specific intellectual areas:

verbal and non-verbal, comprehension, memory, etc. If one accepts the high levels as indicating the potential over-all function, then the child may be considered an underachiever even when achieving at a level appropriate to his intelligence. It is often difficult to be sure about the child's true or basic potential as psychological tests assess only present functioning in a standardized test situation.

4. The organically impaired child shows marked fluctuations in his level of functioning. It is wise, therefore, to ask the parents whether the behaviour we are seeing is typical of the child at his best or at his worst.
5. There is a common tendency to equate hyperactivity with organic impairment. Not all organically impaired children are hyperactive. Not all hyperactive children are organically impaired. Hyperactivity, as it is extremely difficult to tolerate, is often the symptom which brings the child to the physician.

MANAGEMENT

The terms "brain damage" or "brain dysfunction" are highly emotional terms which are frequently interpreted as implying a fixed course and a poor prognosis. This causes some physicians to shy away from such patients whom, they believe, they cannot help.

One need not be so pessimistic. Though these children cannot be cured, both they and their families can be helped considerably by treatment. Early recognition and adequate management of the organic condition can prevent the development of many of the secondary and tertiary signs and symptoms which otherwise cause problems often more serious for the child and family than the brain dysfunction itself. Management must be aimed at the parents or the whole family as well as at the child.

1. *Work with the parents.* First, the parents must be told directly our findings, our understandings of those findings (i.e. the diagnosis), and our concerns. It should be recognized that a diagnosis of brain dysfunction has a high emotional loading, and will be responded to differently by individual parents. To some parents, it implies a "mental defect", something that they may have been worrying about for a long time. Others may conclude that since the child is brain-damaged, he cannot be expected to learn to control his behaviour. Parents react with disbelief, hostility, depression, and further rejec-

tion or overprotection of the child. They may react angrily towards the physician who told them the diagnosis or towards the one who did not. At times their hostility may become more diffused, as they bitterly attack the medical profession, schools, or society in general. They may blame and become angry at each other. These reactions must be understood as part of that family's response to the disappointment and stress inherent in the illness (see Chapter 16).

Still it is necessary that the parents know. They have to make decisions about accepting or not accepting treatment, about bringing the child to a day-care centre, which may be tedious and expensive, or about accepting special education or medication for their child. Sometimes the parents wish to move to a city where treatment is available or to the country where the hyperactive child has more outlets. Most parents wish to obtain a second opinion to confirm the diagnosis and explore possible alternatives to our suggestions. They want to know what the prognosis is and how the child's condition is likely to affect the family.

It is impossible to deal with all these matters in one or even a few sessions. Parents need time and sympathetic support from their physician in adjusting to the diagnosis. Very often a plan to relieve the mother from the care of the child for part of the day gives needed relief and assistance. One must recognize and attempt to relieve parental feelings of guilt and hostility. Parents' questions should be answered honestly and directly. One gives suggestions regarding child management when this is possible, even if the parents are not yet able to use them. When one is asked a question to which he does not know the answer, it is much more helpful to acknowledge this openly than to evade the issues or to play the role of the expert who has an answer, albeit meaningless, for every situation.

2. The next step is helping the parents recognize which symptoms result from the organic child's condition and are likely to persist and which can and should be corrected.
3. This done, one can then counsel the parents towards improving relationships with the child, discuss with them problems of management, help them find outlets for the hyperactivity and other special problems of their child. The rest of the family or at least the parents may need help in learning to cope with their reactions and relationships with the problem child. The parents may require support in understanding their child's special problems and in recogniz-

ing and accepting their negative feelings towards the child. This may be an essential part of preventing rejection of the child by the family.

HELP TO THE CHILD

Psychiatric and psychological assessment are helpful in arriving at a treatment plan. This will vary with the nature of the child's symptoms and with his age.

1. *For pre-schoolers,* a plan of management involves consideration of each of the following:

a) *A structured environment* for part of the day (nursery, specialized nursery, day-care treatment centre), which can provide structure for the child as well as relief for the mother.

b) *Medication* is less useful for pre-schoolers than for school-age children, but in some cases it can be very helpful. If medication is prescribed while the parents are feeling guilty about "poisoning the child", the treatment will fail due to irregular administration or early withdrawal. Any medication is most helpful if used together with other forms of therapy and training of the child. One should use the time before the effect of a particular drug wears off to "get through" to the child while he is slowed down or less anxious. To prevent drug accommodation and to have a regular check on the effectiveness of the medication, one can use "drug holidays" (i.e. Sundays or weekends without medication). It is helpful to have someone in addition to the parents report on the effectiveness of the drug. Parents' guilt feelings often interfere with their taking full responsibility. Any drug will have to be tried and the dosage adjusted for the particular child. All these general principles will have to be discussed thoroughly with the parents.

The usual drugs used include the stimulants and phenothiazines. The phenothiazines may be used for a few months during particularly stressful times, as they often prove helpful for the very anxious child. Stimulants should not be used before three years of age, and while not without side-effects, they may be beneficial over prolonged periods if seen as part of an over-all program of management. A trial of methylphenidate is indicated for the hyperactive child, while phenothiazines represent the drug of choice for the emotionally labile and highly anxious child. Drugs alone, if not combined with an ongoing attempt to use improved relationships to help the child manage more effectively, are contra-indicated. Children with abnormal EEGs may benefit from Dilantin, which may assist not only in the control of seizures but also in the management of associated behaviour disorders. Further details of drug dosage, administration, and side-effects are found in Chapter 23.

2. *The school-age child.* The school-age child often requires remedial teaching and/or special class placement to help compensate for learning difficulties resulting from the brain dysfunction. Should treatment for emotional sequelae be required, a form of therapy offering concrete approaches such as one involving behaviour modification may prove useful. Family or group therapy can often help the child learn to function better in a family or social situation, while in-patient admission at times of crisis may prove helpful. Individual psychotherapy has a more limited application with the child with brain dysfunction, although it may prove helpful with some older children whose damage is limited. (For a further discussion of the techniques and indications for the various forms of psychotherapy see Chapter 22.) Medication, particularly the use of stimulants for those who remain restless, can be especially helpful if used as part of a total program to assist the child in his general development.

3. *The teenager.* The teenager with an organic syndrome is often most difficult to treat. Repeated failures, discouragement, poor self-opinion, denial, hostility, and depression, as well as poor relationships with the parents often make successful treatment impossible. There is a better outlook for those who are more neurotic than antisocial, for those who are well motivated, and for those who can use their parents for support. The therapy can be individual, group or family, out-patient or in-patient, according to need and availability. Drugs are less suitable for this age because of the danger of addiction, misuse, and overdose.

COMMON ERRORS IN MANAGEMENT

1. Failure to share findings with the parents. At times this is avoided out of fear that full and frank sharing would interfere with the parents' relationship with the child. The news media contain frequent descriptions of organically impaired children, and many parents are aware of the diagnosis before seeing their physician. If not told directly, they may believe that the physician has missed the diagnosis.

2. Identifying with the child against the parents. The parents are the key to the child's management. The physician who cannot relate to parents with empathy and understanding should refer the case to someone who can.

3. Giving advice on child management or prescribing drugs before the parents are ready to accept them or before the physician has had time to be sure his recommendations are appropriate.
4. Responding with disappointment or hostility to parents who cannot accept what the physician has to say or offer at a given time. It may take a year for parents to fully accept that their child has a brain abnormality and another year to accept that it will not fully disappear. Each developmental step the child makes—or fails to make—confronts the child and family with another aspect of reality that must be faced.

PROGNOSIS

The prognosis depends largely on the degree of impairment. This is best assessed by clinical and psychological reassessments repeated once a year. In spite of the current tendency to deny its importance, intelligence testing and the component tests still offer the best predictive information at least for school placement and future educational and work planning. Almost no one whose intelligence quotient remains below 50 can lead an independent life.

Those with IQs between 50 and 90 can frequently benefit from special classes in the school system. The response of a given child to this educational program will depend not only on his intellectual level but on his emotional and social adjustment, his work habits, and his motivation. Recent studies of the effect of medication on behaviour suggest that learning handicaps or general intellectual functioning may not improve significantly even if the child's behaviour and concentration improve. However, the child who is more co-operative and better behaved integrates more easily with his environment and, in the long run, is better off.

Those children who have normal intelligence have of course the best prognosis, but may remain troubled for years by their learning, emotional, and social difficulties. Some of them, however, will succeed in becoming highly educated and successful people. In general, it is wise to help the parents think and plan about a year ahead, since during the early years one cannot be too accurate in long-range predictions of future behaviour. An honest reply to parents' questions about the future, including one's own uncertainty, is always the best policy in the long run.

RECOMMENDED FOR FURTHER READING

Since this an introductory textbook, this chapter has focused primarily on generalized or diffuse brain syndromes rather than on those resulting from damage to a specific localized area of the brain (e.g. temporal lobe epilepsy). However, references 1, 2, and 7 will provide further information about localized brain lesions.

1. BENSON, D. F., and BLUMER, D. *Psychiatric Aspects of Neurologic Disease.* New York, Grune and Stratton, 1975.
—this textbook deals with the psychiatric aspects of localized brain lesions, including frontal and temporal lobe seizures.

2. BRAY, E. F. "Temporal Lobe Syndrome in Children: A Longitudinal Review". *Pediat.* 29: 617–28, 1962.
—good review of this syndrome, which results from a localized lesion in the temporal lobe.

4. CHESS, S. "Neurological Dysfunction and Childhood Behavioural Pathology". *J. Aut. Child Schizo.* 2: 299–311, 1972.
—drawing from her experience of more than one thousand consultations over nineteen years, the author discusses the relationship between neurological dysfunction and childhood behavioural disturbance.

5. CLEMENTS, S. D. *Minimal Brain Dysfunction in Children: Terminology and Identification: Phase One of a Three-Phase Project.* U. S. Dept. H. E. and W., Public Health Publication, no. 1415, 1966.
—best single reference with regard to terminology and identification. Brief and well organized with an extensive bibliography.

8. GARDNER, R. A. "Psychogenic Problems of Brain-Injured Children and Their Parents". *J. Amer. Acad. Child Psychiat.* 7: 471–91, 1968.
—discusses both intrapsychic or interpersonal elements of the adaptation of both brain-injured children and their parents, with emphasis on short-term supportive forms of treatment.

9. HIGGINS, J. H.; LEDERER, H,; and ROSENBAUM, M. "Life Situations, Emotions, and Ideopathic Epilepsy", in *Proceedings of the Association for Research in Nervous and Mental Disease,* 137–47. Williams and Wilkins, Baltimore, 1950.
—an attempt to evaluate the psychodynamic significance of the epileptic seizure by the detailed psychiatric study of epileptic patients.

10. KENNY, T. J.; CLEMMENS, R. L.; HUDSON, B. W.; LENTZ, G. A.; CICCI, R.; and NAIR, P. "Characteristics of Children Referred Because of Hyperactivity". *J. Pediat.* 79: 618–27, 1971.
—a clinical evaluation of data on one hundred children referred as hyperactive concludes that hyperactivity is an ill-defined and inconstant phenomenon.

11. VOELLER, K. K. S., and ROTHENBERG, M. B. "Psychosocial Aspects of the Management of Seizures in Children". *Pediat.* 51: 1072–82, 1973.
—attempts to demonstrate that diagnosis and attention paid to the psychosocial situation, personality development, and guidance of the parents may have great therapeutic value in the management of children with seizure disorders.

12. MEICHENBAUM, D. H. *The Nature and Modification of Impulsive Children: Training Impulsive Children to Talk to Themselves.* University of Waterloo Research Report, no. 23, Waterloo, Ontario.
—a discussion of ways of helping hyperactive children learn to modify their behaviour to become less impulsive and difficult to live with, thus improving the "fit" between them and their environment.

15. SCHAFFER, D. "Psychiatric Aspects of Brain Injury in Childhood: A Review". *Develop. Med. & Child Neurol.* 15: 211–20, 1973.
—deals with such questions as: "Does brain injury increase the likelihood of psychiatric disorder? Which factors predispose most towards psychiatric disorder? Are certain psychiatric syndromes pathognomonic of brain injury?"

16. WALKER, S. "Drugging the American Child: We're Too Cavalier about Hyperactivity". *J. Learn. Dis.* 8: 354–58, 1975.
—discusses the widespread abuse of stimulant drugs in children termed hyperactive whose main symptomatology centres around behaviour or learning problems in the absence of true hyperkinesis.

17. WEISS, G.; MINDE, K.; WERRY, J. S.; DOUGLAS, V.; and NEMETH, E. "Studies on the Hyperactive Child. 8: Five-Year Follow-Up". *Arch. Gen. Psychiat.* 24: 409–21, 1971.
—a behavioural, academic, and neurological follow-up of sixty-four severely handicapped children, most with minimal brain dysfunction.

18. WEISS, G.; KRUGER, E.; DANIELSON, U.; and ELMAN, M. "Effect of Long-Term Treatment of Hyperactive Children with Methylphenidate". *Canad. Med. Assoc. J.* 112: 159–65, 1975.
—while there is no doubt that stimulants are effective drugs for many

hyperactive children, as the sole method of management their value is limited.

19. WENDER, P. H. "Some Speculations Concerning a Possible Biochemical Basis of Minimal Brain Dysfunction". *Ann. N.Y. Acad. Sci.* 205: 18–28, 1973.
—critical of the lack of diagnostic precision, Wender defines a "hyperkinetic behaviour syndrome". The criteria he suggests are well operationalized, and their general adoption would do away with much of the confusion resulting from the synonymous or overlapping case of such terms as learning disorders, minimal brain dysfunction, and hyperactivity.

20. WENDER, P. "Minimal Brain Dysfunction in Children". *Pediat. Clin. N. Amer.* 20, 187–202, 1973.
—a good general review of the syndrome as seen in 1973.

21. WERRY, J. S. "The Diagnosis, Etiology, and Treatment of Hyperactivity in Children." *Learning Disorders.* Vol. 3: 173–90. Seattle, Wash., Special Child Publication, 1968.
—a good review of the area of hyperactivity.

22. WERRY, J. S.; MINDE, K.; GUZMAN, A.; WEISS, G.; DOGAN, K.; and HOY, E. "Studies on the Hyperactive Child. Neurological Status Compared with Neurotic and Normal Children". *Amer. J. Orthopsychiat.* 42: 441–50, 1972.
—a comparison of twenty hyperactive children with normal and neurotic controls showing that minor neurological dysfunctions, learning difficulties, and hyperactivity are three fairly distinct clinical entities each with its respective symptomatology.

ADDITIONAL READING

3. CHESS, S. "Diagnosis and Treatment of the Hyperactive Child". *New York State J. Med.* 60: 2379–85, 1960.

6. EISENBERG, L. "Psychiatric Implications of Brain Damage in Children". *Psychiat. Quart.* 31: 72–92, 1957.

7. ERVIN, F.; EPSTEIN, A.; and KING, H. E. "Behaviour of Epileptic and Non-Epileptic Patients with 'Temporal Spikes' ". *Arch. Neurol & Psychiat.* 74: 488–97, 1955.

13. MINDE, K. "Hyperactivity in 1975: Where Do We Stand?" Unpublished review. Presented at International Congress of Child Neurology, Toronto, 1975.

14. *Minimal Brain Dysfunction in Children:* Educational Medical and Health Related Services. Phase Two of a Three-Phase Project. Public Health Service, no. 2015, 1970.

ELSA BRODER

11. The Child Whose Behaviour Is Antisocial

All societies have codes that define behaviour that is acceptable and expected and behaviour that is unacceptable and therefore carries sanctions. The codes vary from society to society and from era to era within a particular society's development. Sanctions can vary from informal acts of condemnation, social isolation, or ostracism to legal and punitive actions. Individual judges vary in their interpretations of these codes and in their selection of sanctions for particular offences. In addition, the social or personal circumstances of an individual who has transgressed the social codes may influence the response of the official agents of control. Thus the consistency and vigour with which existing laws are enforced and the balance between informal disposition as opposed to formal procedures (i.e. laying a charge) can vary significantly, and, in so doing, markedly raise or lower the apparent rate of delinquency and crime.[11, 12, 22, 34, 35, 36]

Children are expected to learn to distinguish between acceptable and unacceptable behaviour, primarily from the family but also from school and other social agencies. Children acquire this ability to distinguish first by sensing the parents' approval or disapproval of specific behaviour and then by associating parental disapproval with a fear of punishment and withdrawal of affection. Later, with the development of conscience, this process of control is less dependent on external figures and more on an inner sense of guilt and discomfort on contravening the mandate.[16] However, children vary in their response to this training and in their willingness to accept it. In addition the trainers, namely the family, school, and others, may convey either mixed and confusing or at times covert antisocial messages. Most children at some time transgress these social codes, usually rarely and at an early age. Some children, however, continue to commit transgressions in ways that bring them into conflict with society. Society then brings to bear a number of forces to help the child come into line or to isolate him for his own protection and that of society.

Delinquency is a legal, not a medical or psychiatric, term. Its definition varies from jurisdiction to jurisdiction within a country, between different countries, and with time. In Canada, at present, "any child who violates any provision of the Criminal Code of any Dominion or provincial statute, or of any by-law or ordinance of any municipality, or who is guilty of sexual immorality or any similar form of vice, or who is liable by reason of any other act to be committed to an industrial school or juvenile reformatory under the provisions of any Dominion or provincial statute" is labelled delinquent and is subject to the jurisdiction of the juvenile and family court.[14] This jurisdiction continues from the time the child turns seven until the sixteenth birthday. Before the age of seven the child is not considered responsible for his behaviour, hence a charge cannot be laid.[8] As soon as the child reaches sixteen, in the eyes of the law he or she is an adult and therefore subject to the laws regarding adults who commit offences. At present in Canada, the possibility of raising the minimal age of criminal responsibility to fourteen is being considered. Simultaneously the upper limit of those to be considered juveniles would be raised to age eighteen, leaving the fourteen-to-eighteen-year-old age group exclusively under the jurisdiction of proposed youth courts.[37]

A child charged with an offence under the present legislation and found to be delinquent by the juvenile court is legally termed an *official delinquent*.[36] The proceedings of most juvenile courts are held in an informal atmosphere, and the names of the juvenile offenders are not released to the public. The purpose of these courts is defined as rehabilitation rather than punishment, and offences committed as a juvenile do not become part of an adult or criminal record. While the term "delinquent" should probably be confined to those who have been so found by a court, it is at times extended to cover all youngsters who have been cautioned or investigated by police and even those whose reported behaviour contravenes laws, whether or not they have been apprehended.

Children can thus be charged with committing acts that, if they were adults, would be dealt with as offences. Children can also be, and at times are, brought before the juvenile authorities in situations that would not apply to adults. As a result, young persons who are neglected or out of control, who have run away from home, or who are "sexually immoral" are also frequently labelled delinquent. Where school attendance is mandatory, children who are repeatedly truant are frequently charged with delinquency, although they share little in common with the stereotype of the official delinquent. In this situation, as in others, children can be charged by the parents and by the schools, as well as by society, which can charge both children and adults. Currently a number of jurisdictions are experimenting with repealing legislation that has heretofore permitted children who are out of control or unmanageable to be labelled and dealt with as delinquent. The movement is to have these children cared for through child-welfare legislation and resources and mental-health facilities.

Epidemiology

The fact that so many disparate groups of children have fallen under this common label of delinquency has made for confusion of management and in interpretation of reported findings. This is particularly so when those reporting fail to define with clarity the precise group of delinquents under discussion. Nevertheless, on reviewing the literature a number of features common to different societies do emerge.

Studies have demonstrated that while everyone has broken the law one or more times, few have been caught. Although large numbers (58 per cent) of young people report behaviour that is chargeable, only a few are repeatedly and seriously delinquent.[11, 12, 22, 34, 35] Of those apprehended only a small percentage (between 3 and 20 per cent) appear before the courts. The majority are, can, and should be dealt with informally through the resources of family, school, and community.

The rapid, recent changes in society have been reflected in changes in the "typical" profile of the officially delinquent youth. A decade ago, eight to ten boys were seen in court for every girl.[7] Those who appeared were predominantly from disadvantaged social classes, and more than likely from a minority group. These were commonly in the older age groups (fourteen to sixteen) and frequently gave a history of academic problems, truancy from school, and membership in a gang. Delinquent boys typically broke the Criminal Code (e.g. breaking and entering, car theft). The girls were more frequently before the court as being in need of care and protection or charged with immoral behaviour (e.g. running away from home, sexual offences). Certain ethnic groups (e.g. Chinese and Jews) characteristically have low rates of delinquency. Other groups, particularly first-generation immigrants regardless of country of origin, produce disproportionately high numbers of official delinquents. Urban areas account for proportionately more delinquent youth than rural ones. Within cities, neighbourhoods that feature social disorganization, transience, migration, and mobility have higher delinquency rates than do other neighbourhoods.[7, 11, 17, 22, 35]

Today, fairly consistently across the Western world, this marked preponderance of juvenile males appearing in court is diminishing. Within the city of Toronto, for example, the ratio of boys to girls appearing in court has remained relatively steady at four to one over the last five years. The nature of the offences is also changing, with more from middle-class and established families being charged than was once the case. More girls are being charged with criminal offences, while more boys are being dealt with as needing care and protection.

There is no typical family structure that predisposes specifically to delinquency. However, family histories of delinquents show a higher than average incidence of loss, separation, disorganization, deprivation (emotional and physical), multiple living situations, and single parenting. These families and their individual members also have a greater number of involvements with social agencies, including mental-health professionals and psychiatrists. Family factors were found by the Gluecks to be the best predictors of future delinquency in boys.[12] School histories reveal a higher than average number of failures and many changes of schools. Academic achievement is retarded an average of two years from the age norm in spite of average intelligence. There are no apparent correlations between delinquency and intelligence, although there are between intelligence and being caught; the less bright are apprehended more frequently.

Studies at the level of juvenile courts and at institutions for juveniles reveal a considerably higher frequency of emotional disturbance in the delinquent group than in the over-all population. Whereas 5 to 10 per cent of school children are consistently found to be emotionally disturbed, in a delinquent group an incidence of emotional disturbance as high as 30 per cent has been reported. Although a single study reports 29 per cent of 150 referrals were psychotic or brain damaged, most investigators report a low incidence of psychosis in the delinquent population.[19] The most frequent diagnosis applied is that of character or personality disorder. A number of studies suggest that girls who are delinquent are much more disturbed than delinquent boys, although this may reflect less on delinquency itself than on the lack of other community facilities, leaving the correctional institution as the only available method of dealing with the situation.[22, 27, 33]

The majority of children who appear in court do not return, but complete their period of probation, if imposed, without further mishap. Of those who go to a correctional institution, an estimated 50 to 58 per cent have no further trouble with the law.[5, 18] The picture for the rest remains grim. They are youth for whom society has not yet any real answer. Some pass through a series of living situations eventually coming to some type of adjustment, while a small but significant percentage ends up in adult institutions.

Within juvenile correctional institutions (e.g. training schools, approved schools, and Borstals), suicide attempts, "carving", self-tattooing, running away, physical aggression, vandalism, homosexual behaviour, and depression are all common. When questioned about this, those involved commonly reply, "Well, what else was there to do?" These behaviours do, in fact, seem to have less serious implications in an institutional setting than if they appeared in the community. They may be more symptomatic of group contagion and the lack of acceptable outlets for feelings in correctional institutions.

Aetiology

There are a number of approaches towards the explanation and understanding of delinquency. Some authorities concentrate on the nature of the delinquent act, while others focus on the development and personality of the delinquent. Still others view the delinquent behaviour as a normal reaction against a socially and economically disadvantaged environment. They regard delinquent acts merely as symptoms of an essentially social problem, and look for its origins and its remedies in the conditions and distortions in society itself.

The behaviour of most delinquents can best be understood as a pattern that has been learned from the socializing group or as a reaction to family and life situations. These young people have been taught values that are discordant with those of the general society, although in keeping with those of that part of society that has been a major influence in their lives. This *subcultural delinquency* is unlikely to drop substantially; in fact it may continue to increase as long as large identifiable groups within the population, and particularly within cities, continue to feel disadvantaged and deprived of the standard of living, educational opportunities, and social status from which they see themselves excluded by the more privileged groups within society. Born into families already struggling under major social and economic stress, often suffering the effects of early malnutrition, exposed only to limited stimulation before school, they enter a school system usually at its weakest and least supported points. Under the influence of the powerful mass media, they and their families are conditioned to a set of expectations that they realize rather early in adolescence they are unlikely to be able to achieve. Their understandable resentment frequently is discharged in actions against society, particularly when such behaviour is condoned, accepted, and even rewarded by peer-group status. Ryan, in his book *Blaming the Victim*, graphically outlines this cycle of those who are disadvantaged by lack of opportunity being blamed for the predicament that is not of their creation.[29] These primarily sociological delinquents need increased training opportunities from an early age accompanied by substantial changes within the society itself, rather than treatment aimed at making them "adjust".

Less commonly, delinquents are emotionally disturbed. In such cases, the delinquency is merely a symptom or method of expressing the underlying emotional problem (see Chapter 6). Even here, however, there is not a one-to-one relationship. Most children who are emotionally disturbed are not delinquent, and even in those who are both delinquent and disturbed, improvement in the emotional problem may or may not alter the delinquency.

Theories of delinquency can be organized into five main groups: constitutional, organic, psychological, sociocultural, and familial.

Constitutional theories include the concept of the born criminal (Lombroso)[20] as well as the attempts to correlate body structure and temperament with delinquency.[12, 30] In twin studies, Shields has found ascending concordance for siblings, dizygotic and monozygotic twins.[31] Mental deficiency has been advanced as predisposing to delinquency but is now considered more related to who gets caught than to who commits delinquent acts. Recently, interest has been shown in an XYY chromosome defect in males, which has been identified and tentatively associated with increased aggressiveness, well above average height, less than average intelligence, and severe long-term social maladjustment.[30] However, the significance of the defect as a contributor to antisocial behaviour in juveniles is questionable and awaits further study.[15]

Organic theories have been supported by studies showing an increased frequency of abnormal and immature patterns on the EEG in delinquent groups. Children diagnosed as hyperactive at an earlier age have a higher incidence of delinquency in adolescence, but here, environmental reactions probably also play a major part. Delinquency is related to alcohol and drug usage. Some drugs such as alcohol and amphetamines increase or facilitate aggressivity, while others such as marijuana do not have this effect. However, many use delinquency to finance the habit. This problem is greater in cities and more prominent in some than others. It also varies according to the fashions, cults, and prevailing mores of youth at a particular time. At present, although the use of chemical compounds continues, alcohol is the drug most commonly abused by young people (see Chapter 14).

Within a *psychological framework*, delinquency has been related to assertion of masculinity, compensation for lack of love, exaggeration of adolescent identity conflicts, defects in conscience (superego), defects in impulse control and judgment (ego defects), overly strong sexual and aggressive drives (id impulses), and defects in the interpersonal maturity level. Delinquency has been related to a variety of defence mechanisms, including turning aggression on the self as part of depression (the "kick me" game described by Eric Berne);[4] a defence against feelings of anxiety, weakness, and inadequacy by behaving aggressively; the projection of angry feelings outwards; a substitution for lack of love. Glueck, Walker, and McGrath all have good reviews of these theories.[12, 35, 22]

One does find frequently in the more seriously and chronically delinquent an early history of severe emotional and physical deprivation. Bowlby, Spitz, and others have linked lack of early mothering to development of character disorders.[6, 32] Berne and McCormick have related delinquency to early "script" messages from parents that convince the child that he has no alternative but to be bad.[4, 21] Learning theorists point to the role of parents in both instigating and reinforcing the child's misbehaviour. Johnson has suggested that parents at times unconsciously encourage children to behave in a delinquent manner as this provides a release for their own repressed aggressive and antisocial tendencies. This concept explains delinquent behaviour in individuals with otherwise "normal" superegos, as opposed to individuals with generalized and explicit antisocial attitudes or impulse-ridden personalities. As the parents are not aware of their encouragement of behaviour to which they are consciously opposed, Johnson postulates that the unconscious communication results from gaps, which she terms "lacunae", in the parents' superego.[13] Role expectation, lack of teaching of impulse control, delinquent models, failure to learn control or to develop successful ways of expressing feeling, and faulty communication regarding standards and expectation have all been advanced as causative factors.

A *sociocultural* perspective calls into question society's norms and laws. Most delinquents are simply misbehaving according to society's standards. In such cases, the judgment is as much a reflection of the labeller's (society's) anger, guilt, disapproval, and frustration as it is of anything else. While there is a large element of chance involved in who gets the label, since the majority ("technical delinquents") are not caught, increasing chronicity and severity of the delinquent behaviour will greatly increase the likelihood of the child being apprehended, charged, and designated an official delinquent.

Perhaps the most broadly accepted cultural theory is that of subcultural delinquency, which has already been referred to. Other cultural theories stress the role of social disintegration, confusion over changing mores, cultural conflict, and the influence of the media, especially television, which glorify crime. The influence of the city has also been seen as favouring the development of delinquency, as has mere opportunity (see Gibbens).[10]

Increasingly the literature emphasizes the importance of the *family* in the development of delinquency. The Gluecks found in attempting to predict delinquency in boys that five social (interpersonal) factors of family life were highly accurate predictors.[12] These include discipline by father, supervision by mother, affection of father, affection of mother, and family cohesiveness. Delinquency can be seen as a manifestation of stress resulting either from malfunction within the family system or as the reaction of the poorly functioning family to external stress. The more rigid and closed the family system, the greater the upset in the usual homeostatic mechanisms in response to stress and the more difficulty the family is likely to have in coping successfully (see Chapter 3).

Parsons and Alexander in their studies of delinquent families note major communication deficits with difficulties in problem-solving.[1] They and Minuchin point to marital conflict, separation, parental inconsistency, and collusion with the delinquent child as frequent contributing factors.[23]

This multiplicity of theories emphasizes that delinquency is not a single condition with a unitary cause. Delinquent behaviour results, rather, from a variety of conditions contributed to by a number of causes which potentiate one another.

Management and Treatment

Faced with the child or young person whose behaviour is antisocial, one must begin with an assessment of the individual's current functioning and relationships as well as a survey of past experience. This assessment includes a review of the total family's functioning, determining whether, where, and how the needs of the child are being met. The child's behaviour may be symptomatic of a greater problem involving the family system. One can be sure that unchecked antisocial behaviour, if it is not already a problem at the time of presentation, will rapidly become one for child and family, leading inevitably to increased tensions, which will tax the family's resources (see Chapter 15). Management must be related to a careful formulation of the needs and capacities of the child, his family, and society, and the resulting plan must be one that is realistically available and likely to be implemented and followed through by the participants.

Kohlberg has studied the development of moral judgment and believes that young children are good because they have to be out of fear of punishment ("big stick" morality).[16] Later they are good because they realize that society expects it and that life is more rewarding if one conforms. At the highest level, one is "good" because of an internalized code of morality, in which one has thought through the implications of personal behaviour and come to the conclusion that to be "good" is best for oneself and for the world. Not all people get beyond even the earliest stages. Many are good because they have to be and will be bad if they can get away with it. A large part of the management program must involve helping the delinquent develop his own code of ethics that is compatible with that of society in general. Through retraining or treatment, one seeks to help the individual move from the earliest type of morality to a higher level, which can be maintained even when he is on his own.

The law, in discussing the management of the delinquent child, states that "the action taken shall, in every case, be that which the Court feels the child's own good and the best interests of the community require".[14] There are many kinds of intervention possible, ranging from doing nothing to the opposite extreme of incarceration. In cases before the court, the juvenile-court judge or probation officer may ask the physician, worker, or counsellor to assist by providing a report summarizing his understanding of the case and any recommendations as to the management of choice. Basically, what is sought is a report which, in a brief and clear manner, devoid of jargon, provides the following:

1. A summary of the relevant history and the clinical (including psychological) examination of the child and family.
2. A clear, concise, down-to-earth, and internally consistent statement of how the clinician or worker understands the case, including factors he sees as contributing to the delinquent behaviour and, if relevant, to the child's disturbance.
3. A statement of what strengths are available to the child and family either from within or from the environment.
4. Recommendations derived logically from the body of the report, ranked in order of preference.

Reports sent to court are frequently read to the child and his parents at some point in the proceedings. One should therefore confine himself to information that pertains to the recommendations and conclusions. Only material that one is prepared to have the family see and hear in an open tribunal should be included. It is advisable in most cases to show or, at the very least, discuss the report with the family prior to submitting it. Failure to do so will likely make continuation of treatment or involvement with appropriate social agencies difficult, as well as increasing the likelihood of the family contesting and rejecting the recommendations.

The child who has committed a minor isolated offence at a young age (for example, taking money from mother's purse), in the absence of other findings and with parents who are genuinely concerned about this, is probably best served by reassuring the parents that such events are not unusual, along with counselling them about ways of handling the situation. The parents should be encouraged to tell the child clearly but without long lectures that the behaviour is unacceptable, why this is so, and, if possible, to suggest what would have been acceptable alternatives. They should be instructed to hold the child responsible for his behaviour should there be a recurrence. A first episode of shoplifting should be dealt with by having the parents take the child back to the store to return the stolen articles. Uncomfortable though this may be for everyone concerned, it is a graphic way of illustrating with actions that the child must control his behaviour or face the consequences. Parental consistency, the definition of reasonable limits, follow-through in support of these limits and reinforcement for desired behaviour are all issues requiring discussion in such cases.[25, 26]

Should the act be of a serious nature or should minor acts persist, one would consider next a variety of interventions including brief family counselling, guidance counselling through the school, interviews with the family physician, the seeking of advice and support of trusted friends and relatives, or consultation with a specialist in work with children, adolescents, and their families.

The discovery of delinquency in a child often precipitates a family crisis but it may also afford an opportunity for effective counselling. It may bring to the forefront major areas of tension which, had the crisis not occurred, the family might be reluctant to acknowledge and begin dealing with. This heightened anxiety that the discovery produces can be used to initiate counselling to identify and delineate issues contributing to the problem and, particularly, to encourage more open communication between parents and child and between parents themselves. The plan of action and its implementation should deal directly with the problems contributing to the disturbance while simultaneously emphasizing and strengthening the healthiest aspects of the child's and family's functioning.[2]

Should the problem not respond to these methods of intervention, referral to a specialized agency (child-guidance clinic, child psychiatrist, or other agency qualified to handle these problems) should be recommended and supported. Wherever possible, such agencies attempt to treat the child and to provide help and guidance to the parents around effective management while still maintaining the child in his own home. Should the behaviour at home, school, and in society not improve, one may have to consider a variety of alternatives that involve removing a child temporarily from his family. These include specialized schools on a day or boarding arrangement, a move to a home of a relative or family friend, or other alternative living arrangements such as foster homes, group homes. Other environmental manipulations such as measures to include the child in supervised community activities, helping the family secure more adequate housing, or involvement of a social agency (e.g. Big Brothers) may also prove helpful.

When and if the child appears before the court, a number of alternatives are available to the presiding officer. Courts have the authority to adjourn the case, to levy a fine, to put the child on probation while living at home or with someone other than his family, to make psychiatric help or counselling a condition of probation, to recommend removal from the home to a foster home, to a residential program or to a correctional institution, training school, approved school, or Borstal.[14] The court may, in making its decision, request the help and advice of a court clinic where one exists, or from mental-health and psychiatric services in the community.[24]

Correctional institutions for children and youth have often been thought of as a place of last resort. They have in most cases been located other than in the child's community, and have had difficulty recruiting and retaining particularly specialized staff while, in general, receiving rather niggardly financial support. They are expected to deal with some of the most difficult children in the population while faced with the pressure resulting from overcrowding and a constant turnover of cases. While they, by their own admission, are far from ideal, in some instances they may represent the best placement for a youth at a particular point in his life. It is an unfortunate reflection on society that some children will experience in a training school, perhaps for the first time in their lives, a guarantee of three square meals, a roof over their head, clothes on their back, and the security of knowing that at least for a period of time somebody is taking the responsibility of caring and providing for their needs.

Training schools are useful for children whose impulse control is minimal and who, for their own and others' safety, require a more structured and containing environment. Alternative situations, including hospitals, rarely have the facilities or the willingness to contain and provide for these omnipotent and impulsive children in conditions of safety. Training schools can provide control and a regular environment and attempt to provide the youth with a set of standards that, if accepted, will make it easier for him to live in harmony with society's expectations. Currently there is a trend away from admission to such institutions. This trend is desirable not only on humanitarian grounds but also on practical grounds; data show that the longer and more frequently the child is in an institution, the poorer the prognosis for social readjustment.[11, 18, 28, 33] Alternative living arrangements, such as supervised group homes, are currently in vogue. Their success will depend on the accuracy of the courts in assessing the needs of individual children and on the availability of special facilities suited to their needs. Community acceptance of these facilities varies; they are, at times, regarded with prejudice and concern. What is needed is a series of accurate measures that would allow for precise decisions about which child would benefit from placement in a foster home or group home, treatment in a residential school, or a stay in a correctional institution, combined with an attention to simultaneously working with the families from which they have come and to which they may return.

Conclusion

Infractions of the law and the standards of society are common occurrences. How the first instance is managed often determines the outcome. Early diagnosis and effective intervention fitted to the child's needs, capacities, and ability to meet expectations are of primary importance. The longer the situation is left unattended, the more difficult becomes the management and therefore the more serious the likely eventual outcome. In most cases, an adequate early response utilizing simple methods of intervention with the family and community can be very gratifying. Many of the remainder require only little contact with the court and correctional services. Only a very few go on to adult institutions and have lasting difficulty in personal and social adjustment.

The problem of delinquency is defined by the society. Psychiatry may do much in helping the individual delinquent, but considerably less in combatting the larger problem of delinquency. The application of psychiatric principles may, in selected cases, aid in the rehabilitation of some of those who seem at present destined for a career in crime through pointing the way towards earlier and more adequate intervention. But if there is a solution to the larger problem of rising delinquency rates, it lies in somehow changing society to eliminate or counteract some of the clear sociological origins of much of the behaviour that is labelled delinquent.

RECOMMENDED FOR FURTHER READING

1 ALEXANDER, J. F., and PARSONS, B. V. "Short-Term Behavioural Intervention with Delinquent Families: Impact on Family Process and Recidivism". *J. Abn. Psychol.* 81: 219–25, 1973.
—describes a study of different styles of family intervention showing that short-term behavioural approach obtained superior results.

2. BARTEN, H. H., and BARTEN, S. S. *Children and Their Parents in Brief Therapy*. New York, Behavioral Publications, 1973.
—series of articles reviewing short-term work with families including principles of crisis intervention.

4. BERNE, E. *Games People Play*. New York, Grove Press, 1964.
—one of the classic books on transactional analysis.

5. BIRKENMAYER, A. C., and LAMBERT, L. R. *An Assessment of the Classification System for Placement of Wards in Training Schools. 1: The Determination of Assessment of Outcomes*. Toronto Ministry of Correctional Services, Planning and Research Branch, 1972.
—hard look at training schools and grounds for placement.

6. BOWLBY, J. "Separation Anxiety: A Critical Review of the Literature". *J. Child Psychol. Psychiat.* 1: 251–69, 1960–61.
—updating of literature that had evolved since Bowlby's original presentation; with critique.

7. BRODER, E. A. "The Delinquent Girl". Unpublished dissertation for Diploma in Child Psychiatry, University of Toronto, 1966.
—review of literature plus study of a group of delinquent girls up to mid-sixties—since then there have been changes in the typical profile.

9. FISHER, S. M. "Life in a Children's Detention Centre: Strategies of Survival". *Amer. J. Orthopsychiat.* 42: 368–74, 1972.
—critical examination of the detention centre for children and adolescents held waiting trial, exploring institutional structure and survival mechanisms of children and staff.

11. GLASER, D. *Strategic Criminal Justice Planning*. Crime and Delinquency Issues, National Institute of Mental Health, Rochville, Md., 1975.
—up-to-date review of current studies and thinking about delinquency.

12. GLUECK, S., and GLUECK, E. *Delinquents and Non-Delinquents in Perspective*. Cambridge, Mass., Harvard Univ. Press, 1968.
—Gluecks have done the largest, most comprehensive study of delin-

quent boys and have developed predictive scales—this book also includes a review of their work to that time.

13. JOHNSON, A. "Sanctions for Superego Lacunae of Adolescents", in Eissler, K. R., ed., *Searchlights on Delinquency*, 225–45. New York, International Univ. Press, 1949.
—classic paper for the understanding of one group of delinquents relating the delinquency to difficulties in the parents.

16. KOHLBERG, L., and GILLIGAN, C. "The Adolescent as a Philosopher: The Discovery of the Self in a Post-Conventional World", in Kagan, J., and Coles, V. R., eds., *Twelve to Sixteen*, 144–79. New York, Norton, 1972.
—excellent review of development of thinking and morality in Piaget's terms.

17. KONOPKA, G. *The Adolescent Girl in Conflict.* Englewood Cliffs, N.J., Prentice-Hall, 1966.
—good review of thoughts of delinquency in girls.

18. LAMBERT, L. R., and BIRKENMAYER, A. C. *An Assessment of the Classification System for Placement of Wards in Training Schools. 2: Factors Related to Classification and Community Adjustment.* Toronto, Ministry of Correctional Services, Planning and Research Branch, 1972.
—further results of Ontario Study of training school wards.

20. LOMBROSO, C. *Crime, Its Cause and Remedies*. New York, Patterson-Smith, 1968 reprint.
—first classical study of a criminal population—fascinating look at thoughts prevalent in the turn of the century.

21. Mc CORMICK, P. *Guide for Use of Life-Script Questionnaire in Transactional Analysis*. Berkeley, Calif., Transactional Publications, 1971.
—part of a larger study comparing the efficiency of transactional analysis, a behavioural approach, and the standard approach in training schools in California. Transactional analysis seems to produce somewhat better long-term results.

22. Mc GRATH, W. T., ed., *Crime and Its Treatment in Canada*. Toronto, Macmillan, 2nd Rev. Ed., 1976.
—good review of various aspects of criminology.

23. MINUCHIN, S.; MONTALVO, B.; GUENEY, B. G.; ROSMAN, G. L.; and SCHUMER, F. *Families of the Slums*. New York, Basic Books, 1967.
—summary of studies of Philadelphia group from which their method

of family therapy was evolved. It includes much data about "normal" families and therapy and the difficulties of doing such research.

24. NIR, Y., and CUTLER, R. "The Therapeutic Utilization of the Juvenile Court". *Amer. J. Psychiat.* 130: 1112, 1973.
—describes a collaborative program between a juvenile court and an adolescent psychiatric clinic that has made it possible to deal successfully with otherwise untreatable court-referred adolescents.

25. PATTERSON, G. R., and GULLION, M. E. *Living with Children.* Champaign, Ill., Research Press, 1971.
—practical manual that can be given to families to read to get across basic behavioural principles of child management.

26. PATTERSON, G. R. *Families.* Rev. Ed. Champaign, Ill., Research Press, 1975.
—small book written for laymen telling how to apply the principles of social learning to family life.

27. PAYNE, W. D. "Negative Labels". *Crime and Delinquency.* 19: 33–40, 1973.
—provocative article on repercussions of labelling gangsters delinquent.

28. PEARSON, J. W. *The Group Home Project: An Exploration into the Use of Group Homes for Delinquents in a Differential Treatment Setting.* State of California Human Relations Agency, Department of Youth Authority, 1970.
—good review of different modes of placement tried in California.

32. SPITZ, R. A. "Hospitalism: A Follow-Up Report on Investigation Described in Volume 1, 1945", in Eissler, R., ed., *Psychoanalytic Study of the Child.* Vol. 2: 113–17. New York, International Univ. Press, 1946.
—classic paper on the topic.

33. SCHUR, E. M. *Radical Non-Intervention: Rethinking the Delinquency Problem.* Englewood Cliffs, N. J., Prentice-Hall, 1973.
—thought-provoking thesis—worth reading and thinking about.

34. VAZ, E. W. *Middle-Class Juvenile Delinquency.* New York, Harper and Row, 1967.
—good review questioning some of our usual preconceptions.

35. WALKER, N. *Crime and Punishment in Britain.* Edinburgh, Edinburgh Univ. Press, 1965.
—thorough, well-documented review of whole area.

ADDITIONAL READING

3. BERG, J. M., and LOWY, F. H. "XYY Syndrome: A Comment". *Mod. Med. Canad.* 30: 692–93, 1975.

8. *Criminal Code.* RSC chap. c-34, s.12 and 13, 1970.

10. GIBBENS, T. C. N., and PRINCE, J. *Shoplifting.* London, Institute for the Study and Treatment of Delinquency Publication, 1962.

14. Juvenile Delinquents Act, 1929, c-46, s.1. *Revised Statutes of Ontario*, B. Johnson, chapter 160, 3507–3524, 1952.

15. KIVOWITZ, J. "The XYY Syndrome in Children: A Review". *Child Psych. Human Devel.* 2: 186–94, 1972.

19. LEWIS, D. O.; BALLA, D. A.; SACKS, H. L.; and JEKEL, J. F. "Psychotic Symptomatology in a Juvenile Court Clinic Population". *J. Child Psychiat.* 12: 660–74, 1973.

29. RYAN, W. *Blaming the Victim.* New York, Pantheon Books, 1970.

30. SHELDON, W. H. *Varieties of Delinquent Youth.* 2 vols. Reprint of 1949 ed., New York, Hafner, 1970.

31. SHIELDS, J. *Monozygotic Twins: Brought up Apart and Brought up Together.* London, Oxford Univ. Press, 1962.

36. WILLIAMS, J. "From Delinquent Behaviour to Official Delinquency". *Social Problems.* 20: 209–29, 1973.

37. *Young Persons in Conflict with the Law*: A Report of the Solicitor-General's Subcommittee on Proposals for New Legislation to Replace the Juvenile Delinquents Act: published by the Communications Division, Ministry of the Solicitor-General: Catalogue no. JS 42-3/1975.

WILLIAM A. HAWKE
STANLEY R. LESSER

12. The Child With a Learning Disorder

In the world of today, at least in the industrialized nations, ever-higher levels of education are an important prerequisite for economic and social success. Thus the child who fails in school is at a disadvantage. The term "learning disorder" refers to a failure to meet society's expectation of academic achievement so necessary not only for social and economic success, but also for the respect of parents and teachers, for prestige among peers, and for the child's own self-esteem.

Although many children identified by schools as having learning disorders are referred to mental-health facilities, this does not mean that all children with psychiatric problems have a learning disorder, or that all those with a learning disorder are emotionally disturbed.

Prevalence

Studies in Great Britain and North America indicate that in the first grade about 25 per cent of children show evidence of significant difficulties in the academic area.[9] This varies widely, depending on socio-economic factors and the criteria of diagnosis. That the average teacher is well aware of this is shown by her dividing her class into three or four reading groups, including one geared to the approximately one-quarter of the class who are slow in developing reading skills. This figure frequently has been misinterpreted and used to suggest that this 25 per cent have specific learning disabilities that will require special educational provisions throughout their academic career. This is misleading, as the figure quoted consists of all those children who are having difficulty developing reading skills at the grade one level. While some of these certainly do have specific learning disabilities, the 25 per cent includes others who are intellectually subnormal and many whose problem stems from chronological, emotional, and social immaturity. For example, in most school systems a child born by December 31 qualifies to enter school in September of a given year, while one born just two days later must wait until the following September. Thus at the point of school entry the first child, who is a full year younger than the second, will normally be more immature in every respect. This relative immaturity naturally will influence his readiness to learn.

Only a fraction of all those children who manifest *learning disorders* at some point in their school career continue to have significant difficulties throughout school. It is the authors' impression that *specific learning disabilities* account for the majority of these persistent learning disorders. The actual prevalence of specific learning disabilities among school children is sometimes given as 5 to 10 per cent,[25, 26] although in the author's estimate this figure may be somewhat inflated. Boys outnumber girls four to one in mild learning disorders and as much as eight to one in severe ones. Male prevalence is even more pronounced in the group with specific disabilities in reading and spelling.

Origin of Learning Disorders

Learning disorders result from a number of causes, the most important of which are the following:

1. INTELLECTUAL FACTORS

a) *General.* Children whose average scores on the Binet or full scores on WISC are below 90 learn more slowly than children of normal ability. (For a discussion of the significance of IQ scores, see Chapter 13.) How fast they learn will depend not just upon their actual ability but also on their organizational skills, their work habits, and their motivation to learn. A child with an intelligence quotient between 85 and 90 who is well organized, well motivated, and supported by a stable family may achieve educational levels barely distinguishable from the average of his age group. However, children with similar intelligence but poor organizational abilities, work habits, and motivation will lag far behind their average peers. Children with intelligence quotients below 85 will find it difficult or impossible to compensate for their lower intellectual ability through application, organization, and motivation.

b) *Specific.* Specific areas of cognitive weakness not sufficient to lessen the over-all intelligence quotient may still interfere with learning. These children, despite intelligence quotients within or above the broad range of normal, have isolated intellectual deficits which significantly affect their learning. They will be discussed in a later section under Specific Learning Disabilities.

2. PHYSICAL FACTORS

Physical factors may affect the learning of the individual in various ways. Four of the most common of these are:

a) A reduced sensory intake, usually deafness and blindness.
b) Involvement of the central nervous system by organic disease, with or without an associated reduction in intellectual ability.
c) Involvement of the central nervous system by organic disease with the production of an organic brain syndrome (see Chapter 10). These children may show hyperkinetic behaviour, short attention span, lack of concentration, and difficulties in the reception and comprehension of language.
d) A reduction in general energy due to chronic illness. Examples would include severe malnutrition, chronic congestive heart failure, chronic nephritis with renal failure, and cystic fibrosis.

3. EMOTIONAL FACTORS

Emotional factors may affect learning either primarily or secondarily. Primary emotional factors are those originally responsible for a learning disability. Secondary emotional factors, while not causing the disorder, intensify the disability, at times interfering even more with learning than the original cause.

The *primary emotional factors* may be considered under two headings: (a) emotional factors in the child; (b) emotional factors in the family.

a) Emotional factors in the child that can interfere with learning include:
   i) *A chronically high level of anxiety or tension* which leaves the child so preoccupied with anxieties and fantasies that he is unable to concentrate in school. So much emotional energy and attention is

diverted into dealing with anxiety that there is little left over to use for learning. Anxiety may also affect learning by reducing short-term memory and organization and by increasing distractibility.

ii) *Certain specific patterns of defence against anxiety* such as hyperactivity and aggressive and antisocial behaviour are unacceptable to most teachers and often cause conflict between child and teacher. This conflict may produce mutual resentment and repeated clashes, thus interfering with the partnership needed for successful learning.

iii) *The child who is chronically depressed* has most of his energy tied up in his depression and unavailable for learning. Academic underachievement is a common depressive equivalent in children and adolescents (see Chapter 7). Children mourning the death of a close family member or a parental separation may, for a time, withdraw their interest in learning.

iv) *Fear of failure* (often resulting from a pattern of repeated failure or, at times, from an exaggerated response to failure) leaves some children incapable of trying for fear of suffering yet another defeat. (See the discussion of the "restricted child" in Chapter 6.)

v) Some children fail to learn due to *resistance and hostility to the expectations of adults in authority*, at first parents, then teachers. These are often stubborn, determined children from equally stubborn and determined families who, in the child's early years, have struggled with each other over many areas of discipline. Where the struggle has been mainly with the mother, it may generalize to all females so that kindergarten and primary grade teachers, usually women, are often faced with considerable resentment displaced from the mother.

vi) A relatively few children with *severe personality disintegration* of a psychotic nature have major learning problems. For most of these, the problems continue throughout the child's entire academic career (see Chapter 8).

vii) *Specific emotional conflicts* may, in a few children, affect the ability to learn. For example, a ten-year-old girl inhibited all curiosity, including the desire to learn, as part of her attempt to deny to herself the repressed knowledge of her mother's extramarital affairs. An eight-year-old boy failed to learn, through fear that his less intelligent but older brother would retaliate should he exceed him at school. (See the discussion of the "constricted child" in Chapter 6.)

The same emotional factors may act in some children as primary factors and in others as secondary. A child afraid of failure, for example, may refuse to answer questions or complete assignments for fear of giving the wrong answer. Another child, whose primary reason for poor scholastic progress is inadequate hearing, may do the same because of a fear of revealing the handicap or because he does not know the right answer. In the former case, the fear of failure is the primary reason for the educational difficulties, while in the latter, it plays a secondary role in maintaining the difficulties.

b) Emotional factors in the family that interfere with learning include:

i) Hidden tensions, open discord with quarrelling between the parents, separation or divorce may so preoccupy children emotionally that they are unable to organize themselves and work effectively in class (see Chapter 20).

ii) Families with excessively high standards and expectations often so emphasize these that children, unable to meet them, feel inadequate and incapable of success.

iii) Families with inadequate controls and discipline not only present poor patterns for identification but produce children with poor work habits and proneness to resisting discipline in the classroom. Often unprepared for the introduction to school and poorly motivated for learning, these children soon learn to expect failure.

iv) Sibling rivalry may contribute to learning difficulties particularly if the siblings are adequate or gifted and the family compares their progress to that of the underachiever. In such situations, some children give up and withdraw, others develop neurotic anxiety, while still others struggle to compete, often refusing to accept their educational limitations.

Secondary emotional factors occur in reaction to a primary disability regardless of its origin. It is the exceptional child with a significant learning disability who does not eventually develop emotional problems secondary to the continued frustration and chronic underachievement.

a) Many of these children are told, and increasingly they begin to feel, they have failed, becoming convinced that they are stupid and incapable of success. These attitudes, often originating in the early grades, may continue throughout the child's academic career, interfering with motivation to learn at all levels. For some, the lack of self-confidence persists into adult life, affecting the individual's employability.

b) Anxiety over academic failure may further block learning by setting up a vicious cycle of fear of failure, reluctance to produce, actual failure, and further confirmation of the fear. Some of these children develop psychosomatic symptoms which they utilize to avoid the pressures of school. Others go further, overreacting to these symptoms with the development of the school refusal syndrome. (For other factors contributing to the development of school refusal, see Chapter 6.)

c) Resistance and hostility to learning may result from the experience of repeated failure. Children in whom these attitudes become fixed often reject any form of assistance and are unable to benefit from remedial programs or tutoring.

d) Continued failure and the associated poor self-esteem lead some children to behave antisocially, first in the school and family and later in the community. Studies of children brought before juvenile courts show a significant number of children with learning disabilities and education retardation (see Chapter 11).

4. CULTURAL OR SOCIAL FACTORS

In recent years it has been recognized that a significant number of children from the poorest social and economic levels—often referred to as disadvantaged—do not learn at the same rate as other more fortunate children. Earlier this was attributed largely to a generally lower intellectual potential. Recent studies, however, indicate that disadvantaged children have normal intelligence levels in infancy and in the preschool years, only to show a gradual drop, particularly in the verbal and language areas, in the early school years. These are precisely the areas of intellectual functioning that correlate most closely with academic success. It is presumed, and probably correctly, that this drop is not related to a change in basic intelligence but to a lack of normal environmental stimulation, especially verbal, during the crucial preschool years. Teachers, who usually have middle-class expectations, often fail to understand and frequently reject the more action-orientated and less verbal patterns of behaviour that these children have learned to use.

The family of the disadvantaged child is likely to compound these difficulties. Frequently the parents are ill equipped to provide the type of environment and stimulation required for learning. Many such children are poorly motivated and, with little family encouragement to accept the structure of the classroom, all too often become truants and drop-outs. The inner cities or "ghettos" from which many such disadvantaged children come include a disproportionately high number of broken families and all of the problems resulting from economic stress. These include the pressures resulting from inadequate income, poor living conditions, family disorganization, chronic parental conflict, and alcoholism—even in those families where both parents are present.

Specific Learning Disabilities

INTRODUCTION

Specific learning disabilities result from precise areas of intellectual or cognitive weakness that exist in some children despite an over-all intelligence within the broad range of normal. They can occur in the absence of a recognizable physical disturbance, primary emotional factors, or social and cultural deprivation sufficient to account for the failure to learn.

Specific learning disabilities first become obvious in the early grades as difficulties in mastering the basic skills of reading, spelling, and arithmetic become apparent. The most frequent disability is *dyslexia,* that is, a difficulty in learning to read. If not overcome, dyslexia will prove disabling in later years as it increasingly interferes with the mastery of all subjects that require the child to read and retain printed material. Associated problems in printing, writing, and spelling often appear as difficulties in completing assignments and in writing essays. Specific mathematical disabilities also occur but less frequently. Achievement tests in children with specific learning disabilities often show levels in one or more subjects well below those expected for a child of the same age and intelligence.

ORIGIN

Learning difficulties in most children are the result of a number of factors acting together. The child with cerebral palsy or deafness, for example, may have an associated intellectual retardation, while the child with a specific learning disability may suffer from a secondary emotional disturbance. Despite the frequently multiple origin, an adequate investigation usually reveals that one factor is the primary reason for the disability, while the others are secondary or reactive.

The primary factor in children with a specific learning disability is a localized deficit in cognitive or intellectual functioning. In the past, this was commonly considered the result of brain damage or, at least, minimal brain dysfunction, since similar cognitive defects occurred in some children with definite organic cerebral disease.* However, the history, neurological examination, skull X-rays, and electroencephalogram of most children with learning disabilities fail to support a diagnosis of definite cerebral damage. Furthermore, the more the families of these children are studied, the more often one detects comparable disorders in parents, siblings, or relatives, thus suggesting an inherited or genetic contribution. In some children, the disability clearly stems from demonstrable brain damage; more frequently it seems to be the result of a constitutional or inherited pattern of intellectual functioning.

1. READING AND SPELLING DIFFICULTIES

Most reading and spelling difficulties appear to fall into one of two different types depending on whether it is the *audiovocal* (spoken) or *visuomotor* (written) area of language that is primarily involved. Audiovocal language (the ability to understand and communicate through speech) is the original language of the human race. Children normally develop it during the pre-school years. Visuomotor language (the ability to comprehend and communicate by some form of written script) was evolved later in the history of the human race. The child begins to acquire it at a later date, around the fourth or fifth year of life.

a) *Disabilities Resulting from Defects in Audiovocal Functioning*

Children with audiovocal difficulties do poorly in tests of verbal functioning on the Binet or the WISC (Wechsler Intelligence Scale for Children), but relatively well on tests of performance in non-verbal areas.

On the ITPA (Illinois Test of Psycholinguistic Abilities), weaknesses are detected in the audiovocal but not in the visuomotor areas.**

*The term "minimal brain dysfunction" implies irregularities in intellectual functioning detectable on psychological tests, while making no statement as to the origin of the disability. The value of the term lies in the implication that the cognitive deficit arises primarily from intrinsic factors, rather than in response to a damaging environment. For further discussion, see Chapter 10.

**The WISC and Binet are standard tests used in assessing children's intelligence. The ITPA assesses language functioning, and is often useful in delineating the specific nature of a defect in the language area. These and other tests are discussed later in this chapter under the heading Diagnostic Assessment.

For example, specific deficits in short-term auditory memory or retention can be demonstrated. There is often a history of delayed speech development and problems in articulation. In the classroom, these children have a poor vocabulary and have trouble in explaining things orally and in writing. They may also have difficulty understanding and retaining verbal instructions given by the teacher. Children with an audiovocal defect typically have great difficulty learning to read phonetically. Although able to sound out individual letters, they cannot remember these sounds long enough to blend them into a word. Thus, while capable of analysing the word letter by letter, they cannot recognize the total word.

By the time the average child enters school, audiovocal language is usually fairly well developed. A significant deficit in mastering audiovocal language by the time of school entry is commonly part of a continuing disability that is likely to cause continued problem in reading even as an adult.

b) *Disabilities Resulting from Defects in Visuomotor Functioning*

Children with visuomotor disabilities have adequate or normal verbal scores in intelligence tests, but do poorly on performance or visuomotor quotients. The ITPA confirms a deficit in visuomotor functioning, and defects in short-term visual memory or visual retention are frequently demonstrated. Children with visuomotor deficits are often detected in kindergarten and the primary grades by their difficulty in matching shapes and forms, and through the extent to which they reverse letters and numbers. While generally able to sound words phonetically, they are poor sight-readers because of their difficulty remembering and recognizing the total word. Although eventually they usually become better readers than children with an audiovocal defect, their reading remains slow and their preoccupation with decoding individual words often causes great difficulty in understanding and remembering the drift of what they have just read. Children with a visuomotor defect commonly have difficulty in spelling. As English cannot be spelled phonetically, their defects in visual memory interfere with their remembering the shape and structure (gestalt) of words whose spelling does not follow simple phonic rules.

Since visuomotor skills develop just around the time when the average child enters school, a number of children will begin school somewhat behind in visuomotor functioning because of normal variations in maturation and development. These children may have reading problems initially. If the primary deficit and the child's reactions to initial difficulties are not too great, and if motivation and work habits are adequate, some such children will mature in this area, and can achieve reading levels that permit success at the secondary school or even university level. For other children with more severe and persistent visuomotor deficits, reading may never get beyond phonetic decoding.

Some children have defects in both the audiovocal and visuomotor areas. They do poorly on both verbal and performance tests of intelligence and show difficulties in both the audiovocal and visuomotor areas on the ITPA. In the classroom, and even on psychological testing, their learning patterns resemble those of the child who is mentally retarded. The prognosis for their overcoming their double deficit and succeeding educationally is limited, as they have both defects to overcome and few areas of strength to build on for successful remediation.

2. DIFFICULTIES IN MATHEMATICS

Mathematical difficulties occur less frequently than those in reading and spelling and, unlike the latter, which occur more commonly in boys, these are more often seen in girls. On psychological tests, these children typically obtain reasonably adequate verbal scores but do less well in the performance area. There are often demonstrable deficits in spatial localization, right-left discrimination, short-term auditory memory, and digit retention, which may affect not just their mathematical skills but also, through multiple reversals, their spelling. The mechanism by which these specific deficits in spatial relationships affect mathematics is not, at present, clearly understood. Difficulties in secondary school mathematics (geometry, calculus) and physical sciences (physics, chemistry) may demoralize them as well as limiting the education and career choices available to them in later years. The suggestion that a cultural expectation may contribute to the predominance in girls has been raised, but not proven.

3. FINE-MOTOR DISABILITIES: PROBLEMS IN PRINTING AND WRITING

Some children, because of a deficiency in fine-motor control, have great difficulty printing and writing. Their awkwardness can be demonstrated on neurological and psychological assessment. Termed *apraxia* or *dyspraxia*, this is thought to result not from a definite lesion involving a specific tract (e.g. the pyramidal or cerebellar tracts) but to a failure in the organization of motor activity at the level of the cerebral cortex. Left-handed or ambidextrous individuals occur with more than average frequency in their families. These children, when carefully assessed, often show confused or mixed laterality (particularly in eye-hand function), poor spatial relationships, and right-left confusion. Because of associated difficulties in gross-motor control, they often do poorly in sports, particularly those requiring eye-hand co-ordination.

In the classroom, even when highly motivated, these children are often slow and sloppy in their written work. Teachers often interpret the lack of neatness or failure to complete assignments as evidence of lack of care and insufficient effort. They may be overly critical, placing unrealistic pressures on these children if they are not aware of the organic factor contributing to their difficulty in carrying out precise motor activities and completing written reports.

SECONDARY FACTORS

Specific learning disabilities may be complicated by any of the secondary factors discussed earlier as intensifying learning disorders. Of particular importance are:

1. The combination of hyperactivity, poor concentration, and inability to focus and maintain attention and to organize behaviour may be seen in conjunction with a specific learning disability.
2. Emotional factors such as anxiety or mortification in child and family that originally results from the impact of the learning disability may greatly compound the interference with learning. Unless these complications are prevented before the child is immobilized by repeated failure, they may keep the child from being able to utilize even an adequate remedial program.
3. The school system's response to the child with a learning disability may either help or aggravate the situation. Prompt recognition in kindergarten or grade one, an adequate diagnostic assessment, and the provision of a remedial program tailored to the child's specific needs provided by a specialized teacher will do much to help the child compensate for the original disability. Tardy recognition or inadequate response by the school will, on the other hand, intensify and fix the difficulties.

DIAGNOSTIC ASSESSMENT

The first suspicion of a learning disability usually occurs when the teacher in kindergarten or grade one notices that a child is falling behind the class in specific subjects or activities.

Formal assessment begins with an appraisal of the child's performance in basic subjects using standardized tests such as the Wide Range Achievement Test of Jastek and Jastek. These give a reasonably clear picture of the level at which the child is functioning in reading, spelling, and arithmetic. They provide a standard score, which compares the actual achievement of the child in a given subject with the achievement of children of the same age without learning disabilities. The mean is one hundred and the standard deviation fifteen.

Other standardized tests may pinpoint specific areas of weakness, such as inability to read using phonics, multiple reversals in writing, printing, and reading, failure to retain basic facts (e.g. multiplication tables) in arithmetic, etc.

One then assesses the child's over-all intelligence to determine whether or not there are significant limitations in general intelligence. In younger children, the Stanford-Binet is often used, while in older children the WISC is usually selected. The results of the latter not only indicate over-all ability (the full quotient, or IQ), but also provide a verbal quotient showing the child's results on tests of verbal language and a performance quotient giving his achievement on tests requiring visual and non-verbal judgments. The verbal and performance quotients may be further broken down to provide specific information about such delineated areas of intellectual functioning as vocabulary, auditory memory, object assembly, block design, etc. (For further discussion of specific areas tested by the WISC, see list of cognitive functions in Chapter 13.)

Next, one generally assesses language function, which, in most clinics, is carried out to confirm and complement the assessment of specific cognitive functioning. The most commonly used test is the ITPA. This test assesses both the spoken (audiovocal) and the written (visuomotor) aspects of language function. It provides quotients comparing functioning in each area to levels obtained in normal children of the same age. Subtests provide additional information about specific linguistic skills essential to learning, such as the reception of spoken or written language, the ability to retain spoken or written language, and expressive ability in both the audiovocal and visuomotor areas.

An adequate physical examination, including a careful assessment of vision and hearing, a neurological examination, and a review of the child's general health are also indicated. It is unfortunately not uncommon for a serious hearing or visual defect to remain unnoticed in a child until grade three or four, while the resulting failure to learn is mistakenly attributed to shyness, lack of motivation, mental retardation, or a response to family or social tensions.

Finally, an assessment of relevant emotional factors should be carried out. This involves taking a social history, assessing the development and personality of the child and exploring the relationships currently existing within the child's family (see Chapter 4).

While a reasonably adequate assessment of a child with a learning disability can often be carried out by a single individual, the current trend is towards a multidisciplinary evaluation through a group or clinic assessment. This minimizes the danger of overlooking a problem in an area with which the principal examiner is unfamiliar. A typical assessment would include the services of a physician, a psychologist, a speech pathologist, and a social worker, with such specialists as ophthalmologists, otolaryngologists, psychiatrists, electroencephalographers, etc., available for consultation if needed. The results of evaluations in each sector are then presented and integrated in a case conference at which a decision is reached as to the origin and type of disability and the form of intervention most appropriate to it.

TREATMENT

1. *Primary Prevention: Early Identification Programs**

Early case identification, early assessment, and early intervention are the key to a rational and effective remedial program. A number of programs are attempting to identify in nursery school or kindergarten those children potentially vulnerable to learning disorders. In some of these, nursery school or kindergarten teachers have been trained to do the preliminary screening. Children considered at risk may then be referred for further investigation by a learning clinic, a psychologist, or a physician. At this stage, the physician will rule out serious chronic illness and obvious problems of hearing and sight. Using his knowledge of developmental norms, he will then take a careful developmental history. The following factors are commonly found in the histories of children at risk: a) a history of birth difficulties; b) a family history of a learning disability; c) a history of neurological diseases, including cere-

*See Chapter 22.

bral palsy, convulsions, etc.; d) a history of difficulty in the development or in the early use of language; e) evidence of deficits in visuomotor functioning and widespread difficulties in fine motor control.

The physician may next initiate referral to a learning clinic or educational psychologist who is better equipped to delineate the nature of the specific disability. While at this point the physician's contribution to the diagnosis may have been made, he may still play a vital role in integrating the contributions of members of the allied professions to diagnosis and management. Also, in his continuing role as family counsellor, he may do much to guide and support the family while helping co-ordinate the separate components of the management program.

These programs have been criticized because not all the children designated at risk have later developed a learning disability. Whatever the accuracy of the programs—and a number of them are being carefully monitored to determine this—they have the advantage of forcing teachers and school systems to recognize that learning disabilities do exist and must be identified in the early years of school. This can pave the way for diagnosis and, potentially, intervention before the child has been exposed to the demoralization of repeated failure, as has been the case so often in the past.

2. *Secondary Prevention*

GENERAL PRINCIPLES In assessing the results of intervention, one must carefully determine not just whether the child's academic functioning has improved but whether there has been significant change in his standard scores.

> When Jimmy was 8 years and 4 months old, he was reading at a grade 2.2 level. After one year in a remedial program, a reassessment showed him reading at a grade 2.9 level. Comparing *grade* levels, he would seem to have benefited, since over the year his reading has progressed by 0.7 grades. However, consider his standard scores contrasted in Table 12-1 below:

Table 12-1

Age	*Expected Reading Level*	*Actual Reading Level*	*Standard Scores*
8 years 4 mos	grade 3.3	grade 2.2	88
9 years 4 mos	grade 4.0	grade 2.9	89

Thus the remedial program did not change Jimmy's standard scores, which means that he continued to learn at the same rate as before his involvement in the program.

Unless a remedial program produces an increase in the standard scores, it has been of doubtful academic value. Even should there be no change in the rate of learning, however, a program may do much to help the child become more comfortable (tertiary prevention). For the first time, he may feel that his learning disability has been accepted and that demands made on him are not beyond his capacity, leaving him free to succeed in the work assigned. Thus the success of remedial programs should be interpreted not only by their effect on academic progress and rate of learning but also by their contribution to the social and emotional development of the child.

For many years, children with learning difficulties were treated with programs which were essentially the same, regardless of the nature and origin of the disability. At present, remedial programs are prescriptive whenever possible, tailored to the needs of a particular child as delineated by an adequate evaluation. Currently, many elementary schools have facilities for children with learning disabilities. The children may be placed in a special class for the remedial program or may remain in a regular class with their peer group for some subjects while being released for remedial help during part of the school day. The amount of time spent in the remedial program will depend on the availability of a suitable program, the severity of the child's difficulty, and the child's response to the program. The importance of the individual teacher to the remedial program cannot be overemphasized. For many children, the personality and interest of the teacher are almost as important as the types of program being provided.

As these children progress into secondary school, they will require comparable programs at that level. Given understanding and the availability of suitable courses, a selected group of these children should have sufficient ability and motivation to move into tertiary programs at the community college level. Here, also, there is a need for programs that take into account the basic educational disabilities and make special provision for them.

Any remedial program, to be successful, will require effective co-operation between teacher and child and between parents and teacher. The closer the co-operation between school and family, the more parents will understand the basic disability and the more effectively they can support their child's involvement in the remedial program at home. Conflicts between the child and teacher or between teacher and parents will adversely influence the results obtained by any form of remediation.

SPECIFIC PROGRAMS

a) The child with an audiovocal deficit is given a program planned to help him learn to express himself more adequately. Since defective auditory retention interferes with learning to read phonetically—and this deficit has proven extremely resistant to known forms of intervention—most of these children must learn to read almost entirely through a visual approach (e.g. the use of videotapes, film strips, television, movies, etc.). While such techniques facilitate learning, these children tend to have a fairly significant handicap in the later years at school.

b) Those children with a visuomotor deficit are usually taught to read phonetically and because of their good auditory retention are able to develop phonic skills. Because they are such slow readers, spending so much energy in the decoding of words, they often have difficulty understanding and retaining the meaning of the material. In later years, they often learn to summarize material, reducing the amount of necessary reading as much as possible. Many of them learn through tape recorders, preparing their own taped summaries of an area of study. In evaluating their learning, teachers may need to examine them orally because of their difficulty expressing themselves in writing. Similarly, their problems in spelling should be recognized, accepted, and not penalized.

Although various techniques have been used in attempts to improve visual memory, the results to date have not been particularly satisfactory.

3. *Medication*

In recent years, medication is being used increasingly to decrease the activity and improve the concentration of the hyperkinetic, distractible child. *Methylphenidate* is the usual drug of choice. There is a wide variation in recommended dosages. (See Chapter 23 for a discussion of suggested dosage schedules and other issues related to the administration of this and other drugs mentioned in this chapter.) While the drug is widely used, there is considerable controversy regarding its effect upon learning, with some studies suggesting that behaviour alone is improved while others report an increased ability to learn, secondary to improved concentration and attention.

Particularly for the anxious, timid child, *phenothiazines* may prove helpful in reducing anxiety interfering with classroom functioning. Some hyperkinetic children who fail to respond to methylphenidate may also benefit from a trial of phenothiazine. The *amphetamines*, one of the original groups of drugs used in treating the hyperkinetic child, are rarely used today because methylphenidate and other drugs have proven as effective, freer of side-effects and less addictive.*

4. *Motor Training*

Programs of motor training, proposed originally in the hope that an improvement in motor skills would be accompanied by an increased capacity to learn, have both their proponents and opponents. Current thinking holds that such programs improve motor skills and may enhance self-confidence, which may then be reflected in improved motivation and, secondarily, better school work. This is also considered true of the programs fashionable several years ago in which intensive work was done in ocular training with exercises devised to improve ocular control. There is currently little support for the hypothesis that improving either basic motor or ocular skills will directly increase the learning capacity.

5. *Psychotherapy*

The emotional factors affecting learning must be considered as part of any remedial program. For some children, remedial teaching and realistic expectations with reduced pressure may be sufficient, and the emotional component may not need to be confronted directly. In others feelings of failure, discouragement, and resentment may be so intense that they may make it impossible for the child to benefit from even the most appropriate program of remedial teaching. In such cases, it may be necessary to involve the child and family in some form of psychotherapy as part of the total program. While the form of intervention might vary depending on the needs of the case (see Chapter 22), the therapeutic program for a child with a learning disability would not, in general, differ significantly from the program designed for a child with psychoneurosis or a behaviour disorder. Specific topics that would need to be dealt with in therapy would include the reaction of the child and family to the disability and the child's feelings about the more successful siblings and peers.

6. *Residential Programs*

A number of children with learning disabilities have emotional problems serious enough to warrant admission to a special treatment setting. Such a referral would be based on two factors: the removal of the child from the family setting could in itself be helpful, and specific assistance could be given for both the emotional and for the educational problems. Both parents and the learning-disabled child resist placement in institutions planned primarily for emotionally disturbed children. For this reason, specific residential schools have been developed which provide a program combining treatment for the emotional problems and an individualized teacher program for the learning disability. The separation of a child from his family is not to be undertaken lightly. Residential programs should be considered primarily for those children for whom an adequate out-patient program attempting to deal with both the educational and the emotional components of the problem has proved unsuccessful.

7. *Recent Therapies*

At the present time, a number of additional therapies based largely on biochemical concepts are at times recommended for children with learning disabilities. One such program recommends a low-glucose diet on the ground that given normal amounts of dietary glucose some children respond with a rebound hypoglycaemia, which leads to fatigue and interferes with learning. Another approach, considering hyperactivity a manifestation of an allergic reaction to certain dyes and other food additives, relies on a rigorously controlled diet. Still another, the so-called "megavitamin therapy", holds that a number of these children have unrecognized vitamin deficiencies, despite what are considered by most physicians adequate diets. It therefore consists of the regular administration of multiple vitamins in extremely high doses.

Unfortunately, most of these therapeutic approaches have not had carefully controlled studies, so that their value is at best unproven. Megavitamin therapy has been tested repeatedly under controlled conditions by respected researchers. These studies have been consistently unable to duplicate the results claimed by its enthusiastic supporters. So one-sided is the existing evidence that the Canadian and American

Psychiatric Associations have gone on record as stating that megavitamin therapy is scientifically unproven, not indicated as a treatment of choice, and not without attendant dangers.

PROGNOSIS

Most, if not all, children with a learning disability can be helped. However, this does not necessarily mean that the learning disability can be corrected, as the improvement may be less in the educational than in the social and emotional areas of the child's life. With increased experience, it is becoming evident that many children are left with persistent educational deficits that, as yet, we do not have a way of correcting. In many cases, therefore, one must accept limited academic progress while seeking to bring about significant improvement in other areas of function (i.e. tertiary prevention).

In a given child the prognosis depends on a number of factors, the most important of which are:

1. The child's over-all intellectual ability. The more intelligent the child, the greater the capacity to compensate for the deficit.
2. The type of deficit. The prognosis is better for those with a visuomotor language deficit than for those whose deficit is in the audiovocal language system.
3. The severity of the deficit as determined by the diagnostic assessment as well as by the academic progress.
4. The emotional stability and motivation of the child, the emotional stability of the family, and the support given to the child are all particularly important in older children.
5. The early detection of the disability and the prompt provision of an adequate remedial program before secondary psychological reactions occur and become fixed.

RECOMMENDED FOR FURTHER READING

There are numerous references to learning disabilities in the medical, psychological, and educational literature. It is important to recognize that many articles hold sharply contrasting opinions, and that many of the earlier publications present points of view that are no longer generally accepted. Much of the material prepared for this chapter was based upon the clinical experience of the authors. Nevertheless, the following references appear pertinent, and may contain in their bibliographies references appropriate for one seeking to penetrate further this very complex area.

1. ADAMS, J. "Clinical Neuropsychology and the Study of Learning Disorders". *Pediat. Clin. N. Amer.* 20–3: 587–98, 1973.
—this review of clinical neuropsychological studies does not support the notion that learning disorders represent behavioural disorders of brain dysfunction, although methodological and conceptual limitations do not rule out the possibility of more complex neurophysiological disorders than those studied so far. The best rule of thumb is to disregard any diagnosis unless its use provides clear treatment or educational implications for the child.

2. ASHER, E. J. "The Inadequacy of Current Intelligence Tests for Testing Kentucky Mountain Children". *J. Genet. Psychol.* 46: 480–86, 1935.
—one of the original articles dealing with the impact of culture on intellectual functioning.

3. BRUTTEN, M.; RICHARDSON, S.O.; and MANGEL, C. *Something's Wrong with My Child.* Harcourt Brace Jovanovich, Inc., 1973.
—a book for parents about children with learning disabilities.

4. COHEN, A.K. *Report of the National Institute of Mental Health on Juvenile Delinquency to the United States Congress.* February 1960.
—a clear statement of the disadvantages faced by the lower-class child on being exposed to a basically middle-class school system.

5. CRICHTON, J.; KENDALL, D.; CATTERSON, J.; and DUNN, H. *Learning Disabilities: A Practical Office Manual.* Victoria, B.C., Canadian Pediatric Society, 1972.
—another textbook.

6. DAVIE, R.; BUTLER, N; and GOLDSTEIN, H. *From Birth to Seven: The Second Report of the National Child Development Survey.* Humanities, 1972.
—recommended for those interested in reading more about the prevalence of learning disorders in the general community.

7. De HIRSCH, K. *Learning Disabilities: An Overview.* Bulletin, New York Academy of Medicine: April 1974.
—describes methods of predicting future reading disabilities in young children.

8. De HIRSCH, K.; JANSKY, J.J.; and LANGFORD, W. S. *Predicting Reading Failure*. New York, Harper and Row, 1966.
—an excellent review article.

9. EISENBERG, LEON. "Reading Retardation 1: Psychiatric and Sociologic Aspects". *Pediat.* 37: 352–76, 1966.
—a special article dealing with both the psychiatric and sociologic sources of reading retardation.

10. HAWKE, W. A. "A Six-Year Study of Development of Jamaican Children" (in preparation).
—illustrates problems in using tests of intellectual function with children raised in a different cultural environment.

11. KINSBOURNE, M. "School Problems". *Pediats.* 52: 697–710, 1973.
—very clearly written and at times controversial article. The author feels that the terms "minimal brain damage" and "dyslexia" are potentially harmful. He stresses the harm that can be done through group assessments of intelligence, the importance of the concept of developmental lag, of deriving a management program suited to the specific difficulties and areas of strength of the particular child, discusses techniques of assessing neurological development and the selective use of medication.

12. KINSBOURNE, M. "The Hyperactive and Impulsive Child". *Ont. Med. Rev.* 42: 657–60, 1975.
—maintains that it is not the hyperactivity *per se* but rather the impulsivity and inability to attend—i.e. the distractibility—that interfere most with both learning and socialization. Stresses the important role of stimulants in increasing the child's accessibility to behavioural intervention.

13. KAPPELMAN, M. M.; LUCK, E.; and GANTER, R. L. "Profile of the Disadvantaged Child with Learning Disorders". *Amer. J. Dis. Child.* 121: 371–79, 1971.
—in-depth study of 100 disadvantaged children, attempts categorizing the causes of learning disabilities. Discusses the contribution of family adequacy and family motivation.

14. HELLMUTH, J., ed., *Learning Disorders*. Vol. 1 (1965) to Vol. 4 (1971); Special Child Publications, Seattle.
—a good periodic review of the area.

15. LESSER, S. R., and EASSER, B. R. "Personality Differences in the Perceptually Handicapped". *J. Amer. Acad. Child Psychiat.* 11: 458–66, 1972.
—children whose development from birth has not followed normal pathways because of perceptual handicaps are bound to be psy-

chologically affected by their different experience. Presents the need for a greater understanding of the psychological consequences of primary perceptual handicaps.

16. MULLIGAN, W. "A Study of Dyslexia and Delinquency". *Acad. Ther.* 177–87, 1969.
—discusses the high correlation between dyslexia and delinquency, stressing the importance of early identification and remedial treatment of the dyslexic child.

17. MYKLEBUST, H. R., and JOHNSON, D. J. *Learning Disabilities: Educational Principles and Practices*. New York, Grune and Stratton, 1967.
—a sound textbook.

18. MYKLEBUST, H. R., ed., *Progress in Learning Disabilities*. Vol. 1 (1968) to Vol. 3 (1975). New York, Grune and Stratton.
—also a comprehensive periodic review of the field.

19. PAGE-EL, E., and GROSSMAN, H. J. "Neurologic Appraisal in Learning Disorders". *Pediat. Clin. N. Amer.* 20: 599–605, 1973.
—discusses the neurologic indicators of learning disorders, suggesting both standard tests and special procedures which will assist in an office evaluation. Questions the usefulness of the term "soft" neurological signs.

20. *Report of the Conference on the Use of Stimulant Drugs in the Treatment of Behaviorally Disturbed Young School Children.* Sponsored by the Department of Health, Education and Welfare, Washington, D.C., January 11–12, 1971.
—a brief, tightly organized summary which touches upon the lack of clarity in diagnosis, and then raises a number of concerns related to the use of stimulant drugs before concluding that "there is a place for stimulant medications in hyperkinetic behavioral disturbance, but these medications are not the only form of effective treatment".

21. ROHWER, W. D. "Learning, Race, and School Success". *Review of Educational Research.* 41: 191–210, 1971.
—attempts to differentiate school success from intelligence. Presents some of the problems black children face in our school system.

22. SAFER, D.; ALLEN, R.; and BARR, E. "Depression of Growth in Hyperactive Children on Stimulant Drugs". *New. Eng. J. Med.* 287: 217–20, 1972.
—dextroamphetamine and ritalin caused suppression of growth in weight and height in a group of twenty-nine hyperactive children. The growth inhibition was greater with dextroamphetamine, and rebound weight gain occurred when medication was abruptly stopped.

23. SCHULTZ, C. B., and AURBACH, H. A. "The Usefulness of Cumulative Deprivation as an Explanation of Educational Deficiencies". *Merrill-Palmer Quart. Behav. Devel.* 17: 27–39, 1971.
—explores these questions: Do the learning disabilities of disadvantaged children represent deficiencies in skills and knowledge required by school or are they the result of a genuine arrest of intellectual development? Is this arrest permanent? Does the lower-class environment merely correlate with the learning retardation or cause it?

24. SPRAGUE, R. I., and SLEATOR, E. K. "Effects of Psychopharmacologic Agents on Learning Disorders". *Pediat. Clin. N. Amer.* 20: 719–35, 1973.
—Cites figures indicating that in some areas up to 25 per cent of all children are given stimulants for so-called hyperactivity.

25. THOMPSON, L. J. "Learning Disabilities: An Overview". *Amer. J. Psychiat.* 130: 395–99, 1973.
—another competent overview of the field.

26. WALZER, S., and RICHMOND, J. B. "The Epidemiology of Learning Disorders". *Pediat. Clin. N. Amer.* 20: 549–65, 1973.
—this epidemiological study stresses the contribution of biological, socio-cultural, and psychological factors, stressing the degree to which these are concentrated in the socio-economically disadvantaged child.

27. WEISS, G.; KRUGER, E.; DANIELSON, U.; and ELMAN, M. "Effect of Long-Term Treatment of Hyperactive Children with Methylphenidate". *Canad. Med. Assoc. J.* 112: 159–65, 1975.
—consistent use of stimulants in hyperactive school children over a five-year period, while decreasing impulsivity, hyperactivity, and aggression, did not result in improved psychiatric, academic or psychological functioning as opposed to a no-drug control group.

WILLIAM A. HAWKE

13. Psychiatric Aspects of Mental Retardation

The problems of mentally retarded children stem primarily from the deficits in intellectual and cognitive ability implicit in the diagnosis. In addition, these children are subject to stresses and emotional and social problems similar to, or even greater than, those experienced by children of normal and superior cognitive ability. The retardation, however, limits their ability to deal effectively with these problems. Although the degree of emotional disturbance is not directly related to the intellectual handicap, some mentally retarded children are able to cope with stress better than others. Also mentally retarded children experience stresses that children of normal intelligence do not, such as family reactions to their retardation, be it overt or covert rejection or overprotectiveness. The influence these factors have on the retarded child varies with the child's age and developmental capacities and with the obviousness of the defect. Often it is the emotional and behavioural problems of the retarded child that cause the greatest difficulties for the family, the school, and society. These problems, rather than the retardation itself, may be the reasons that institutionalization of the child or his removal from the home is sought. The first person with whom the family discusses these problems is usually their family practitioner or paediatrician, rather than a psychiatrist. Thus, it is the primary physician, rather than the psychiatrist, who will be expected to help them deal with their difficulties and added responsibilities.

The condition that causes a child's retardation may be primarily responsible for the emotional problems he presents. Thus, if retardation results from structural or organic brain damage, it may be accompanied by behaviour associated with the specific area of the brain involved. Temporal lobe lesions may result in aphasia, lack of emotional control, or specific learning difficulties. Pathology in the frontal lobe may be accompanied by disorganized behaviour, poor memory for both recent and past events, and a general lack of social judgment and concern. In retardation resulting from progressive organic deterioration, associated behavioural problems increase as the disorder becomes more advanced. Cases of so-called cultural deprivation will show many of the problems inherent in being raised in an environment that is inadequate or distorted socially, intellectually, and emotionally. There are, however, problems common to most children with mental retardation, and it is to these that this chapter will primarily address itself.

Over the past three decades there has been a major shift in the concepts of retardation and in the resources available for the management and support of the retarded child and his family. In the past, many retarded children were placed in institutions as soon as the diagnosis was made from intelligence testing. The institutions were usually in remote areas, understaffed, and able to provide only benign custodial care for the large numbers thus dumped upon them. Nowadays the trend is to maintain the child in his own home and community wherever possible, and to reserve institutionalization for those cases in which all other measures have proved inadequate to the needs of the child and his family. Thus, today it is possible for most retarded children to remain at home in the care of their families with the help of resources such as nursery schools, educational programs for the school-age child, and training and special workshops for the older retardate. There is a move well under way to phase out the large institutions and, as an alternative, to provide special facilities of a group-home nature in the child's home community.

In the area of education as well, substantial changes have occurred. Despite the fact that educational programs were once considered to have little to offer the retarded child, experimental demonstrations have showed that many such children can improve their social adjustment *and* their basic educational skills when handled with special techniques geared to the child's cognitive ability and applied with patience and repetition.

Again recently, there has been increased attention paid to the emotional problems of the retarded and their families. Parents now have available opportunities for education on how to support the child as well as help in dealing with their own feelings about having a retarded child and practical methods of management and handling. This social network, still developing, is greatly reducing the problems associated with the management of the retarded child in the past, allowing the child to remain in his own family and rapidly diminishing the need to fall back on institutional care.

Definition

An individual who receives an intelligence quotient of 70 or less on a standardized test of intelligence is defined as mentally retarded. Descriptive terms currently in use appear in Table 13-1.

Table 13-1

Intelligence Quotient (IQ)	*Descriptive Term*
50–70	high-grade retarded
25–50	educable retarded
less than 25	trainable retarded

These terms, with their implication of hope, have replaced the earlier terms "moron", "idiot", and "imbecile".

Factors that May Produce Problems in Adjustment for the Retarded Child

1. FACTORS IN THE CHILD HIMSELF

a) *The general level of intellectual ability.* One would expect that the lower a child's intellectual ability, the greater his vulnerability to problems in adjustment. This is not always true. Often the grossly retarded child adjusts more easily than the high-grade defective, who wishes he could be like normal children but is aware he cannot. He may then handle continual frustration through disturbed behaviour in the home, at school, and in the community.

b) *Special areas of cognitive or intellectual weakness.* As well as having deficits in their general level of ability, retarded children may show specific handicaps in circumscribed areas of intellectual functioning. A child may show a specific weakness in verbal or performance functions, in auditory or visual perception or in perceptuo-motor functioning, any one of which would cause learning disabilities even in children with normal ability. In retarded children these specific deficits often contribute not only to academic deficits but to problems in social adjustment as well.

> John, a child of six with an IQ of 50, has a mental age of three years. Theoretically, he has the intellectual capacity to utilize speech for communication. He has, however, almost no expressive speech. This is due not to his general level of intelligence but to a specific weakness in expressive language and verbal fluency.

> Jean, a fourteen-year-old girl with an IQ of 50 and a mental age of seven years, is unable to learn to read. This is due not to her general level of ability but to a specific weakness in spatial orientation and visual motor skills.

The number of these specific cognitive functions is unknown, perhaps because psychologists approach intelligence in different ways using a variety of special abilities. However, areas of cognitive function in which specific and circumscribed defects have been identified include the following:

1. *Word fluency:* the ability to express oneself in language;
2. *Auditory perception:* the ability to perceive and then comprehend what has been heard;
3. *Auditory memory:* the ability to remember what has been heard;
4. *Visual perception:* the ability to perceive and then comprehend what has been seen;
5. *Visual memory:* the ability to remember what has been seen;
6. *Spatial ability:* the ability to orientate oneself in space and to discriminate right from left;
7. *Mathematical ability:* Cultural expectations may contribute to this weakness, which, unlike the others mentioned above, is more common in girls than boys;
8. *Judgment and reasoning:* The innate ability one hopes to assess in intelligence testing.

A weakness in any of the above areas of cognitive function will be reflected in a specific and circumscribed deficit which will affect the individual child's functioning.

In the 1930s, intellectual functioning was considered the direct result of intelligence, and psychological assessment was assumed to indicate a child's true or native ability. It is now recognized that an individual's level of intellectual functioning depends both on his innate ability, which is inherited, and on his life experience since birth. The concept of an environmental influence on intellectual functioning has been supported by studies of children raised in very deprived homes and nurseries, by studies of children brought up in the inner city, and by studies of children living in underdeveloped or underprivileged nations. The results of any assessment of intelligence will be affected by a number of factors, including:

1. *The attitude of the individual to the test.* Anxiety, fatigue, tension, shyness, hostility, and lack of co-operation may all adversely affect performance.
2. *The language in which the individual has been raised.* Since most tests are standarized on individuals whose primary language is English, children raised in another language may have scores that are artifically lower.
3. *The physical health.* Intelligence tests can be influenced by disturbances of general health, of hearing, and of vision.
4. *The cultural background of the individual.* Children raised in a disadvantaged situation tend to function at a lower level than those experiencing a normal environment. Some of these children may achieve significant gains on formal tests of intelligence following exposure to a more stimulating environment.

The results of intelligence tests—and particularly the results of any single test performance—should therefore be accepted with some degree of caution. This is especially true if any of the above factors which may be affecting the result are evident. It is not uncommon for children who are not innately retarded to test in the 50 to 70 IQ range because of environmental factors or their response to the test situation. If these children are then labelled and educated as retarded, their innate potential may never be realized.

c) *The personality or temperament of the child.* This will significantly affect how the child deals with the limitations imposed by his retardation. It is now generally accepted that a number of basic personality traits are to a degree inherent (constitutionally determined) and are evident even in infancy. These basic traits, however, are significantly influenced by the way the environment responds to the child's behaviour. Behaviour that has a strong constitutional basis is more difficult to modify than behaviour resulting largely from environmental influences. The following behaviour patterns seem particularly important in the retarded:

1. *The basic drive.* This involves the child's basic aggressiveness or passivity. The aggressive child may struggle against his limitations by acting out or fighting with the environment to achieve his goals. Passive children, on the other hand, typically withdraw under pressure and often fail to achieve their potential.
2. *The basic activity pattern.* The hyperactive child is continually on the go, testing limits and requiring constant supervision and control. This pattern, particularly evident in the pre-school years, is often extremely upsetting to the family. The hypoactive child, on the other hand, presents fewer problems for the family and is less difficult to manage but, as a result, may fail to receive the environmental stimulation and involvement he needs to realize his potential.
3. *Attention span and concentration.* A short attention span, relatively poor concentration, and difficulty in organization are frequently found in the retarded child who is also hyperkinetic. If present, they intensify the problems of dealing with the hyperactive behaviour in the early years, inevitably creating major problems when the child enters a formal learning situation.
4. *The ability to handle anxiety and pressure.* Some children tolerate pressure without excessive anxiety, while others, under minimal pressure, become extremely anxious and disorganized in their behaviour. This is of particular importance in school, where the overly anxious child, overwhelmed by the program, may function at a level far beneath his potential.
5. *The ability to accept limitations.* Some children accept without difficulty the limitations imposed on them by their retardation. Other, usually more aggressive children are constantly frustrated and struggling against them. The ability to accept limitations permits the child to handle frustration, to accept substitutes for desired goals when necessary, and, in the case of the retarded, to do without gratification for a considerable period of time.
6. *The ability to control impulses*, especially anger and hostility. Some children, despite retardation, have adequate emotional controls and avoid conflict with the environment. Others, who have major difficulty controlling their emotions, have their lives characterized by extreme swings of mood, frequent tantrums, and repeated conflict.

Since many of the emotional problems of the retarded stem from excessive environmental expectations, children with identical IQs may function quite differently in school and in the community. Those with a good attention span and satisfactory organization and work habits will learn much better than those of comparable intelligence who are distractible, poorly organized, and lacking motivation. Expecting the latter children to achieve at the same level as the former will only create emotional problems through excessive environmental pressures. In setting goals and planning a program of management for a given child, one must take into account both his innate intelligence and his specific strengths and weaknesses if destructive pressures are to be avoided.

2. FACTORS IN THE FAMILY

The family of the retarded child will do much to determine whether or not the child achieves to his potential or develops emotional problems. Their relationship with the child, their expectations for him, their ability to accept his limitations, and the way they deal with problems as they arise will all have an important bearing on his adjustment. The following familial factors play a key role in influencing the adjustment of the retarded child.

a) *The reaction of the family to the realization that the child is retarded.* This reaction usually begins during infancy or in the early pre-school years, but may occur suddenly either without preliminary warning or after the family has been prepared for the possibility. Learning the diagnosis comes as a profound shock. All hopes and dreams for the child are destroyed. Usually, the shock is accompanied by grief, as the family begins to mourn for the normal child they have just lost. The duration of the resulting depression may vary depending on the personalities of the individuals involved and the presence or absence of other family problems.

In some cases, the depression may be warded off temporarily by denial that the child is retarded. The parents may refuse to accept the diagnosis and frantically search for developmental evidence or a second opinion to refute it. Such a request is reasonable and may be necessary to help the family deal with their grief. Some families, however, cannot accept even a second opinion and shop around from doctor to doctor, searching for someone who will give a more favourable prognosis. Occasionally they will find someone who will tell them, for example, that the child is not retarded but just perceptually damaged. In time, however, the truth can no longer be avoided, and there is a return of the previous depression, often to a more intense degree. In the meantime, time goes on and the parental denial—and the distress that lies deep to it—may interfere with appropriate planning and management.

Many parents react with anger on learning that their child is retarded. "Why did this have to happen to me?" they ask. Others feel intense but irrational guilt, as if the retardation were a punishment from God for sins and inadequacies on their part. It is not hard for the parents of a retarded child to find some personal flaw, real or imagined, on which to anchor their guilt. In some cases, these attitudes in the parents may be masked by anxiety, depression, or rage. This free-floating rage may be directed against any number of irrelevant persons or situations. They may lash out at the physician who made the diagnosis, at those providing a program of management, or at the educational system for failing to teach their child to function at the desired level. Many physicians and others are bewildered and upset when their attempts to counsel the parents and derive an adequate program for the child are met with hostility. This hostility may become more tolerable if one recognizes that this rage is a distorted derivative of the parents' grief and that he is only one of many to whom this hostility may be deflected.

Fortunately these days, with earlier diagnosis, with frank discussion of the diagnosis, prognosis, and future management, and with the opportunity to work through their feelings with a social worker, most parents are able within a reasonable period of time to accept their disappointment and, despite their sadness, to carry on with their lives using good judgment in planning for the child. If they are unable to do so, they may live for years weighed down by chronic depression, anxiety, hostility, and guilt.

b) *Parental acceptance or rejection of the child.* Parents often respond ambivalently to their retarded child, showing a mixture of acceptance and rejection. The greater the parental rejection, the more likely the child is to show behavioural problems. There is probably nothing so detrimental to a child's development as the feeling that he is unwanted by his parents. Sometimes the rejection may be obvious to all; in other cases it may remain covert, usually in response to parental guilt and fear of community criticism. Covert rejections should be suspected in cases of severe overprotection or where there are continued unrealistic demands for the child to achieve beyond his potential. But while over-protection may represent an overcompensation for unwanted or unrecognized feelings of rejection, it may also arise out of genuine concern and affection and a desire to protect the child from his inherent limitations. Fortunately most parents are able in time to accept their child with his abilities and potential. Helping parents face and resolve their feelings of rejection often leads to greater acceptance in the long run and a much more suitable climate for the child. If the parents differ in their ability to accept the child with his limitations, the child may be faced with two contrasting sets of demands and systems of discipline. This may result in confusion and inconsistent training, which further interfere with the child's learning socially appropriate patterns of behaviour. Unfortunately, in many such cases, each parent feels his approach to the child is correct and tries to compensate for the attitude of the other. The greater their polarization, the greater the confusion of the child caught in between in his struggle to sort out what is expected of him.

c) *Basic stability of the family.* The general stability of the family and their ability to deal effectively with the problems of family life will affect significantly their dealings with the retarded child and his ultimate adjustment. Families with considerable tension, discord, or conflicts over child-rearing, separation, or divorce are ill equipped to handle the additional stress presented by a retarded child, thus providing an atmosphere detrimental to his development.

d) *The relationship of the retarded child to the siblings.* Some retarded children, particularly those with higher levels of ability, are keenly aware of the normal pattern of life and future of their siblings. They may be intensely rivalrous, struggling to achieve beyond their capacity and responding to repeated frustration with a variety of disturbances. Some normal children, particularly adolescent girls, may be so sensitive to the presence of a retarded sibling in the home that placement of the retarded child outside the family to spare the feelings of the normal siblings may have to be considered. On the other hand, the following illustrates just how well some families can do in providing a suitable environment for a retarded child.

> Karen, a girl with Down's syndrome, was the daughter of a deeply religious professional family in Northern Ontario. When the diagnosis was confirmed, the parents stated that if God willed that their daughter should remain a child all her life

they and their children would accept this. They undertook to provide her with all the love and affection they could in order to help her develop her full potential.

On reassessment twelve years later, it was obvious that both parents and siblings had been able to accept Karen and provide a warm, understanding, and supportive environment. Karen appeared a happy girl, who related well to the family and in the community, presenting no problems either in the home or in the special day school that she attended.

Common Problems Noted in the Retarded

1. In the early years, major problems generally involve the parents, reaction to the diagnosis and their difficulty dealing with the feelings stirred up by their child's retardation. Parents' complaints at this stage centre around the child's failure to develop, such as his failure to stand or walk, to acquire speech, or to develop appropriate social relationships.
2. In most pre-school and some older children, family complaints centre around hyperkinetic and undisciplined behaviour often associated with a short attention span, lack of concentration, and distractibility. Such children require almost constant supervision, and their short attention span causes much difficulty and frustration for those teaching them to control their behaviour and respond to discipline. The parents may be left feeling hopeless and overwhelmed by the child's inaccessibility to discussion and reasoning. The hyperkinetic behaviour pattern, no longer considered pathognomonic of organic brain damage, fortunately seems to settle gradually as the child grows older (see Chapter 10).
3. Some retarded children have marked mood swings with explosive behaviour, poor impulse control, and a lack of flexibility and consistency in solving any problems that face them. Their behaviour presents difficulties particularly in an educational setting, where it disrupts the class, often stimulating other children to behave similarly.
4. Some retarded children in their early years show behaviour patterns very similar to those seen in the autistic child of psychotic origin (see Chapter 8). Autistic children are unresponsive when picked up or cuddled and seem unable to build a warm relationship with the parents, who frequently report that "he is living in his own world" or "I can't reach her." These children typically show delays in achieving the

normal developmental milestones, but their language development is often far behind what one would anticipate from their own general rate of development. In infancy, it is difficult to distinguish the child who is primarily retarded with some autistic features from the child whose autism is psychotic in origin. Occasionally, the diagnosis can be made from the fact that the psychotic child has islands of behaviour well above his own general level of function, while the retarded child's functioning is uniformly depressed. As many of these primarily retarded children grow older, the autistic patterns decrease and they begin to relate to people, eventually appearing as retarded children with no autistic behaviour.

5. In some families, inadequate training and discipline within the home create problems in habit-training so that the child does not learn to behave acceptably in nursery school or school. Inadequate stimulation in the home may produce a further reduction in the level of functioning. Parental overprotection often blocks optimal development by infantilizing the child. This may interfere less with his intellectual functioning than with his social function and adjustment to others.

6. Parents who make excessive demands and rigidly seek to enforce them may do well with a retarded child who is basically passive, while a more aggressive child is likely to rebel. In many such cases, a power struggle between the determined parent and an equally determined child may go on for years, eventually leading to victory by the child, who can, after all, devote himself fully to the struggle, while the parent is faced with the additional demands of the care of the family and everyday life.

7. Improper school placement may create problems if a child, regardless of tested IQ, is placed in a class whose level of functioning significantly exceeds his own. Such an inappropriate placement may result either because school authorities have failed to recognize the presence or significance of specific learning disabilities or because the parents, unable to accept the child's retardation, insist on placing him beyond his capacity. No matter how hard he tries he finds the work increasingly difficult. Although teachers may misinterpret his failure to achieve as evidence of laziness, disobedience, or lack of effort, his specific response, depending on his basic personality, may range from almost complete withdrawal to acting-out and occasional truancy. Since the recent development of an increasing range of educational facilities for retarded children, these problems are less frequent than they once were.

8. Resistance to discipline, refusal to conform, and rebellion are frequently related to parental rejection expressed through excessive expectations or continued pressure and non-acceptance. Often correctly, the child interprets these as a refusal to accept him as he is (i.e. with his limitations) rather than as a specific reponse to a particular failure.

9. As the retarded child of higher ability grows older, he senses the gap between himself and normal children. This often results in his feeling different and developing a poor self-image. In the community, retarded children make friends with children of their intellectual age who are chronologically younger, but within a year or two these children have outstripped their development, and they are left to search for new friends within an even younger age group. This pattern, repeated over the years, frequently results in their giving up trying to make friends in the community, thus restricting their friendships to family or school, where they are associated with the same children over a period of years. This may be a source of great concern to parents sensitive to the loneliness and isolation of their children.

10. Many parents of retarded adolescents become concerned that their child has normal sexual drives without the normally available judgment and controls. These concerns may or may not have a basis in the behaviour of the child, but are frequently exaggerated in parents who are having difficulty coping with their own sexual drives.

Many, if not most, retarded adolescents are rather immature in their sexual behaviour. Exposure of their genitals or observing the genitalia of others, activities that would be more commonly seen in a latency-age child, are not unusual. In the older child, sexual drives are more frequently discharged through masturbation than through sexual intercourse. Parents of attractive retarded girls, however, may be so concerned lest their daughter be seduced that they frequently attempt to arrange to have her undergo tubal ligation. Similarly, parents of retarded boys who have not been involved in any sexual activity have been known to request that their son be castrated in an attempt to reduce his sexual drive and to protect themselves should he be accused of sexual activity. As might be expected, such extreme requests usually reflect serious personal or sexual maladjustment on the part of the parents. Many mildly retarded adolescents are more capable of learning to regulate their sexual behaviour and of using responsibly appropriate methods of birth control than many of their peers whose intelligence is normal.

11. Many parents, especially in the later years, are concerned about the future care of their retarded children. They wonder where they will live and who will be responsible for them when they, as parents, are unable to care for them or have died. An extreme illustration of this is the father who, on learning that he was expected to die of a malignancy within six months, killed his retarded son because he could not face the fact that the child might not be adequately cared for after his death. Such problems are less common in recent years, now that the community is providing more care for the adult retarded in small homes close to their families.

Prevention of Psychiatric Complications of Retardation

From the point of diagnosis and throughout the life of the child, preventive programs as outlined below significantly reduce the behavioural complications already described. Although adequate community resources have already greatly reduced the emotional sequelae of retardation, some retarded children will always continue to show signs of emotional disturbance. The types of community programs that should be available to all the retarded and their families include the following:

1. All parents should have access to parental counselling, particularly after the diagnosis has been made. On hearing the diagnosis, parents often remember little except that their child is retarded and his future is significantly blighted. There should be an opportunity for reviewing at a later date the facts presented at the point of diagnosis. This makes it possible to determine what, in fact, the parents have heard—which may differ significantly from what was said—and gives them a chance to reassess and discuss the facts. At this time, one can begin eliciting from the parents their feelings about the diagnosis and its implications. Ideally, one would continue these contacts over a period of time, allowing the parents a gradual opportunity to face and learn to deal with their feelings. Not all parents, however, can tolerate such an involvement. Many withdraw either because they wish to handle the situation themselves or because they find the discussions too painful. It has been shown that in a number of chronic handicaps (e.g. cerebral palsy) parents are more easily involved in counselling when the organization providing the counselling is also delivering a specific program for the child. Many parents who cannot accept counselling at the point of diagnosis will utilize it later if it is presented as part of a pre-school program planned for their child.

2. As habit-training and discipline may present particular problems for the family of the retarded child, parents should have access to advice regarding the day-to-day management of their child in the home. In many cases, all they will need is help in devising a program of management appropriate to the child's mental age. For example, the child of six with a mental age of three (IQ of 50) will require a program of home management similar to one normally used for a child of three. Other parents may need concrete suggestions around the handling of problems specific to their particular child.

In many programs for the retarded, the physician plays a key role in the initial diagnosis and the correction of specific physical problems. Later, however, the major role is commonly assumed by the educator and the social worker, although the physician may still be asked to deal specifically with some of the behaviour problems.

3. The community should develop and make available programs that can relieve pressure on the family, as well as ones that will help with the child's socialization, habit-training, and, as far as possible, education. Nursery-school facilities for the retarded pre-schooler are essential, although the age at which the child enters them will vary. Some such settings expect the child to have a capacity to involve himself in the program, while others waive this expectation to free the family from the continued pressure of caring for a grossly retarded child. When the child outgrows the nursery school, he goes on to a more formal program with some of the structure of a normal school. Here he will be encouraged to improve his social relationships, as well as to develop whatever capacity he has in the areas of reading, writing, and arithmetic. Between the ages of sixteen and twenty, the adolescent may move on to a sheltered workshop, where he may either be prepared for simple work in the community or remain throughout his adult life. The sheltered workshop trains him to do jobs that can be done by the retarded, including packaging, sorting, etc., for which he is paid. The complexity of the work will vary with the ability and skills of the individuals involved. There is liaison between the workshop and industries in the community, which provide work to be done on a contract basis. Many sheltered workshops are developed in association with a residence for the retarded. Such residences typically accept a limited number of individuals, with house parents, and if necessary house assistants, available to assist them in their day-to-day living.

In addition to the above facilities, the optimal community

program will provide opportunities for short-term care for the retarded to assist the family during illness or to allow them to go on holidays free from the stress of the retarded child. Some communities also have available a residential centre, whose primary goal is the development of good work habits and training in specific activities that would lead to employment in a sheltered workshop. Cases in which there is marked overprotection or inadequate structure and discipline within the home may need such a facility if the child is to be prepared to function adequately even in a sheltered workshop.

Treatment of Established Psychiatric Complications of Retardation

Where psychiatric complications develop in spite of adequate facilities in the community and attempts at prevention, the results of therapy may be limited by the additional handicaps that have hindered the child's adjustment to family and community. Therapeutic programs to be considered would include the following:

1. Specific counselling of the family, usually by a social worker or occasionally by a psychiatrist, around ways that the family can deal most effectively with the behavioural problem.
2. Psychotherapy for the child may prove helpful, particularly in children with higher levels of intellectual functioning. Since communication through language may be severely limited, however, successful psychotherapy with the retarded child may prove impossible. In such cases, the only remaining approach to a therapeutic program is through modification of the behaviour within the family or in the community.
3. Behaviour modification is a technique that is now being used with many of the retarded. Behaviour modification may include *negative reinforcement*, which involves some discomfort or punishment for undesired activities, or *positive reinforcement*, which implies a reward or praise after desired behaviour. With retarded children, the second form of behaviour modification, termed "operant conditioning", seems more effective than the more aversive or punitive approach. For selected children, a systematic program of behaviour modification will prove effective in bringing about behavioural changes that may become an integral part of his way of relating and functioning. (For further discussion and examples of clinical applications of behaviour modification see Chapter 22.)
4. Drug therapy, when useful, is directed not at the retardation itself but towards associated symptoms. Where the retarded child is also hyper-

kinetic or suffers from convulsions or poorly controlled anxiety, the appropriate use of medication may help control difficult behaviour, thus making the child more accessible to direction and control. Drugs in children must never be used *instead of* other care, but always as *an addition to* care based on human relationships. (For further discussion, see Chapter 23.)

Indications for Residential Care

As mentioned earlier, most retarded children now remain in their families unless there are specific reasons for their entering residential care. Among the most important factors to be considered in deciding whether or not a residential program is necessary are:

1. *The level of ability of the child.* The more gross the retardation and the greater the child's limitations, the more likely residential care is to be required at some point.
2. *Complications associated with the retardation.* Retarded children with associated deafness, blindness, cerebral palsy, or severe convulsive disorders may present increasing management problems as they grow older. While many can be maintained at home during their early years, as they grow larger the problems of physical care may eventually lead to consideration of a residential program.
3. *Patterns of behaviour in home and community.* Some of the hyperactive, impulsive, aggressive, or self-destructive children who fail to respond to any program of therapy may produce so devastating an impact on the family that there is no practical alternative to placement outside the home.
4. *The physical health of the family* is an important consideration, particularly as the parents grow older and are less able to meet the physical or emotional needs of the retarded individual.
5. *The general level of stability in the home.* This includes the emotional health of the family, their intellectual and emotional ability to comprehend and cope with the retarded child, and the quality of relationships among various family members. Should the family structure be vulnerable to disintegration under the pressure of the retarded child, an alternative placement is indicated in the interests of survival of the total family.
6. *The impact of the retardation on the siblings.* In some cases, siblings are so sensitive to the presence of the retarded child in the family that placement must be considered. This is particularly a problem for some

adolescent girls who consider retardation as evidence of a family stigma and are concerned that no one will marry them and take the chance of having retarded children. Fortunately, with greater understanding of the causes of retardation and increased opportunities for counselling the families of the retarded, such feelings are usually able to be resolved without having to resort to institutionalization.

These, then, are some of the major psychiatric aspects of mental retardation for the child and his family. It must be reiterated that both for diagnosis and help regarding management it is to the family physician, paediatrician, educator, or social worker rather than to the psychiatrist that the family is likely to turn for assistance in understanding and managing the problems presented by their retarded child.

RECOMMENDED FOR FURTHER READING.

1. BAKER, B. L. and WARD, M. H. "Reinforcement Therapy for Behavior Problems in Severely Retarded Children". *Amer. J. Orthopsychiat.* 41: 124–35, 1971.
—good examples of behaviour therapy are contained in this description of a project in behaviour modification of severely retarded children.

2. BAKWIN, H. and BAKWIN, R. M. *Clinical Management of Behavior Disorders in Children.* Philadelphia, W. B. Saunders, 1966.
—deals primarily with the management of the behavioural difficulties presented by some retarded children to their families and others.

3. CLARKE, A. M., and CLARKE, A. D. B. *Mental Deficiency.* 3rd ed. New York, Free Press, 1975.
—a major reference work.

4. CYTRYN, L., and LOURIE, R. S. "Mental Retardation", in Freedman, A. M., and Kaplan, H. I., eds., *Comprehensive Textbook of Psychiatry,* 817–56, Baltimore, Williams and Wilkins, 1967.
—provides a summary of the genetic and biochemical abnormalities often associated with syndromes featuring severe retardation, as well as discussing psychiatric aspects of retardation and the diagnostic process. Good discussion of primary, secondary, and tertiary prevention.

5. EYSENCK, H. J. *Uses and Abuses of Psychology*. Harmondsworth, England, 1966.
—a useful discussion of the content, selection, and limitations of psychological testing.

6. FOTHERINGHAM, J. B.; SKELTON, M.; and HODDINOTT, B. A. "The Effects on the Family of the Presence of a Mentally Retarded Child". *Canad. Psychiat. Assoc. J.* 17: 283–90, 1972.
—this thoughtful but technical presentation considers the presence of a retarded child within a family as a source of ongoing stress, and considers the various mechanisms and resources the family may use to cope with this stress.

7. FOTHERINGHAM, J. B.; SKELTON, M.; and HODDINOTT, B. A. *The Retarded Child and His Family*. Toronto, The Ontario Institute for Studies In Education, Monograph Series 11, 1973.
—focuses on the two main alternatives for the retarded child's care—home and institution—examining the advantages and disadvantages of each for both the retarded child and his family.

8. FRANCIS, S. H. "The Effects of Own-Home and Institution-Rearing on the Behavioural Development of Normal and Mongol Children". *J. Child Psychol. Psychiat.* 12: 173–90, 1971.
—compares both normal children and mongols who live at home with those in institutions. Discusses reasons for behavioural differences and the lower developmental level of the institution-reared children.

9. HILLIARD, L. T., and KIRMAN, B. H. *Mental Deficiency*. 2nd ed. Boston, Little, Brown, 1965.
—a general textbook.

10. KOCH, R., and DOBSON, J. C. *The Mentally Retarded Child and His Family*. New York, Brunner/Mazel, 1971.
—an integrated but multidisciplinary approach directed towards all professionals involved with the retarded child and his family. Deals authoritatively with such areas as educational training, psychosocial aspects of retardation, the supporting role of community services.

11. MASLAND, R. L.; SARASON, S. B.; and GLADWIN, T. *Mental Sub-Normality*. New York, Basic Books, 1958.
—a general textbook.

12. MENOLASCINO, F. J. *Psychiatric Approaches to Mental Retardation*. New York, Basic Books, 1970
—deals primarily with the psychiatric consequences of retardation for child and family.

13. *Mental Retardation: A handbook for the primary physician.* A report of the American Medical Association Conference on Mental Retardation held in Chicago, 1964. Published by American Medical Association, Chicago, Ill.
—an excellent general handbook.

15. *The Paediatrician and the Child with Mental Retardation.* Prepared by the Committee on Children with Handicaps, published by the American Academy of Paediatrics, Evanston, Ill. 1968–71.
—another useful handbook for the paediatrician or primary physician.

16. POTTER, H. W. "The Needs of Mentally Retarded Children for Child Psychiatry Service". *J. Amer. Acad. Child Psychiat.* 3: 352–74, 1964.
—reviews the historical background of retardation, the interference of anxiety with the adaptation of the mildly retarded child, and the general lack of availability of psychiatric services for these children.

17. STONE, N. D. "Effecting Interdisciplinary Coordination in Clinical Services to the Mentally Retarded". *Amer. J. Orthopsychiat.* 40: 835–40, 1970.
—advocates shifting the focus from the microcosm of the restricted clinical team to include the patient and his network of significant relationships as an integral part of a therapeutic system for the mentally retarded. The importance of clear role definition is stressed.

18. TARJAN, G.; WRIGHT, S. W.; EYMAN, R. K.; and KEERAN, C. V. "Natural History of Mental Retardation: Some Aspects of Epidemiology". *Amer. J. Ment. Def.* 77: 369–79, 1973.
—an overview of current care of the retarded, emphasizing the prevalence, the process of institutionalization, and recent trends in management.

19. WORTIS, J. *Mental Retardation and Developmental Disabilities: An Annual Review.* Vol. 5. New York, Brunner/Mazel, 1973.
—covering developmental disabilities as well as mental retardation, this annual review deals with clinical, educational, employment, sexual behaviour, and other areas related to the management of the retarded child.

ADDITIONAL READING

14. MURPHY, A., and POUNDS, L. "Repeat Evaluations of Retarded Children". *Amer. J. Orthopsychiat.* 42: 103–9, 1972.

SAUL LEVINE

14. Adolescents and the Drug Scene

Drug use has permeated all societies, all age groups, and all centuries in the history of man. *Drug use* is a firm and accepted part of our culture; indeed, we are a drug-oriented society. People of all ages utilize a variety of prescription and non-prescription chemicals to alter symptoms, feelings, moods, or mind-states. *Drug abuse* applies to taking drugs in a manner that is organically or psychologically destructive, either because of the nature of the drug used or the quantity consumed. The term "abuse" unfortunately has been used pejoratively at times to criticize any drug use that is threatening, for real or imagined reasons, to the dominant society and its mores. Drug abuse is not a phenomenon restricted to contemporary youth; the significant point of distinction between the generations is that each has its "own" favourites. Alcohol, nicotine, tranquillizers, sedatives, stimulants, and pain relievers—traditional drugs—are as susceptible to use and to abuse as are the drugs more commonly favoured by the younger generation.

The drug scene waxes and wanes over the years, even changing markedly and unpredictably within weeks and months. But even in a time of relative quiescense and stability, a fairly sizable proportion of high school and college students experiment occasionally with "illicit", chemical, mind-altering substances. If we include alcohol and nicotine in this classification, the percentage of young people utilizing these drugs at least occasionally reaches astronomical proportions (over 90 per cent). This is *not* to say that anyone who uses any of these drugs has a problem. Before a psychiatric or a medical label is affixed, it is important to know a number of facts about the drug user and the particular drug used:

1. *The user.* This entails learning about the individual as a person, not merely as a drug-swallowing machine. How successfully is he handling the major areas of his life? How does he get along with his family? If he is no longer living at home, was his separation from the family painful and chaotic, or natural? Does he have friends, and what is known about the quality and stability of his friendships? How comfortably and successfully has he worked out his relationships with girls, or she with boys? How does he respond to authority? Is he responsible and productive in his work and school performance? What do we know about his moods, his energy level, his interests, his feelings, and the way he handles these? What are his ideas, values, and aspirations? Does he seem to have a goal and a sense of direction in his life, or does he seem to be drifting aimlessly or changing direction erratically? How important a role do drugs play in his life and the life of his group of friends? Why does he use drugs, and what does he feel they do for him?

2. *The Drug.* In assessing the extent of a "drug problem", it is extremely important to know the exact drug or drugs being utilized. This may involve chemical analysis, because street samples are notoriously prone to adulteration. Aside from the specific *substance,* it is necessary to learn *how long* the individual has utilized the particular drug, in what *dosage,* by which *method* (ingestion—"popping"; intravenously—"cranking, shooting, hitting"; nasally—"snorting"; etc.), and with what *frequency* it has been used. Find out what *other drugs* the individual has utilized and the age of onset of drug use. In addition, one should attempt to determine the social context of the drug taking—alone or with friends, at home or outside, etc. Where does the user get his supply—from friends, underworld, peer-group dealers, etc? How did he get involved initially?

The majority of young people who use drugs do so only occasionally and not because of any serious psychopathology, utilizing minor substances (e.g. marijuana) with no ill effects. Further, in many cases where drugs are being abused, the abuse is symptomatic of other, more relevant problems. Indeed, in most cases in which serious emotional problems are evident, they preceded the onset of drug use. The use of any substance to excess can denote psychological problems. The specific chemical involved is merely one of the variables to be considered.

Reasons for Drug Use

The reasons for drug use are many and varied: there are almost as many motivational considerations as there are different drugs. The question of motivations for drug use can be divided roughly into *social* and *personal* categories:

I. SOCIAL FACTORS CONTRIBUTING TO DRUG USE

1. Pressures of Living in Contemporary Society

No matter where people are living today, few are immune to the effects of rapid change on traditions, life-style, stability, and predictability. All societies are feeling the brunt of rampant technological growth, often accomplished in a blind quest for materialistic acquisition or expansion without sufficient concern for the quality of life. The population explosion is a real concern, especially in light of Earth's limited resources and deteriorating ecological equilibrium. The intact, cohesive, extended family is a thing of the past, and we may even be witnessing the demise of the nuclear family. At the very least, the stresses upon it are enormous. There is a growing feeling of alienation in crowded, dehumanizing environments, which increases when the pace of life exceeds thresholds tolerable for physical or emotional health. People of all ages, not only youth, are reacting to these multi-stimulating pressures and searching for relief of some kind. Drugs offer temporarily at least the illusion of such relief.

2. Cultural Ethic

The world has been utilizing chemicals for mind-alteration for centuries. The fact that we are a drug-oriented society should come as no surprise. But never has there been as much popularization in the media and as much public preoccupation with drug use. Never have as many substances, both legal and illicit, been available. The ongoing redefinition of the work ethic and the pursuit of pleasure as a more acceptable philosophy make experimentation with drugs difficult to prohibit.

There is also a well-defined counter-culture made up in part by those who have reacted to the pressures and instabilities of the outer world by turning inward and becoming preoccupied with subjective experience which is elaborated at times to an extent that approaches the mystical. This has generated its own art and literature, its own music and its own gurus (e.g. Alan Watts, Timothy Leary), many of them philosophically committed to the principle of pharmacological mind-alteration and "consciousness expansion". Within this subculture, certain groups value "tripping", and subtle pressure is put on individuals who wish to be accepted to join in these activities.

II. PERSONAL FACTORS RELATING TO DRUG USE

Each person who uses drugs does so for his own reasons, some of which are listed below. While any of these reasons may indicate psychological problems, the latter four are more usually associated with emotional disturbance. It should be obvious that one cannot simply categorize an individual or his motivational state merely on the basis of drug use or even abuse.

1. *Intellectual curiosity.* Some adolescent drug use is in response to the urge to experiment and to participate in new experiences, that is, "to see or feel what it's like".

2. *Recreation.* Many youth will "light up a joint" just as many adults would take a drink at a cocktail party as a way of enhancing the social experience.

3. *Ignorance.* This includes situations in which drugs are "slipped" to an individual, or ones in which the individual is unaware of the implications of particular drug use.

4. *Philosophy.* Here the individual is using drugs for consciousness-expansion or in the search for truth in keeping with his own or others' theoretical rationale.

5. *Ritual.* Here the drug is intended to provide a mystical experience, which at times may have religious implications.

6. *Self-awareness.* Some adolescents will attempt to achieve an understanding or resolution of recognized personal problems by attempting to increase their self-awareness or free themselves emotionally through drug use.

7. *Rebellion.* For some adolescents, parental or societal prohibitions make the taking of illicit or illegal drugs even more attractive. In such cases, the drug use is an acting-out of feelings of resentment against authority.

8. *Escape.* Drugs can be used in an attempt to find relief from intoler-

able real or imagined stresses or situations. They are thus used in an unrealistic attempt to discover a personal Utopia or to avoid personal problems.

9. *Compulsive.* With some drugs (alcohol, heroin, etc.) true addiction can occur. The compulsive reliance on even non-addictive drugs to meet an individual's neurotic needs may reach the point of psychological dependence (habituation).

10. *Self-destructive.* The repetitive use of drugs in spite of knowledge of the potential danger involved may represent a conscious (or unrecognized) suicide attempt or equivalent.

The Drugs

The following is a brief review of the various substances under discussion. Technical terms used are defined later in the section "Potential Deleterious Effects of Injudicious Drug Use". More details are available in the bibliography.

Alcohol

The abuse of alcohol constitutes by far the greatest drug problem in our society, both in the frequency with which it occurs and in the short- and long-term deleterious physical, emotional, social, and economic effects of alcoholism. Social condoning and even glorification via advertising make alcohol attractive to most susceptible to irresponsible use. Alcohol is addicting and dangerous; one can develop a physical dependence, tolerance, and abstinence syndrome in withdrawal. Alcohol is more widely used and abused among the young than are any of the drugs about which our society is so much more concerned.

Marijuana and Hashish

These are the second most popular intoxicants among high school and college students, although their use seems to have levelled off. They do not cause physical dependence, and no significant degree of tolerance is developed. Reports of physical damage after use have not been substantiated. There is no particular association with crime or violence, but the "amotivational syndrome" causes many in society concern. Much more serious than any of the possible direct drug effects are the legal consequences, which, though gradually easing, remain in some jurisdictions harsh and stringent.

Heroin (and Other Opiates)

These have a relatively low incidence of use, although the proportion of users who become dependent is high. While there has been some increase in their use among middle-class youth, heroin still appeals primarily to relatively socio-economically deprived young males. While they frequently are involved in minor crimes to support their habit, most addicts have a history of antisocial behaviour preceding opiate use, and violent crime is less common than with alcohol or amphetamines. The best forms of therapy thus far are with (a) replacement medication (Methadone), or (b) milieu (Synanon), or (c) medical dispensation of opiates. Methadone treatment is not without danger. Methadone is more highly addictive than heroin and should be reserved for true addicts under strict controls.[5] Milieu therapy involves intensive confrontation ("emotional karate") and a belief-system bordering on the religious. The medical dispensation of opiates is a British form of treatment not practised in North America.

Barbiturates (Long- or Short-Acting)

Barbiturates are addictive substances, dangerous and ubiquitous. Their use is on the increase, partly due to their being prescribed liberally by physicians as sedatives. Barbiturates are frequently used in suicide attempts and completions. There is cross-dependence and potentiation with many other drugs, especially alcohol. An extremely strong psychic dependency develops in addition to a true (physiological) addiction. Though the over-all effect is that of a central-nervous-system depressant, these particular chemicals are often associated with violence, as their initial effect is to lessen behavioural inhibitions.

Amphetamines

The abuse of amphetamines varies from time to time and place to place. Many governments have instituted strict controls, and have successfully curtailed middle-class abuse via physicians' prescriptions for the "wrong" reasons (obesity, depression, fatigue). Strong psychological dependence often develops, although there is no evidence of physical dependence. Chronic use, especially intravenously, is particularly debilitating and is often associated with cachexia, intercurrent infections, exhaustion, depression, and paranoid tendencies, which may reach psychotic proportions and violence.

LSD and Other Hallucinogens (MDA, STP, Mescaline, Peyote, Psilcybin, DMT, etc.)

Use of these chemicals which has been limited to middle-class, largely senior high school and university students, seems to have peaked. They have been employed mainly for purposes of self-exploration or experiencing a psychedelic "high". Occasional rather than habitual use is the rule even among "heads". There is little evidence of any kind of dependence developing; those that do become habitual users show evidence of obvious disturbance before beginning taking hallucinogens. There have been instances of drug-induced panic, which can precipitate a psychosis or suicide attempt, and, rarely, toxic reactions. There is a great deal of unresolved controversy—and ignorance—regarding the long-term effects (psychological, physical, and genetic) of their prolonged use.

Solvents (Glue, Gasoline, Nail-Polish Remover)

A "high" or disorientating effect is achieved via inhalation ("sniffing"), often with a plastic bag for purposes of concentration. Their use is largely restricted to lower-class youngsters (age eleven to fourteen). Repeated inhalation can cause brain damage, toxic delirium, and an acute brain syndrome. The prevalence of their use seems to wax and wane periodically. Strict controls and the addition of noxious chemicals to solvents are important preventative procedures.

Tobacco

Nicotine is found in all cigarette tobacco. Psychic dependency commonly develops, and physical dependence (addiction) occurs in many smokers. The most pernicious physical effects (lung cancer, arteriosclerotic changes, etc.) are caused by the inhalation of smoke, with or without nicotine. In spite of extensive advertising about the dangers inherent in smoking, the incidence of smoking in adolescents is steadily increasing.

"Legal" Tranquillizers, Sedatives, Stimulants

These are mainly abused by adults (users) and their "pushers" (doctors). Many are addicting or more subtly destructive; further, many do not accomplish their desired effect. Of late, some (especially diazepam) have been increasingly utilized by adolescents with or without alcohol to accomplish a unique type of "high", a dully "stoned" feeling, not entirely pleasant. Much stricter controls, and more judicious prescriptions, are in order.

Potential Deleterious Effects of Injudicious Drug Use

1. *Bad trip* means a sense of personal discomfort—fear, anxiety, depression, mild confusion, etc.—while under the influence of drugs. Calm but firm guidance in a quiet room and minor tranquillization usually suffice to "bring the tripper down".

2. *Freak out* refers to varying degrees of psychological decompensation, which may reach the point of acute psychosis with its attendant loose cognitives associations, inappropriate affect (often panic), feelings of derealization and depersonalization, lack of insight, poor judgment, disorientation. There is a continuum ranging from moderate confusion all the way to an acute brain syndrome. Hospitalization may be necessary, and psychotropic medication is indicated. The exact drug taken must be known, as the wrong medication may prove harmful. Treatment is complicated by the fact that street samples frequently are adulterated.

3. *Physical effects.* Each drug can be accompanied by a variety of specific side effects. Further, addiction and/or long-term use can cause specific organic damage to various systems of the body.[2, 5, 6, 8]

4. *Habituation* is a term utilized to connote psychic dependency on a particular drug. Because of personality or neurotic needs, the individual relies continually on the drug to diminish anxiety and unpleasant feelings and to avoid dealing with the intrapsychic and/or external source of his or her problems.

5. *Addiction*—of narcotics, barbiturates, alcohol—means very specifically all of the following:

a) Physiological dependency results. There is a chemical "need" by body cells of the drug, and a subjective feeling of "craving" for the substance;

b) Physical tolerance develops—increasing doses are needed to satisfy;

c) Potentially dangerous withdrawal symptoms (the abstinence syndrome) develop upon the sudden removal of the drug from the user's system.

6. *Social consequences and their management.* Frequently, though none of the above pertain, we are still faced with a major crisis within the family. Parents confronted with evidence of their teenager's use of drugs are often shocked, disappointed, confused, and frightened; they

may even feel stunned and betrayed. The youngster in many instances feels shame, confusion, embarrassment, and guilt. Alternatively (or concomitantly) he might display hostility, aggressive behaviour, or bravado.

The equilibrium of the family is upset, and this affects all members of the household. Like most crises, such a situation need not prove eventually destructive; rather, it is an opportunity for clarification of issues, mobilization of resources, and problem resolution, which can lead to increasing the cohesion and growth of the individual and the family (see Chapter 15). The drug use more often than not turns out to be a subsidiary issue, but a valuable one in that the "real" sources of tension or conflict in the user or in the family are through it made manifest.

Following clarification of the total situation, management might proceed in a number of directions. At times, reassurance and education may be all that are needed. In such situations the family physician or paediatrician can provide crucial input and be most helpful in clarifying the issues and aiding in their resolution where the problem is a relatively minor one that is being aggravated by anxiety and loss of perspective. In other situations, the family clergyman, a respected friend, drop-in centre, free clinic, etc., might provide the kind of support and guidance that are required. In those cases in which even minor drug use precipitates violent arguments or significant tension that fails to be resolved, a mental-health worker's intervention can prove invaluable. Psychiatric consultation should be considered when the young person is obviously disturbed, when the family continues in a state of disequilibrium, or when other attempts at resolving the crisis have been tried and have failed.

RECOMMENDED FOR FURTHER READING

1. BLUM, R. H. *Society and Drugs.* San Francisco, Jossey-Bass, 1969.
—interesting.

2. BRECHER, E. M., and Consumer Reports, eds., *Licit and Illicit Drugs.* Toronto, McClelland and Stewart, 1972.
—the best single reference as of the date published.

3. CROWLEY, T. J. "The Reinforcers for Drug Abuse: Why People Take Drugs". *Comprehen. Psychiat.* 13: 51–62, 1972.
—shows multiple reasons for drug abuse.

4. FORT. J. *The Pleasure Seekers: The Drug Crisis, Youth, and Society.* New York, Grove Press, 1970.
—a fascinating, iconoclastic view of the drug world.

5. GOLDSTEIN, A. "Heroin Addiction and the Role of Methadone in Its Treatment". *Arch. Gen. Psychiat.* 26: 291–97, 1972.
—excellent in its sphere.

6. GRINSPOON, L. *Marijuana Reconsidered.* Boston, Harvard Univ. Press, 1971.
—grass is not necessarily greener . . .

7. LEDAIN, G. (Chairman), *A Report of the Commission of Inquiry into the Non-Medical Use of Drugs: (1) Cannabis, (2) Treatment, (3) Heroin.* Ottawa, Information Canada, 1972.
—excellent, informative, comprehensive.

8. LEVINE, S. V.; LLOYD, D. O.; and LONGDON, W. H. "The Speed User: Social and Psychological Factors in Amphetamine Abuse". *Canad. Psychiat. Assoc. J.* 17: 229–41, 1972.
—for those particularly interested in *one* drug scene.

9. NICHTERN, S. "The Children of Drug Users". *J. Amer. Acad. Child Psychiat.* 12: 24–31, 1973.
—interesting presentation of the many problems surrounding drug users' children and adolescents.

10. PROSKAUER, S., and ROLLAND, R.S. "Youth Who Use Drugs: Psychodynamic Diagnosis and Treatment Planning". *J. Amer. Acad. Child Psychiat.* 12: 32–47, 1973.
—classifies adolescent drug users into three groups (experimental, depressive, and characterological) as a basis for appropriate provision of clinical services.

11. *Resource Book for Drug Abuse Education.* National Clearinghouse for Mental Health Information. U. S. Public Health Publication no. 1964, Chevy Chase, Md., 1969.
—dry but factual.

12. WELL, A. "The Natural Mind: A New Way of Looking at Higher Consciousness". *Psychol. Today.* 6: 52–96, October, 1972.
—fast, fascinating, reaching.

UNIT FOUR: **Psychological Crises for Child and Family**

PAUL D. STEINHAUER
DAVID DICKMAN

15. Psychological Crises in the Child and His Family

This chapter is intended to provide a guide to the understanding and management of psychological crises in children and their families.

The definitive work in the areas of crisis theory and crisis intervention has been that of Gerald Caplan,[5] who has drawn upon the observations and basic principles of sociology, social work, psychology, psychiatry, and preventive medicine in arriving at his conceptual model of a crisis. Caplan suggests that to understand a given crisis, one must approach it simultaneously from two points of view:

1. From the longitudinal perspective, one must understand the ongoing factors that, over a period of years, have moulded the personality of the individual and the structure of the family, predisposing them to breakdown in crisis at a particular point in time.
2. From the short-term point of view, one strives to learn the meaning (to the patient or family) of a particular crisis or of a pattern of repeated crises, each of which is associated with sudden changes in typical patterns of behaviour.

Caplan's conceptual model assumes that in order to avoid becoming mentally disordered, a person needs continual "supplies", that is, adequate sources of incoming gratification. These supplies may be of three basic types:

1. *Physical supplies*, for example, the cuddling of a young child or a physical expression of affection between husband and wife.
2. *Social supplies*, such as a mother indicating her approval of a child's good behaviour or satisfactory school achievement; the admiration

of a child's peer group for his/her athletic prowess, physical appearance, or social acceptability; the respect of one's business or professional colleagues or fellow workers.

3. *Psychological supplies*, for example, the feeling of the young child that he/she has been a good boy or girl; the feeling of the older child or adolescent that he is satisfied with the way he has handled a situation, a relationship, or, better still, life in general.

The nature and amount of gratification each person needs at any given time will vary with a number of factors. These will include:

1. *Age*. The infant is dependent almost entirely on physical supplies to maintain his sense of well-being. As he grows older, social supplies (the approval of his mother and others) and, even later, psychological supplies become increasingly important.
2. *Stage of development*. The mature fourteen-year-old will meet many of his own needs through psychological supplies, while the child who may be chronologically fourteen but is emotionally at the level of a five-year-old will be much more dependent on social supplies (constant gratification from others) to maintain a sense of well-being.
3. *Feelings of deprivation*. These are related to the intensity of the individual's inner demands for gratification. While constitutional differences in basic needs do exist, demands can be inflated if in the past there has been actual deprivation, marked overindulgence, or an inconsistent shift from one to the other. One is dealing not just with the quantity of supplies (e.g. amount of time spent with parents) but also with the quality of the contact (e.g. the freedom of the parent to understand and respond to the needs of the child in time spent together).
4. *Basic character structure*. By the end of latency, the basic character structure is usually fairly well established. This results in a characteristic balance between how much gratification the individual will continue to demand and how much of other's demands for control he is able and prepared to permit.
5. *The number and extent of external pressures with which the individual must cope at a given time*. Failure in school, marital dissatisfaction or divorce, final examinations or business failure, death of relatives, or separation may temporarily greatly increase an individual's need for supplies, if his self-esteem and sense of well-being are not to be adversely affected.
6. *Source of gratification available*. The same thing that for some people

may be a provider of gratification and supplies may, for others, be a draining source of stress and frustration. The areas of work, marriage, and parenting are examples of such situations in adults, while school and relationships with peers and parents can be sources of either gratification or frustration for children.

7. *Variety and effectiveness of defences available.* All of us, from time to time, experience periods of frustration, stress, conflict, and anxiety. The greater the variety and the effectiveness of the defences we have available to us, the less likely that these stresses will deplete our reservoir of supplies to a point that endangers significantly our sense of well-being and our ability to continue to function effectively.

All of these factors will combine to determine the amount of incoming supplies and gratification any individual needs at a given time.

Caplan has defined a crisis as an "upset in the steady state", meaning by this a marked change in the person's habitual pattern of behaviour. But normal development consists of a succession of differentiated phases, each qualitatively different from those that precede and follow it. Between these phases are transitional periods of differentiated behaviour characterized by cognitive and affective upsets. Thus each new developmental advance or demand will, initially, cause additional stress, which may temporarily upset one's balance, leading to a temporary period of disorganization and disequilibrium. Generally, the child, with the help of his family, will soon develop newer and more effective ways of dealing with the stress (i.e. he will learn to successfully defend himself against it) and his equilibrium will then be restabilized at a more advanced level of development. These transitional periods, characterized by stress and disequilibrium, have been termed "developmental crises" by Erikson.[8] Similar periods of psychological and behavioural upset can be precipitated in adults by life hazards involving a sudden loss of basic supplies. Examples would include failure to receive an expected promotion, a couple's suddenly facing the recognition that their marriage is not providing them with the satisfaction they had hoped for, etc.

In Chapter 3, the concept of the family as a system in equilibrium was introduced and developed. When a family's equilibrium is functioning successfully, the individuals involved and the family as a unit will operate in a consistent, characteristic, and effective manner with minimal self-questioning or sense of strain. The equilibrium will be tested if faced by any force or situation that demands an alteration in its previous method of functioning. Thus, if one introduces a stress or problem to the system, the ability of that system to adapt is thereby taxed. An example would occur where, within a marriage originally undertaken in traditional terms, the wife significantly began to redefine her role. This would strain considerably the existing equilibrium and would constitute a demand for adaptation. If the husband could and would meet the demand, a new equilibrium would be established. If not, the couple would be faced either with a continuing disequilibrium or with a breakdown of the system.

The essential factor in determining whether or not a crisis will occur is the balance between the difficulty or importance of the stress or problems with which the child and family are confronted at a given time and the adequacy of the supplies, external resources, and defences immediately available to deal with the problem. In a crisis, the equilibrium is disrupted because the individual or family is faced with stresses that are so great that the usual adjusting (i.e. defence) mechanisms are unable to contain them within the required period of time. Thus a crisis is characterized by a number of rapid developments squeezed into so short a period of time that the existing defences are overwhelmed. As a result, when a new equilibrium is eventually achieved, it may differ significantly from the previous one. For many people, lasting and significant shifts in personality development and over-all functioning seem to have occurred during fairly short periods of crisis.

For all practical purposes, a crisis is any situation that the family or community define or respond to as a crisis. While certain forms of behaviour (e.g. stealing, running away from home, sexual promiscuity, drug use) are more likely than others to precipitate crises, it is the family or communal reaction rather than the behaviour *per se* that will determine whether or not a crisis exists. Thus one family may be plunged into a crisis on learning that their seventeen-year-old, who seems to be doing well in every way, has experimented with marijuana, while another may show no apparent response to a long-standing pattern of clear drug abuse. Thus it is not the precipitating event—nor is it the importance that we as professionals place on that precipitating event—that constitutes the crisis. Rather it is the nature and extent of the response to that event that will determine whether or not a crisis exists.

Classification of Child-Centred Crises

Child-centred crises can be classified into three main groups.

GROUP 1: THE PSYCHOPATHOLOGICAL SYNDROMES

Although in this group the psychopathology of the child is the single most striking feature, one is nevertheless dealing with a psychosocial crisis rather than a disease entity. Almost any child-psychiatric syndrome may contribute to the development of a crisis in a vulnerable family. Other families will tolerate the same illness in a child without significant decompensation of the family's equilibrium. One study of 109 consecutive emergencies suggested that over two-thirds of what were orginally presented as child-centred crises could be described more accurately as social or family crises.[18]

GROUP 2: DEVELOPMENTAL CRISES

Reference has already been made to those transitional periods of stress and disequilibrium termed "developmental crises" by Erikson. These may arise from a sudden but normal increase in environmental demands occurring routinely in the course of development. Examples may include the demand that a child toilet-train, that he separate from mother to attend school, that he learn to read in grade one, etc. Alternately they may originate from a child's difficulty in dealing successfully with a normally occurring increase in his internal (biological) drives, for example, the physiological increase in sexuality and aggressiveness following puberty. For a more detailed discussion of developmental crises, see Chapter 5.

GROUP 3: SITUATIONAL CRISES

In a situational crisis, what is presented as a crisis in the child turns out, on examination, to be a basically healthy child's response to a seriously disturbed family or social situation. Similarly, minimal latent psychopathology in the child may be temporarily activated when the family or social situation deteriorates. Examples of situations which may precipitate crises include: (1) parental illness, physical or emotional; (2) parental loss, through death, divorce, or imprisonment; (3) marital maladjustment; (4) the addition of a step-parent to a family; (5) relocation or financial crises; (6) examinations; (7) hospitalization.

Even in the absence of overt conflict between the parents, marital maladjustment should be suspected in a family seeking help for a crisis centring around a child. The child's symptoms may be the only overt sign of distress within a seriously disturbed family system. Any child-centred crisis, regardless of the nature of the presenting symptoms of the manner of presentation, can reflect or mask chronic disturbance within the family or community, a disturbance that may or may not primarily involve a child. Should such a situational crisis occur simultaneously with a normal developmental crisis, the combined impact may result in a crisis of major proportions leaving long-lasting effects.

Natural History of a Crisis

The typical crisis consists of four overlapping phases:

PHASE 1. Tension increases as the individual or family seek to solve the problem in old ways.

PHASE 2. As the old methods fail to bring a solution or relief, a further increase in tension results.

PHASE 3. This mounting tension leads to the mobilization of emergency problem-solving methods, as child and family seek new ways to define the problem, relate it to previous experience, and resolve it. These may include focusing on heretofore neglected aspects of the problem, setting aside others as irrelevant or unmanageable, trial and error (in thought or in action), or active resignation and giving up. These may or may not lead to resolution of the crisis and re-establishment of the same or a modified level of equilibrium.

PHASE 4. Should the problem not be resolved, tension continues to mount beyond the limit of tolerance. If relief is not available at this critical point, there is very real danger of major and lasting disorganization in child and family.

Thus a crisis can be viewed as a transitional period presenting the individual and family with, on the one hand, an opportunity for growth and redirection and, on the other, a risk of adverse effects resulting in a chronically increased vulnerability to subsequent stress.

How do we assess the meaning of a childhood crisis in order to derive that sort of understanding that will point to an appropriate plan of intervention?

1. APPROACH TO THE CRISIS—APPROPRIATE TIMING

Crises are complex situations laden with tremendous anxiety, relief of which is sought urgently and immediately. The anxiety may be highest in the referring agent such as the school principal, public-health nurse, or in the parents or relatives.[5] The doctor must allow enough time for his initial assessment so that he can see all the participants in the crisis at a time and in a situation in which he does not feel unduly pressured. Much anger and frustration is generated when a hurried professional tries to deal with a crisis while under pressure from other sources or service demands. Unless time is set aside, the anxiety engendered by the crisis will be aggravated by a waiting room full of other patients or by delayed social commitments.

2. HANDLING THE TELEPHONE REFERRAL

Very often, by the time a message about a family crisis reaches the doctor, it has been distorted by anxious intermediaries. Frequent calls or messages should warn of a mounting crisis. One should not give advice over the telephone under pressure. An agreement to return the call with the prospect of fuller discussion allows both some time to think and an opportunity to deal with the matter at a time when one is less harassed.

Just giving the referring person or family a definite time at which they will be seen—even if it is not immediately—often goes a long way toward reducing the anxiety which is usually greater in adults than in the child.

3. MOBILIZING SUPPORT FOR THE CRISIS

The doctor or worker himself often needs support in handling the crisis. If possible, community workers, case aides and interpreters should be mobilized, especially if they have had previous involvement with the family. Then assistance may help decrease the pressure on the professional, thus allowing for a more adequate assessment and deposition.

If the family has to wait for an extended period, provision of a separate room (coffee, etc.) is helpful. Waiting in a busy public emergency section often makes the family feel that they are a burden and generally increases their anxiety.

Identification of Contributing and Precipitating Causes

In nearly every case, the designated patient and his parents (or the foster parents and social worker for wards of a Child Welfare Association or a Children's Aid Society) should be seen as part of the emergency assessment. It is always dangerous to accept as the whole truth any one participant's description of a conflict situation. All of us, husbands or wives, parents or children, tell the truth as we see it. Without realizing it, parents may seek to manipulate their physician or worker into taking sides in a family conflict, unconsciously selecting or slanting their data to gain the professional as an ally against another family member with whom they are in conflict. The physician or worker who sides with a teenager against his parents or with the parents against their child risks losing his potential for helping at a time when his objectivity is badly needed. To avoid this risk, an increasing number of primary physicians and other workers in the mental-health field are learning to assess family conflict situations through interviewing the family as a unit. The techniques of family diagnostic interviewing go beyond the scope of this chapter, but can be mastered by the average primary physician or mental-health professional. Once learned, they should prove invaluable diagnostic and therapeutic adjuncts.[11, 12, 14, 15, 16]

The primary physician or allied professional is frequently consulted about the symptomatic behaviour of the child. The doctor who confines his investigation to the child and who fails to determine whether the child's symptoms are primarily a reflection of pathology and distress involving the entire family is in danger of misinterpreting and responding inappropriately to the situation. A framework is necessary for clarifying the often confused and confusing situation. Inquiry should focus on the following five areas:

1. THE CHILD AND HIS OVER-ALL ADJUSTMENT

First one must determine to what extent psychopathology in the child is a contributing factor. With what pressures, either internal or interpersonal, is the child struggling to cope through his symptomatic behaviour? In addition to exploring the nature of the presenting symptom, one must survey the over-all adjustment of the child. How does he function within his family? Are there either academic or behavioural difficulties at school? Is he able to make and keep friends? Can he deal appropriately with his feelings? Are there other evidences of disturbance that either he or the parents recognize? Does the precipitating behaviour seem an isolated event or just one more manifestation of what seems to be a fixed or habitual pattern of behaviour?

One cannot answer these questions just from the nature of the presenting complaint, a situation not unique to psychiatry. A patient with a persistent cough could be suffering from any one of a number of related or diverse pathological condition, all of which could produce the symptom in question. But just as one cannot intelligently treat a patient's cough without understanding the pathology that is giving rise to it, similarly one cannot manage appropriately a behavioural symptom without understanding the psychopathology of child and family that are contributing to it. Thus the more clearly one can understand the child's symptomatic behaviour, the more accurately one can focus intervention. There may, of course, be overlap. A variety of remedial teaching techniques can help children with learning problems, but the specific techniques indicated for a child with a serious perceptual problem would differ from those one would use with the child in whom severe neurotic problems were interfering with an otherwise intact learning potential.

2. THE FAMILY

How does the crisis reflect—and in what way is it affecting—the day-to-day functioning of the family? What conflicts or tensions within the family are contributing to the symptoms of the child they identify as the patient? How are the family, as individuals and as a unit, being affected by the symptoms and behaviour of the identified patient?

In some cases, the crisis will seem clearly related to such obvious threats as serious physical or emotional illness, marital separation, loss of job or financial security, etc. In others, the precipitating factors, while more obscure, may be no less important. When one asks *why now* and cannot find an answer, consider the possibility that essential information is being withheld, either deliberately or because the family does not consider it related to the behaviour that concerns them. For example, a family may fail to mention a serious marital problem either out of deliberate or unrecognized defensiveness or because they never connected it with their son's beginning to steal. If, however, the stealing was in fact the child's way of handling his distress at their marital conflict, the key to understanding could come from identifying what had changed in the family to disrupt a previously tolerable equilibrium.

3. THE COMMUNITY

Stress resulting from community pressures and expectations may precipitate the breakdown of an already fragile family situation. These pressures may stem from relocation, changes in community tolerance towards certain types of behaviour or confrontation between school system or police with the child or family. Peer-group pressure on children from a middle-class family now living in public housing may be a source of extreme pressure. The effect of crowded apartment living on a rural family lately moved to the city and the loss of social supports (e.g. church or extended family) may be other contributing factors.

4. THE CHILD'S DEVELOPMENT

How is the crisis related to—and how does it affect—the ongoing development of the child? Is this what has been referred to earlier as a developmental crisis, or has there been sufficient internalization of the disturbance to indicate the presence of either a psychoneurosis or a neurotic behaviour disorder requiring ongoing treatment?

It should not be forgotten that parents continue to develop as well and that crises in adult development may change parent-child relationships significantly, precipitating a crisis in the family as a whole.

5. THE PRECIPITATING FACTOR

What is the event that has disrupted the family's customary equilibrium (steady state) and led to the crisis? An analysis of the precipitating event is always important in getting to the heart of the matter.

Intervention

A family is particularly accessible to intervention during the period of disorganization and suggestibility at the height of crisis. Excessive haste or delay is to be avoided. Generally, frequent support is needed. The family may need to have the physician, the primary worker, or one of his associates available at least by telephone until the crisis settles. For some families, the need for support may activate a fear that to accept help is to acknowledge intolerable weakness. In such cases too much help—or help given in a way that intensifies the parents' fears of dependency and feelings of inadequacy—may be as harmful as too little.

Intervention involves a continual reassessment, analysis, and treatment of the factors contributing to the crisis. The main causes—and the precipitating factor may either be one of these or merely the straw that broke the camel's back—must be identified, sorted, and, if possible, resolved. Not all of the causative factors will prove equally accessible to treatment. One is concerned not just with areas of weakness but with the family's strengths, with which factors most need to be modified, which are most accessible to intervention, and how this can be undertaken to best ensure family co-operation while minimizing the threat of further decompensation. Adequate short- and long-term follow-up should be a regular part of the protocol to provide a realistic assessment of its effectiveness. What follows is a description of some of the methods used.

Methods of Management

1. REVIEW AND RETURN

When, following an adequate assessment, one reaches a diagnosis of a developmental problem in a basically normal child, then a wait-and-see attitude is justified. Many such children, in time find more successful ways of dealing with the temporarily increased tension level. One should, however, avoid giving unqualified reassurance because not all such children succeed in developing healthier ways of adapting to the stress. Some, instead, rely increasingly on their neurotic or behavioural defences to the point where what was once a transient response to unaccustomed stress, becomes a fixed and habitual mode of response shaping the child's character and dominating his dealing with life. When pathological responses have become automatic and internalized, the terms *psychoneurosis,* or *neurotic behaviour disorder,* which imply significant entrenched psychopathology, are in order. Should this occur, definitive psychotherapeutic intervention is indicated. The aim of psychotherapy in such cases is the resolution of the child's internal conflict, thus freeing him to live more fully, more productively and more comfortably.

2. REASSURANCE

There are undoubtedly situations in which having understood the child's behaviour in the family and developmental context one can safely say, "He'll grow out of it." Helping overconcerned parents regain their perspective in such situations may be invaluable. But at other times an anxious parent attempts to mask his anxiety by a seemingly casual request for reassurance in a situation that, if all the facts were known, would obviously demand further investigation. Premature, inappropriate, or unqualified reassurance may be damaging instead of helpful in such cases, as it may postpone dealing with a problem that is still reactive (i.e. before the process of internalization has been completed). While it is true that most boys, at some point, experiment with stealing, one must avoid categorically reassuring a mother that her son's stealing is normal until the pattern and its determinants are sufficiently understood to rule out the possibility that this child's stealing is a symptom of signifcant underlying disturbance. Also to respond to a fourteen-year-old's anxiety about a homosexual experience by lightly reassuring him that such things are normal for teenagers may do more to relieve the physician's or worker's embarrassment than to address the boy's need, which, if the extent and duration of the homosexual behaviour and the degree of the associated concern were understood, might be recognized as a serious problem with which he was struggling.

3. SYMPTOMATIC TREATMENT

When, based on an adequate understanding of the total situation, one is confident that there are no major underlying problems in either child or family, symptomatic treatment (e.g. imipramine for enuresis or a change of living arrangements for a teenager in conflict with his parents) may be indicated. Here again the situation is analogous to that in other areas of medicine. One would not, for example, suppress a cough symptomatically before ruling out the presence of serious pathology requiring direct treatment. Indeed, suppression of a cough could prove harmful if it led to the neglect of an underlying imflammatory, obstructive, or neoplastic condition. Similarly the family's preoccupation with the presenting symptom may serve as a decoy, distracting them from a recognition of the true nature and extent of the underlying sources of conflict and tension. To offer only symptomatic treatment in such a situation would be to risk ignoring and possibly aggravating significant and often treatable sources of distress.

4. BRIEF THERAPY

The general physician is often the first one to whom the family will turn for advice and help. If he has treated the family for some time their confidence and trust in him will give him an unequalled opportunity for helping at the point of crisis.

The aim of intervention, wherever possible, should extend beyond just relieving the presenting symptoms to using the crisis as an opportunity to improve the coping or functioning capacities of the child or family. Viewed in this way, the family crisis provides a useful occasion for relatively brief intervention. It allows them to examine patterns of maladaptive behaviour and to increase their ability to deal successfully with stress. This can be achieved by encouraging the ventilation of pent-up negative feelings with the physician serving as a safety-valve and a source of encouragement. The physician or other counsellor can serve as a catalyst to improve communication that may have broken down, thus helping members understand one another's position and providing a basis for problem-solving and badly needed negotiations. He can also help in clarifying and identifying important areas of conflict and distress by eliciting proposed directions of action and by supporting the more appropriate alternatives. Not that the physician can solve all the family's mental-health problems, even though the family, drawing on the medical model, may expect him to do so. But a crisis allows an opening for the alert and concerned physician to help child and family not just weather the current crisis but learn from it to avoid—or, at least, to deal more successfully with—similar situations in the future.

Successful brief therapy demands that the counsellor intervene at a superficial level using actions derived from a deeper understanding of the factors causing and maintaining the crisis. Therapist and family agree upon a series of short-term goals towards which they contract to work for a predetermined number of sessions. It is important that the agenda be closely adhered to, and that any temptation to allow the therapeutic goals to be diffused be resisted. If desired, therapist and family can always recontract to work together for an additional period towards a new set of goals.

5. ROLE OF MEDICATION

Occasionally a child's behaviour may be so out of control and his anxiety level so high that tranquillizers or sedatives may be indicated temporarily. Recognize, however, that a heavily sedated person—child or adult—is not likely to avail himself of the opportunities for adaptive change available at the time of crisis intervention. Details of drug use will be found in Chapter 23, "The Role of Drugs in the Treatment of Disturbed Children".

6. REFERRAL

This family brings us to a discussion of referral for psychiatric or specific mental-health consultation. Situations in which a referral for psychiatric consultation is indicated include:

a) When the primary physician, workers, or counsellors, having done all they can to clarify the situation, still remain unclear as to the nature of the problem and the type of management needed.

b) When, despite treatment, the situation fails to show sufficient improvement.

c) When the extent of the crisis (e.g. serious suicidal threats, massive and continuing behavioural problems) goes beyond the family's ability to cope or demands more time and involvement than the primary physician or counsellor feels he can spare.

d) If a sense of personal discomfort begins to intrude, the physician or counsellor is well-advised to use consultation to obtain an objective assessment of the ongoing involvement or to consider asking a psychiatrist to undertake treatment.

e) When in doubt, it is wiser to obtain a consultation than to wait until a crisis deteriorates beyond the point of redemption.

There is no point trying to force psychiatric consultation on a family: one can only recommend it. The referral will prove pointless if the family accepts it merely out of obedience to the doctor's or counsellor's suggestion rather than because it makes sense to them. Parents frequently balk initially at the idea of seeing a psychiatrist. The suggestion may mobilize considerable anxiety and guilt, aggravating pre-existing feelings of inadequacy. Following a direct and clear discussion of the issues, the decision whether or not to accept the referral should be left with the parents, which may mean seeing people temporarily go without the help they need. This situation, however, is preferable to forcing the issue. It is to be hoped that over a period of time there will be other opportunities to help the family see their need in perspective.

The management of the process of referral is frequently crucial to the success of the consultation and may do a great deal to determine the psychiatrist's potential for being of help to the family and the referring professional. Children should be told directly to whom they are being referred and for what reasons. The more clearly a child understands the purpose of a psychiatric referral, the more likely he and the family will benefit from it. If the parents are helped to deal with their anxieties around the referrral, they can usually find ways of preparing the child so that he knows why they are seeking additional help.

It is helpful in the course of practice to develop a working relationship with a few psychiatrists or psychiatric facilities to whom one refers. In making a referral, it is important to state clearly whether this is a case on which a consultation is sought (i.e. the physician is prepared to continue actively treating the family) or one in which the psychiatrist is being asked to take over the treatment of the case. In seeking consultation, it is essential that the consultant have a clear picture of the areas that are not understood and the problems in management around which his views are requested.

RECOMMENDED FOR FURTHER READING

1. ALEXANDER, J. F., and PARSONS, B. V. "Short-Term Behavioural Intervention with Delinquent Families: Impact on Family Process and Recidivism", in Francks, C. M., and Wilson, G. T., eds., *Annual Review of Behavior Therapy: Theory and Practice*. Vol. 2: 472–85, New York, Brunner/Mazel, 1974.
—provides a model for short-term behavioural intervention towards clearly defined goals.

2. BARTEN, H. H., and BARTEN, S. S. *Children and Their Parents in Brief Therapy*. New York, Behavioral Publications, 1973.
—illustrates the technique of "thinking deeply but acting superficially" that plays a major role in much crisis intervention.

3. BOYCE, M. "Crisis of later Adolescence and Early Adult Life". *Canad. Psychiat. Assoc. J.* 17: 117–22, 1972.
—discusses and classifies the crisis typical of late adolescence and early adult life.

4. BRANDON, S. "Crisis Theory and Possibilities of Therapeutic Intervention". *Brit. J. Psychiat.* 117: 627–33, 1970.
—a good theoretical presentation of the issues involved in the development and management of crisis.

5. CAPLAN, G. *Principles of Preventive Psychiatry*. New York, Basic Books, 1964.
—presents Caplan's basic conceptual model and a guide to management.

6. DARBONNE, A. "Crisis: A Review of Theory, Practice, and Research". *Internat. J. Psychiat.* 6: 371–79, 1968.
—highly condensed but tightly organized. Extensive bibliography up to date of publication.

7. EISLER, R. M. and HERSEN, M. "Behavioural Techniques in Family-Orientated Crisis Intervention". *Arch. Gen. Psychiat.* 28: 111–16, 1973.
—the application of behaviour therapy to crisis intervention.

8. ERIKSON, E. H. *"Identity and the Life Cycle: Selected Papers". Psychological Issues.* Vol. 1, No. 1. Monograph No. 1, 1959.
—the original description of developmental crisis.

9. HEARD, D. H. "Crisis Intervention Guided by Attachment Concepts: A Case Study". *J. Child Psychol. Psychiat.* 15: 111–22, 1974.
—following summaries of Caplan's concepts of crisis intervention and Parkes's concept of psychosocial transition presents a case study of a suicide attempt in a young adolescent boy and applies the principles discussed to treatment. Technical but useful.

10. HILL, R. "Generic Features of Families Under Stress", in Parad, H. J., ed., *Crisis Intervention: Selected Readings,* 32–52, New York, Family Service Association of America, 1965.
—good description of the production of crisis.

11. KEITH, D. V. "Use of Self: A Brief Report". *Fam. Proc.* 13: 201–6, 1974.
—brief description of the effects of crisis in a family and of a way for the family therapist to help family members express their feelings and free themselves from rigid attitudes.

12. LANGSLEY, D. G., and KAPLAN, D. M. *The Treatment of Families in Crisis.* New York, Grune and Stratton, 1968.
—a guide to understanding and management of the family in crisis.

13. MAZER, M. "Characteristics of Multi-Problem Households: A Study in Psychosocial Epidemiology". *Amer. J. Orthopsychiat.* 42: 792–802, 1972.
—describes a study of sixty-three families with multiple psychiatric and psychosocial predicaments. Such families are commonly in, or on the verge of, crisis.

14. Mc PHERSON, S. R.; BRACKELMANNS, W. E.; and NEWMAN, L.E. "Stages in the Family Therapy of Adolescents". *Fam. Process.* 13: 77–94, 1974.
—outlines the role of the crisis as therapeutic opportunity in the course of family therapy. Presents eight crisis points (stages) which can provide special opportunities for growth and change and their relation to therapeutic intervention.

15. MORRISON, G. C. "Therapeutic Intervention in a Child Psychiatry Emergency Service". *J. Amer. Acad. Child Psychiat.* 8: 542–58, 1969.
—good description of child-orientated crisis intervention service. Stresses the importance of prompt but flexible intervention. Bibliography up to date of publication is excellent.

16. PARAD, H. J., ed. *Crisis Intervention: Selected Readings*. New York, Family Service Association of America. 1965.
—a framework for understanding and approaching families in crisis.

17. ROSENTHAL, A. J. and LEVINE, S. V. "Brief Psychotherapy with Children: Process of Therapy". *Amer. J. Psychiat.* 128: 141–46, 1971–72.
—examines techniques and content of brief psychotherapy with children, suggesting that brief psychotherapy is highly effective in dealing with a situational crisis.

18. STEINHAUER, P. D.; LEVINE, S. V.; and Da COSTA, G. A. "Where Have All the Children Gone?: Child Psychiatric Emergencies in a Metropolitan Area". *Canad. Psychiat. Assoc. J.* 16: 121–27, 1971.
—a study of 109 consecutive psychiatric emergencies involving children and young adolescents in a large metropolitan area.

19. TUCKER, G. J. "Psychiatric Emergencies: Evaluation and Management," in Freedman, D. X., and Dyrud, J. E., eds., *American Handbook of Psychiatry*. Vol. 5: *Treatment*. New York, Basic Books, 567–92, 1975.
—the classification, evaluation and management of psychiatric emergencies.

PAUL D. STEINHAUER
DAVID N. MUSHIN
QUENTIN RAE-GRANT

16. Psychological Aspects of Chronic Illness*

When parents bring a sick child to a physician, they come with a number of questions and one overriding request.

The questions, in their language, are simple. What is the matter with my child? What has caused it? What can the physician do to help? What can the parents do? How long will it last? Will he be completely cured? But the hope is that, by medicine or by magic, the child will be rapidly, uneventfully, and successfully returned to complete health. This is frequently asking, however, more than the physician can deliver.

With improvements in the treatment of the infectious diseases and our ever-increasing ability to sustain life even when we cannot restore health, the practising paediatrician is increasingly relied upon to aid in the management of the child who is severely and chronically ill. Here, contrary to parental expectations, he cannot cure. But there are a number of things, all of them important, that he can do. He may be able to control the rate of progression or the frequency and severity of complications of the disease. He may do a great deal to help the child compensate for some of the more destructive effects of his illness. Finally, and equally important, he may be able to help child and family face the limitations, anxieties, and discouragements which accompany the disease, to develop a plan of management which can serve as an

*First published in SYMPOSIUM ON CHRONIC DISEASES IN CHILDREN, a special issue of *Paediatric Clinics of North America,* vol. 21, no. 4, Philadelphia, W. B. Saunders, 1974.

Table 16-1 Emotional Responses to Acute and Chronic Illness

	Acute Illness	*Chronic Illness*
Onset	Sudden	Sudden or insidious
Duration of Illness	Brief	Prolonged
Treatment	Often effective	Palliative or none
Outlook	Frequently excellent	Generally poor
Crisis identity	High	High
Crisis duration	Brief	Prolonged
Family reactions	Anxiety ↓ Relief	Denial and disbelief, anxiety, depression, guilt and responsibility, resentment
Physician's reactions	Relief	?

antidote to feelings of utter helplessness, and to rise above the feelings of resentment and despair which could otherwise crush and overwhelm them.[9, 22]

Any illness of a child represents a crisis for the family. The degree to which this crisis can be sustained or resolved depends on the answers to the above questions and on the pre-existing strengths of the family unit. Even an acute and rapidly responsive illness may lead to further decompensation in an already precarious family situation. It requires on the other hand great strength, stability, and support to sustain a severe chronic illness in one family member.

This chapter deals with the emotional responses to chronic illness (Table 16-1), the responses of patients, their parents, and their siblings to the hardships imposed by the disease. It also deals with our role as physicians, and the contribution we can make towards helping the family minimize the destructive effects of these responses.[22]

Since the child is a developing individual with different needs and capacities depending on his stage of development, the nature and extent of disruption occurring during illness will vary according to the stage at which it occurs. Either the illness itself or restrictions imposed during its management may affect the child's function and disrupt normal living. By and large, the common acute illnesses of childhood leave few major or lasting emotional sequelae. Although their behaviour while in the hospital may present problems, few children show long-term effects following short-term hospitalization unless they previously showed evidence of maladjustment.[31]

Chronic illness, however, is associated with defects and ongoing problems. The prolonged disruption in life experience may have lasting effects on the cognitive and emotional development of the child. To manage chronically ill children and their families, one must understand the child's premorbid personality and needs, his stage of development and its vulnerabilities, his perception of the illness and its management, the nature of the illness itself and its potential effects on child and family, the nature of management procedures, and the potential for support of the child from family and medical staff.

Premorbid Personality and Needs

A child's development and adjustment prior to becoming ill will influence his responses during the illness. The child who has difficulty separating from parents may have problems coping with hospitalization. The previously phobic child is likely to develop inordinate fears of minor procedures, while the hyperactive child will have difficulty tolerating forced immobilization. The child who already fears and resents authority figures can be expected to rebel against doctors and nurses, whereas a previously shy and withdrawn child whose illness involves some deformity is prone to extreme self-consciousness which may seriously interfere with his relationships. A child from a previously depriving environment may, through the demand for enforced isolation, fall even further behind in his intellectual development.

Circumstances at the onset of illness may influence the child's adjustment to his disease. Thus a young child who was severely burned during a phase of jealousy following the birth of a new sibling might ascribe infrequent parental visits to the parents being more interested in the new sibling than in him. He might interpret the burn as a punishment for hostile and rivalrous feelings towards the sibling. An independent and secure child would probably cope better with a chronic illness than one who is immature, insecure, and inhibited. There is some evidence, at least in acute illness, that certain children's emotional adjustment may be improved with successful handling of their illness.

Nature of the Illness and Management and Potential Effects on the Child

The child's adjustment will be affected by a number of factors which, separately or in combination, may be present during the course of an illness. Consider the following:

Separation from Parents

This is particularly upsetting for children between six months and four years of age, but may also cause problems for older children who have had prior separations. Three stages are described in the child's adverse reactions to separation. First is the *stage of protest* where the child demands the parents, and tearfully and angrily resists attempts to care for him. When the child has lost hope of forcing the return of the parents, he withdraws and loses interest in his environment and even in food. Following this *stage of despair*, the child may become more alert, regain appetite, and relate to people, but avoid attachment to any one person and ignore the parents if they visit. This is called the *stage of detachment* or *denial*. While the first two stages are reversible on being reunited with parents under appropriate circumstances persistent defects in the ability to form relationships and in intellectual functioning may result if the third stage is reached. The child who is institutionalized for long periods is particularly vulnerable to these complications of separation. Repeated actual or threatened separations may produce frequent and irrational anger and anxiety in the child, which will cause difficulty in his management.

Separation problems can be alleviated by regular, predictable visiting by the parents, and by ensuring that the child is looked after by a small number of staff whom he gets to know. Infrequent and sporadic visiting by parents and care from many adults with only superficial contact increase the traumatic effects of separation.

Restriction, Sensory Impairment, and Isolation

Some illnesses may require that the child experience periods when mobility is restricted, or that he be isolated from familiar people and objects. In addition, certain illnesses can impose sensory restrictions upon the child: blindness, deafness, and the decreased tactile stimulation that accompanies the treatment of the burned child. Cognitive development, particularly in young children, depends partly on physical exploration of the environment. All children require stimulation from the environment and an ability to take in such stimulation. From the emotional point of view, restrictions on play may remove the safety valve a child needs to drain off anxiety and unpleasant feelings, while sensory impairment may interfere with explaining proceedings to the child, as well as interfere with his relationships with parents and medical personnel. When such avenues are blocked, the child may withdraw into excessive fantasy as a means of coping, this tendency being enhanced by isolation. This may lead to an escalation of fears and unrealistic expectations regarding the illness and management.

Dependency and Lack of Consistency

In dealing with sick children, adults tend to gratify dependency needs in an attempt to help the child feel more secure and to comfort him. While to some extent this additional support is needed, prolonged and excessive gratification of these needs may prove so satisfying that the child may resist giving it up. This may interfere with the normal striving towards mature independence, thus blocking the development of self-confidence and initiative. Such problems are more marked in children who for any reason (including congenital illness where parental guilt fosters overprotection) have prior dependency problems. Rehabilitation and the achievement of maximal functioning in spite of residual physical problems may be impeded. The aim in management is to maintain a balance between allowing dependence during the acute phase and gradual encouragement towards independence whenever possible.

Pain and Deformity

A child's response to pain will vary with the way he perceives the pain as well as with the amount of pain accounted for on a physiologic basis.[8] Pain interpreted as punishment or maltreatment (e.g. reaction to injections) may be accompanied by anxiety, which will intensify the pain. Other children may perceive pain as pleasurable, leading to passive devotion to the medical staff who inflict it. The young child who imagines adults are all-powerful and capable of removing all pain may interpret their failure to do so as an expression of anger towards him. This may be reinforced if the adult becomes angry at the child's persistent complaints or apprehensions regarding procedures.

The threat of surgery and deformity is greatest in the late preschool and early adolescent years. Toddlers see surgery as a punishment with potentially dire consequences, for in this age group the least scratch is blown up to the proportions of a major wound. In the adoles cent, deformity and fears of mutilation are the result of an increased concern with body image, a need to be the same as peers, and fears of being a defective and hence inadequate person.

Threat of Death

A full discussion of this topic is beyond the scope of this article and is discussed by writers such as Kubler-Ross.[13] It is not until age nine or ten that the child fully understands death as being both universal and permanent. Prior to that, he views death as similar to sleep or as a separation. Parents' feelings about imminent or threatened death may interfere with their ability to relate to the child. This will increase the child's anxiety. The child may interpret his parents' depression as anger, leading to a feeling that he is letting the parents down. Similar problems may occur between the child and medical staff, for example, when the surgeon avoids his dying patient after an unsuccessful operation.[13]

Medication

Certain forms of medication may affect the child's alertness (e.g. barbiturates) and behaviour (e.g. corticosteroids). Such effects should be considered in prescribing these drugs. Drugs having physical side effects (e.g. cytotoxic drugs) may cause anxiety through disturbance of body image. Prolonged and regular use of drugs (e.g. insulin) or diets may be accepted at younger ages but rebelled against in early adolescence where it is seen as an imposition by authority figures. Acceptance of such regimens may be seen as a sign of weakness, a constant reminder of the illness, and a symbol of dependence and inadequacy which the child would often rather forget.

Absence from School

Multiple absences not only may contribute to the child's falling behind in school work, but also may seriously interfere with his peer relationships. These may be of crucial importance to the older child and adolescent. Relaxed visiting privileges and provision for continuing his schooling while in hospital or at home may do much to minimize the seriousness of these potential complications.

Problems Specific to Certain Illnesses

Certain illnesses may directly influence behaviour and cognitive development. Various causes of mental retardation affect intellectual development. Certain forms of brain damage may be associated with hyperactivity, poor impulse control, and poor attention span. These may affect perception, and thus learning, in a child with normal intelligence. Children with temporal lobe epilepsy may exhibit a wide range of psychological problems ranging from behaviour disorder through episodes of depersonalization to hallucinations, and it is feasible that some psychoses in children, for example, types of autism, have at least in part a physiologic basis. In such conditions, the specific effects of the illness interact with the general problems described above.

The Effect of the Illness on Development

Illness may impair the child's ability to overcome the problems which occur during normal development. Thus the toddler who is learning to walk and to develop bowel control will have this movement towards normal independence disrupted by forced confinement to bed and chronic diarrhoea. Such a child, in seeking mother's help during the illness, may substitute the gratification this brings for the advantages of autonomy. At a later age, the danger is that the child will remain overly dependent rather than learning to rely on his own resources. Unresolved problems at an earlier stage of development (e.g. separation problems) can affect development at later stages (e.g. development of an independent identity as an adolescent).

Family Reactions

Faced with the diagnosis of a severe and chronic illness, the entire family is confronted with a series of stresses and demands that will tax relationships both within and beyond the family unit. The degree and nature of the stress will vary, as will a particular family's ability to meet it. The following factors will influence the family's response to the illness.

The severity of the illness, the likely prognosis, and the availability of an effective treatment. The more debilitating the illness and the poorer the prognosis, particularly in a previously healthy child, the greater the stress on the family. This is especially true if the clinical course is one of relentless progression. In such cases, the parents face the constant threat of losing their child. The resulting strain is intensified if sudden death is a possibility (e.g. some forms of congential heart disease, Riley-Day syndrome, some severe asthmatics).

Whether the disease is congenital or acquired. Illnesses in which congenital factors have been implicated (e.g. fibrocystic disease, the muscular dystrophies, congenital heart disease, some forms of mental retardation) are likely to intensify parental feelings of guilt and responsibility.

The age of onset of the illness, and of diagnosis. If the diagnosis is made at birth, the family will never have experienced the child as normal. Their concept of him will always have included expectations altered because of his illness. If, however, the illness appears or is diagnosed after the child's personality has developed and his place in the family is established, family members will have had time to think of him as a normal child, so that an even greater sense of loss and depression will be experienced when they are forced to scale down their hopes and expectations in view of the illness. Illness striking first in adolescence is resented by both child and family as a particularly painful cheating of someone about to experience all the supposed freedoms and opportunities that go with adult status.

One must also consider the effects of parental expectations on the ongoing process of development. The more the child is able to be seen and treated like a normal child, the less his development will be interfered with. However, the earlier the diagnosis is made—and the more the parents see the child as fragile, handicapped, or limited—the more likely the parents are to grossly overprotect and overindulge the child, thus distorting the parent-child relationship and the normal process of development.

Presence of pre-existing emotional disturbance within the family. The greatest psychological or social problems are likely to develop when serious chronic illness occurs within an already disturbed family situation. While the entire family will inevitably affect—and be affected by—severe chronic illness in any family member, there are two situations in which this poses a particular threat to the family's emotional equilibrium. One occurs when chronic disease develops in a child whose relationships are already disturbed. The other is seen when the parents' marriage is already strained almost to the limit of tolerance.

The nature and effects of the illness itself. Pain or malaise resulting from the child's illness or a resented treatment program may cause the child to be cranky, irritable, unpleasant, or demanding. These same traits will present additional pressures and evoke feelings of resentment, guilt, and inadequacy in the parents, especially the mother. If the illness is clearly apparent and frequently elicits reactions of disgust or aversion from others (e.g. congenital amputations or deformities, severe scarring from burns, conspicuous mental retardation), the continued confrontation with the discomfort of others will prove a serious blow to the normal parental desire to have an attractive, healthy child who will reflect well on them. This may also be so if failure to thrive secondary to the disease rather than a more obvious deformity deprives the parents of the beautiful, healthy child they long for.[17]

Effects of program of home management and restrictions on family life. Some illnesses involve a demanding program of home management and restrictions, for example, fibrocystic disease, with its daily regimen of inhalations, positive pressure, postural drainage, and frequent medications, and juvenile diabetes with its dietary restrictions, regular testing, and daily insulin injections. These demands, despite their absolute medical necessity, may be resented and vigorously resisted by the child they are intended to help. Even with appropriate explanations of the purpose and importance of the regimen, the child may not be able to accept the need for unpleasant restrictions or treatments. Indeed, excessive compliance on the part of the child is more likely to indicate pathologic passivity and depression than mental health. Even normal resistance, however, will result in additional work and emotional strain for the parents who are struggling to administer the prescribed regimen. If they respond with excessive impatience, resentment, and guilt—or, alternatively, if they back off and provide only inconsistent care—both physical health and emotional relationships are bound to suffer.

A moderate amount of self-assertion and opposition to parental authority is an essential feature of the normal child's progression towards independence. In the child who is chronically ill, the oppositional behaviour may become concentrated around opposing the unwanted treatment regimen, which will then become a daily battleground, resulting in developmental distortions and resentment and guilt in both parents and child that may spread to contaminate not only their relationship but the emotional tone within the family as a whole.

Presence or absence of other affected siblings. The parental reaction may be very much affected by whether or not this is the first child to have been affected by the illness. The presence of other healthy children—especially in situations in which a congenital factor has been demonstrated—may serve to mitigate the parents' feelings of inadequacy and distress. Alternatively, parents who have more than one afflicted child—or who have lost a child to the disease—can be expected to have even more than usual difficulty adjusting to the illness of a subsequent afflicted child.

Repeated hospitalizations and surgical procedures. Should the disease be one requiring frequent hospitalizations, painful treatments or repeated surgery (renal failure, severe burns) additional pressures will be brought to bear on the parents. Children, especially toddlers, often find coming into the hospital upsetting. They may not understand why they have to leave the family or the reason for frightening or painful procedures. As a result, they may feel punished or abandoned by their parents, whose uncertainty and guilt will be intensified if the child is miserable and resentful. At times (e.g. the severely burned child) parents may see their child suffering but be totally unable to comfort him. Even worse (e.g. the parents of a child with congenital heart disease) they may be forced to make decisions which can literally determine whether their child lives or dies, without any assurance that they are deciding correctly.

Cost of the illness. In estimating the cost of the illness, there is no avoiding, even in state-underwritten systems, the hidden dollars-and-cents cost (e.g. doctor and hospital bills, medications, special diets, needed equipment and appliances, etc.). For families with limited incomes, these expenses may prove additional sources of pressure and anxiety. They may necessitate the mother going out to work or the father having to take on a second job to make ends meet. Drained and exhausted, the parents then come home to the demands of administering or supervising a vigorous and unpopular program of management or restrictions. The cycle is vicious. Emotional needs of both parents and children frequently go unmet. The rate of family breakdown in families with severe chronic illness is high.[8, 22, 28]

Specific Emotional Reactions

These include the following (Fig. 16-1).

Denial. All parents to some extent react with denial in response to the shock of their child's illness. While denial may help the parents through the initial trauma and subsequent disorganization, normally—but by no means always—their use of denial should gradually decrease as the family's ability to come to grips with the reality of the illness increases. Denial is probably never completely abandoned, certainly not at any single point in time. Persistent massive denial in the face of obvious illness will interfere with the family's learning to live with their reactions to their child's illness and with their successfully meeting the day-to-day needs of the child, thus perpetuating the crisis precipitated by the illness. It is this denial, closely related to their need for hope, that may lead parents to misinterpret what their physician is saying, or to go from doctor to doctor in an attempt to find one who will give them the diagnosis—and prognosis—they want to hear.

Figure 16-1 Family Reactions to Severe Chronic Illness

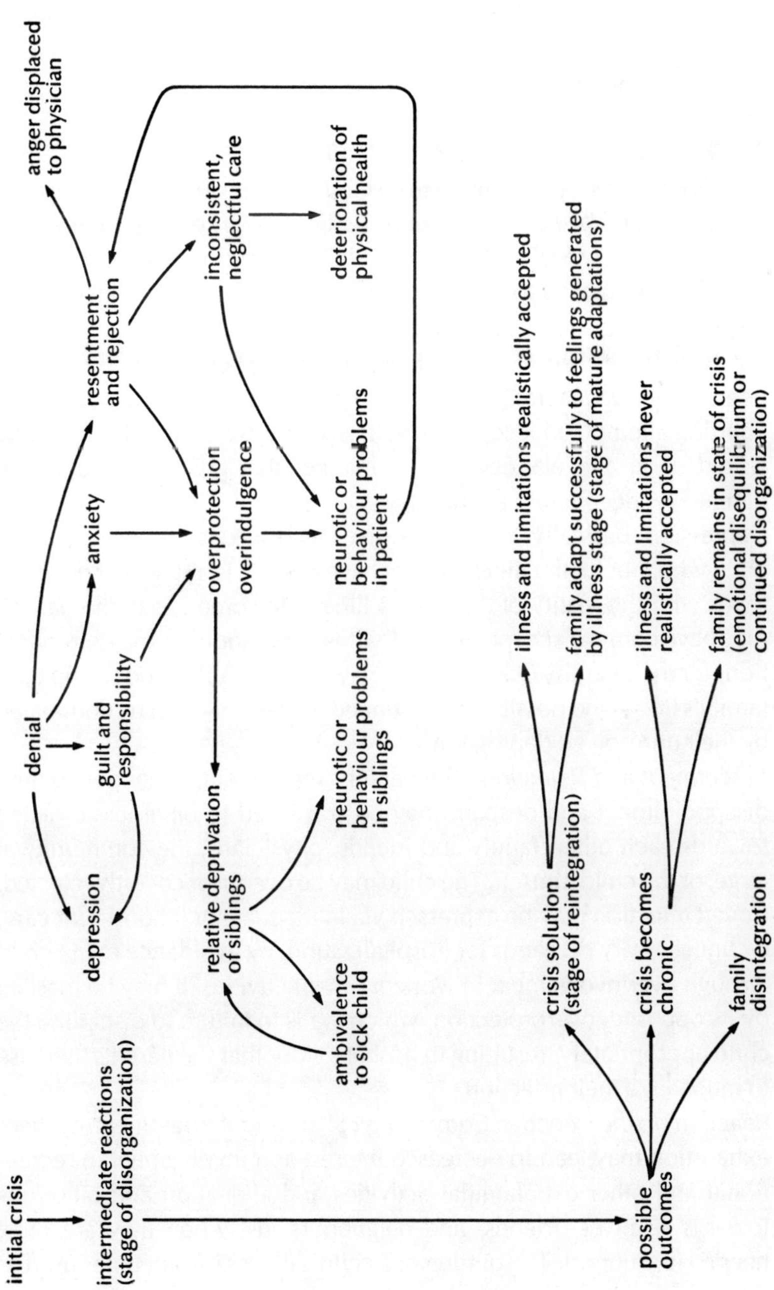

Anxiety. To a greater or lesser degree, the parents are chronically anxious about the health—or the very survival—of their child. If the parental anxiety is excessive, either because of a realistic possibility of sudden death or because of a neurotic overreaction, it may lead to overprotection, overindulgence, and difficulties in disciplining the child.

Feelings of Guilt, Responsibility, and Self-Blame. Some parents see their child's illness as a punishment from God for their sins, while others will feel victimized by Fate. Still others, particularly if the disease is a congenital one, may feel that the child's illness is proof of their inadequacy (i.e. their inability to bear a normal child). Although these feelings of responsibility are totally irrational, attempts to use logic to argue parents out of them are likely to fail. Each of us has his or her own secret sins and personal inadequacies, and these (e.g. an unwanted pregnancy, an abortion attempt, unacceptable feelings towards the sick child) may be seized upon and elaborated in a manner that grinds the depressed parent ever deeper into the rut of despondency.

Depression. Basically, the depression experienced is a mourning for the child who, but for the illness, might have been. It is a stage in coming to terms with the reality of the child's illness. In some cases, the parents may have come to accept the child's illness or handicap and its implications for their family. Other parents may never be able to do so and their family's life—and possibly its continued existence—will be dominated by their unresolved depression.

Resentment and Rejection. The parents' resentment, a reaction to their disappointment and despair, may be converted to bitterness directed towards each other, family and friends, physicians, the community at large, or the child himself. The child may be overtly or covertly rejected. Covert rejection may be expressed via inadequate or inconsistent care, by unnecessary demands for hospitalization, by avoidance of the child through overinvolvement in work or other activities. It may be masked by its opposite, overprotection, which leads to failure to discipline the child appropriately, resulting in misbehaviour that the parents then use to rationalize their rejection.

Reactions to the Extended Community. Shame, embarrassment, or sheer exhaustion may lead to decreased interest and involvement in recreational and other extrafamilial activities and alienation and bitterness towards relatives, friends, and neighbours just when they are most needed for support. The burden of a child's illness is sometimes used as the reason for failure to advance vocationally or professionally.

Sibling Reactions. The sibling of the sick child has no easy task to handle. He will frequently react with jealousy and resentment towards the child who draws off so much of the attention and energies of the family. The parental preoccupation with the sick child and their own reactions to his illness may result in the other children experiencing a moderate to severe degree of emotional deprivation. But in some families it is not "right" to feel jealous of a sick or dying child. If the parents cannot allow the other children to express openly their resentment towards the sick child or their feelings of being shortchanged, the guilt they feel secondary to their resentment will be intensified. This will frequently result in their hostility going underground, to be expressed covertly by pathological withdrawal, underachievement in school, behaviour problems or delinquency, or neurotic reactions. The case of Nina, discussed on p. 143, is an example of the effect on one child of severe chronic illness in a sibling.

Cain et al.[4] have studied children's disturbed reactions to the death of a sibling which they found related to factors such as the nature of the death; the child's pre-existing relationship with the dead sibling; the immediate and the long-term impact of the death upon the parents; the child's cognitive ability to understand death; the parents' handling of the immediate impact of the death on the surviving child; the impact of the death upon the total family structure. Pathologic reactions, when they occurred, took the form of excessive and prolonged guilt reactions; depressions; blaming the parents for the death of the sibling; distorted concepts of illness and death; disturbed attitudes towards doctors, hospitals, and religion; death phobias; and identification with the dead child. The need to recognize the impact of a child's death on the surviving siblings if these disturbed reactions are to be avoided cannot be overstressed.

Physicians' Reactions to Chronic Illness

Physicians and other attending staff may react emotionally to chronic fatal illness in a child. The physician who is unable to tolerate being unable to provide a cure may feel increasingly helpless, hopeless, and guilty. This may lead him to withdraw from patient and family, leaving them to face the stress of the disease without his support. He may overidentify with the parents, or in his anxiety may say too much too soon, that is, before the parents have overcome their initial shock and denial to the point where they can hear what he is saying. Physicians may resent parents, sometimes in response to parental hostility but at other times in reaction to parental dependence which merely underlines the physician's feeling of helplessness. Garrard and Richmond[9] have stressed the importance of the physician maintaining an awareness of his own separateness from the family, while recognizing just how difficult this may prove to be. They stress that what families need is empathy, not sympathy; detachment rather than avoidance. Pakes[22] has drawn attention to the extent to which physicians' reactions to their chronically ill patients often parallel those of their parents.

Management

1. Successful management of the emotional aspects of chronic illness is based on a recognition that illness in one child will have major implications on mental health, relationships, and possibly even the continued existence of the family.

2. The more successfully family members (especially parents) are able to resolve the feelings of anxiety, depression, responsibility, and resentment aroused by the illness, the more able they will be (a) to meet the physical and emotional needs of the child and (b) to resolve the crisis created by the diagnosis and the additional strains imposed by their child's illness with minimal damage and disruption to the family as a whole.

On the other hand, failure to resolve the emotional sequelae of the illness will substantially diminish the family's ability to satisfy the emotional needs of all its members and will increase the likelihood of family breakdown.

3. Only when parents have been given a clear and definitive diagnosis can they begin to deal with reality first at the level of practical planning. Only then can they begin the arduous but no less important task of emotional acceptance.

4. The diagnosis of a severe chronic illness will precipitate a state of crisis in the family. If the physician recognizes the potential for disorganization this will inevitably produce in both instrumental and emotional functioning, he may play a major role in minimizing the destructive effects and aiding in the reintegration and mature adaptation of the family as a whole.

Often if one looks for them, the family's past history of adjustment will give clues that will allow one to anticipate the nature of potential difficulties. An assessment of previous family responses to stress is helpful. An awareness of marital problems would indicate the need to communicate with both parents to help them face problems together. Prior peer, school, and behaviour problems may indicate possible difficulties for the child and staff during management. Observed interaction between the child and his parents is a guide to possible reactions to medical staff.

5. It is essential that the attending physician recognize that what the family *hear* and *understand* may differ considerably from what they have been *told*. Parents can assimilate only what they are emotionally ready for. In their distress, they may hear what they need to hear, selecting or distorting what has actually been said either to obtain false reassurance or to confirm their worst fears. Be simple and direct, avoiding unwarranted optimism or excessive pessimism. Timing may be important here. While saying too much too soon may cause unnecessary anxiety, more commonly too little is said too late, and in too ambiguous a manner. One important reason for maintaining regular contact with the family is to explore with them what they *have* heard regarding diagnosis, prognosis, and management, and how they are coping, in terms of both day-to-day management and emotional adjustment.

6. It is desirable that the physician review periodically with the parents their concept of the child and his over-all management. Severe overprotection and unnecessary restrictions on activity, failure to provide age-appropriate expectations and to supply discipline, the presence of obvious behaviour or academic problems in a sibling or mounting tension within the marriage, and a major and continuing discrepancy between physician and parents around what the child can do may be as serious an indication that the family is in trouble as is evidence of inadequate or inconsistent care.

7. Similarly, through his ongoing contacts with the child, the physician is in a position to explore the child's understanding of the nature of his illness and help him deal with his feelings about it. By asking questions about how the child sees himself and his illness, the child can be encouraged to express his concerns. Often the parents in their anxiety cannot allow the children, including the sick child, to raise openly any of their anxieties. Helping the parents face and master their own anxieties, thus preparing them to tolerate and deal with the concerns of the children, can be crucial in minimizing serious and long-

lasting emotional damage. What is spoken and acknowledged is often less threatening than that which is known but not talked about. The conspiracy of silence which leads to avoidance of any mention of consequences of the illness—including hospitalizations, operations (especially when they involve mutilation, for example, amputations) or approaching death—is usually a pretense, trying for all, but especially for the child, who is the central character. This topic deserves far more discussion than is possible here, and is discussed in more detail by Cain,[4] Patterson et al.,[23] and Kubler-Ross.[13]

8. School and peer relationships are extremely important in the life of the child. In chronic illness there may be significant absence from school, requiring tuition during hospitalization. The assistance of the child's teacher should be sought in co-ordinating schooling. Despite hospitalization, the child should be encouraged to maintain contact with peers either through visits or by mail. The child's embarrassment and shame regarding illness and deformity may in fact contribute to an alienation from the peer group which, under the right circumstances, could be a source of support for the child. With the older child, alertness on the part of the physician to a refusal to contact peers may help him to discuss the child's worries regarding his friends.

9. Physicians are frequently the undeserving objects of hostility. This is not intended as, and should not be construed as, an attack on them personally even though it may be expressed in very personal terms. Rather, it is a displacement of the parents' resentment that this (the child's illness) has occurred, and a reaction against the one who, out of necessity, confronts them with painful realities they would rather not hear. If the physician responds with hostility or by withdrawing from and rejecting the family, he will lose the opportunity to provide needed services at this time of great distress. If the feelings are too intense to be resolved right at the moment, it is probably advisable to have the parents back in to discuss the situation again in the near future. Some parents may need a chance to vent their emotional reactions before they will be able to listen and take hold, make the necessary practical decisions, and co-operate regarding management. If the physician can approach the parents with continued empathy and objectivity, he may be able to help them deal with their distress more appropriately and move on to the problems of practical management.

10. The management of the chronically ill child and his family requires the resources of a team of professionals. Adequate paths of communica-

tion should exist between team members for co-ordination of management. A frustrating family, by increasing demands and creating tension between team members, may cause friction and breakdown of team co-ordination. Disagreements among team members may be taken out on the patient. Under such circumstances, team meetings can help place problems in perspective, and will allow team members to support each other at times of stress.

11. Restrictions on activity are often inevitable. While pre-schoolers generally limit their own activities, older children, because of their need to conform and to prove their social adequacy, may tend to overtax themselves. The physician may be helpful in defining and explaining necessary activity restrictions, as well as in arbitrating between parent and child about them. Realistic restrictions because of illness, however serious, may not be as crippling as those constructed or fantasied by parent or child. By highlighting areas of satisfactory function and potential strengths, the physician may do much toward helping the family towards an acceptance of the child's real strengths along with his realistic limitations.

Children need and use play as an avenue for expressing their feelings and as a vehicle for resolving conflicts. Young children require play materials for such purposes, and puppets, painting materials, and toy medical equipment can be used. Such play also provides a means of activity and an area of independence for the immobilized child. Occupational therapy and play therapy are important in this regard for all such children.

12. Any major decision (around surgical intervention, around whether or not to hospitalize) or any necessary but disappointing statement regarding prognosis may unleash a severe and unpleasant emotional reaction, or may be greeted with docile passivity. In either case, one should realize that the obvious parental reaction may be very different from what the parents are struggling with within themselves. Some parents may need active encouragement if they are to express feelings which have been held in but are tearing them and their family apart. In making important decisions, the family needs help in recognizing and weighing the facts of the situation, and reassurance and encouragement once a decision has been made.

13. Physicians differ in their ability to help families cope with their emotional reactions to chronic illness. While each family needs on an ongoing basis someone who can help them with their emotional re-

sponses to the illness, this might or might not be their physician. Should the demands of meeting the emotional needs of the families of chronically ill patients seem excessive (i.e. extending beyond what the physician is in a position to provide) there is always the alternative of referring the family to someone geared to helping them deal with the emotional sequelae of the illness. A child psychiatrist, a social worker, a pastoral counsellor, or an association of parents who have experienced a similar problem could be of major assistance to the family and to the physician. In making such a referral, it would be important to distinguish clearly between whether the physician is planning to continue to play a major role in helping the family with their emotional difficulties and is seeking a consultation, or whether he prefers the referral agent to take over the management of the emotional aspects of the case in continuing consultation with regard to overall management.

14. Episodes of hospitalization may represent acute or chronic crisis situations. When hospitalization is necessary, hospital staff may be at the receiving end of parental criticism or overinvolvement. Parents may indeed be demanding, critical, and competitive with nursing staff. But hospital staff may need reminding that *their* patient is *still* the parents' child and that the parents' reactions are a response to anxiety and a displacement of their resentment at having a seriously ill child. This may help hospital staff maintain some understanding and empathy for parents, instead of responding with hostility and rejection. This serves only to aggravate the parental distress as friction and antagonism between parents and hospital staff escalate. By anticipating, recognizing, and mediating such conflicts as they appear to arise, the physician may be of great help to all in avoiding or breaking the vicious circle of recrimination.

RECOMMENDED FOR FURTHER READING

1. AISENBERG, R. B.; WOLFF, P. H.; ROSENTHAL, A.; and NADAS, A. S. "Psychological Impact of Cardiac Catheterization". *Pediat.* 51: 1051–59, 1973.

2. ANTHONY, E. J., and KOUPERNIK, C., eds., *The Child in His Family.* Vol. 2: *The Impact of Disease and Death.* New York, Wiley and Sons, 1973.
—a highly recommended collection of papers dealing with the reactions of children and parents to disease, death, and mourning.

4. CAIN, A. C.; FAST, I.; and ERICKSON, M. E. "Children's Disturbed Reactions to the Death of a Sibling". *Amer. J. Orthopsychiat.* 34: 741–52, 1964.
—deals directly with psychological reactions of children to sibling loss.

5. CLINE, F. W., and ROTHENBERG, M. B. "Preparation of a Child for Major Surgery: A Case Report". *J. Amer. Acad. Child Psychiat.* 13: 78–94, 1974.

6. DANILOWICZ, D. A., and GABRIEL, H. P. "Postoperative Reactions in Children: 'Normal' and Abnormal Responses after Cardiac Surgery". *Amer. J. Psychiat.* 128: 185–88, 1971–72.
—acute responses in sixty-eight children undergoing cardiac surgery were divided into four main groups: anxiety, anger, co-operation, and compliance. The need for evaluating a child's adjustment before and after surgery and for adequate preparation for surgery is stressed.

7. FREEDMAN, A. M.; HELME, W.; HAVEL, J.; EUSTIS, M. J.; RILEY, C.; and LANGFORD, W. S. "Psychiatric Aspects of Familial Dysautonomia". *Amer. J. Orthopsychiat.* 27: 96–106, 1957.
—good description of the effects that parental anxieties and guilt have on child rearing and on the development of disturbed patterns of behaviour.

10. GATH, A. "The Mental Health of Siblings of Congenitally Abnormal Children". *J. Child Psychol. Psychiat.* 13: 211–18, 1972.
—investigates evidence that a congenitally abnormal child may adversely affect the mental health of siblings. Discusses the serious problems a handicapped child living at home may present to his family.

12. KAUFMAN, R. V. "Body-Image Changes in Physically Ill Teenagers". *J. Amer. Acad. Child Psychiat.* 11: 157–70, 1972.
—describes how a few patients imagine change in their body image resulting from chronic illness such as diabetes.

13. KUBLER-ROSS, E. *Questions and Answers on Death and Dying.* New York, Macmillan and Company, 1974.
—the classic discussion of the psychology of death and dying.

14. LANSKY, S. B. "Childhood Leukemia: The Child Psychiatrist as a Member of the Oncology Team". *J. Amer. Acad. Child Psychiat.* 13: 499–508, 1974.
—preliminary report of an ongoing study of the leukemic child and his family. Discusses the psychological impact of prolonged anticipation of death on child and family, recommending that a child psychiatrist serve as part of the treatment team.

16. MC KAY, R. M. "Coping with a Family-Shattering Disease", in Patterson, P. R.; Denning, C.; and Kutscher, A. H., eds., *Psychological Aspects of Cystic Fibrosis*. New York, Columbia University Press, 1973.

—useful discussion of how chronic illness can wreak havoc with the family of the involved child.

18. MANNINO, F. V., and SHORE, M. F. "Family Structure, Aftercare, and Post-Hospital Adjustment". *Amer. J. Orthopsychiat.* 44: 76–85, 1974.

—confirms the important effect of family variables on post-hospital adjustment and treatment outcome in an after-care program. Has important implications for program planning.

21. NOVER, R. A. "Pain and the Burned Child". *J. Amer. Acad. Child Psychiat.* 12: 499–505, 1973.

—discusses pain as a central factor which influences the behaviour of the burned child. Relates the child's experience of pain to the degree to which the pain is charged with psychic meaning. Good.

24. PLESS, I. B., and ROGHMANN, K. J. "Chronic Illness and Its Consequences: Observations Based on Three Epidemiologic Surveys". *J. Pediat.* 79: 351–59, 1971.

—describes three surveys of children with chronic physical disorders, relating the type, duration, and severity of the disorder to the frequency of secondary handicaps in behaviour, psychological maladjustment, and educational deficits.

26. SELIGMAN, R. "A Psychiatric Classification System for Burned Children". *Amer. J. Psychiat.* 131: 41–46, 1974.

—classifies normal and pathological responses of children to severe burns, which if adopted, could facilitate research into the prevention of serious psychological complications.

27. SIGAL, J. J.; CHAGOYA, L.; VILLENEUVE, C.; and MAYEROVITCH, J. "Later Psychosocial Sequelae of Early Childhood Illness (Severe Group)". *Amer. J. Psychiat.* 130: 786–89, 1973.

—severe early childhood illness may result in "the vulnerable child" syndrome, which may cause later disturbances in the parent-child relationship.

29. TURK, J. "Impact of Cystic Fibrosis on Family Functioning". *Pediat.* 34: 67–71, 1964.

—discusses the impact of chronic illness on affected families.

ADDITIONAL READING

3. BOWLBY, J. *Attachment and Loss.* Vol. 2: *Separation: Anxiety and Anger*, 3–24. New York, Basic Books, 1973.

8. FREUD, A. "The Role of Bodily Illness in the Mental Life of Children", in *The Psychoanalytic Study of the Child*. Vol 7: 42–50, 1952.

9. GARRARD, S. E. and RICHMOND, J. B. "Psychological Aspects of the Management of Chronic Disease and Handicapping Conditions in Childhood, in Lief, H. I.; Lief, V. F.; and Lief, N. R., eds., *The Psychological Basis of Medical Practice*, 370–403. New York, Harper and Row, 1963.

11. GLASER, H. H.; HARRISON, G. S.; and LYNN, D. B. "Emotional Implications of Congenital Heart Disease in Children". *Pediat.* 33: 367–79, 1964.

15. LEFEBVRE, A. "Problems of Patients with Cystic Fibrosis in Adapting to Adolescence and Adulthood". *J. Amer. Acad. Child Psychiat.* In press.

17. MADDISON, D., and RAPHAEL, B. "Social and Psychological Consequences of Chronic Disease in Childhood". *Med. J. Aust.* 2: 1265–70, 1971.

19. MEYEROWITZ, J. H., and KAPLAN, H. B. "Familial Responses to Stress: The Case of Cystic Fibrosis". *Soc. Sci. Med.* 1: 249–66, 1967.

20. NATTERSON, J. M., and KNUDSON, A. G. "Observations Concerning Fear of Death in Fatally Ill Children and Their Mothers". *Psychosom. Med.* 22: 456–65, 1960.

22. PAKES, E. H. "Child Psychiatry and Pediatric Practice: How Disciplines Work Together". *Ont. Med. Rev.* 41: 69–71, 1974.

23. PATTERSON, P. R.; DENNING, C.; and KUTSCHER, A. H., eds., *Psychological Aspects of Cystic Fibrosis*. New York, Columbia Univ. Press, 1973.

25. ROSBERG, G. "Parental Attitudes in Pediatric Hospital Admissions" *Acta Pediat. Scand.* Supplement no. 210, 1971.

28. SOLNIT, A. I., and GREEN, M. "Psychological Considerations in the Management of Deaths on Pediatric Hospital Services. 1: The Doctor and the Child's Family". *Pediat.* 24: 106–12, 1959.

30. VANLEEUWEN, J. J. "Child Psychiatry and Pediatric Practice; Dialysis-Transplantation". *Ont. Med. Rev.* 41: 71–73, 1974.

31. VERNON, D.; SCHULMAN, J.; and FOLEY, J. "Changes in Children's Behavior after Hospitalization". *Amer. J. Dis. Child.* 3: 581–93, 1966.

JAMES VAN LEEUWEN

17. Hospitalization and Its Meaning to the Child and His Family

Hospitals are of indisputable value. The majority of patients, adults as well as children, are admitted for good reasons. Nevertheless, the criteria for the hospitalization of children are not always clear. Obviously, certain medical and surgical procedures can be performed only in a hospital, but many children are admitted for observation, minor treatments, and laboratory investigations merely out of custom or for the convenience of the physician or the parents. There are risks in treating a sick child at home, whereas hospital treatment offers a sense of security, which some physicians need more than others. Styles of medical practice differ in terms of readiness to make house-calls and in terms of office or hospital orientation. Not only reasons for admission but also the average duration of hospitalization for identical illnesses vary from hospital to hospital and from physician to physician. Cultural factors seem to influence the choice as to whether certain procedures such as tonsillectomy and circumcision will be carried out. Similarly, the dying child is often routinely hospitalized because there seems to be a cultural intolerance to death taking place at home.

While questioning the need for hospitalization, one must not forget that certain families offer inadequate child care, which can be hazardous to children with relatively minor illnesses. In such cases, admission to hospital may be preferred as the lesser of two evils, even though the medical condition does not ordinarily warrant in-patient care. Hospitalization can avert acute disaster in the life of children whose self-destructive behaviour, suicidal gestures, panic states, or somatic complaints are recognized as early warning signs of their potential disintegration under the stress of life.

In general, the psychiatrist does not discourage hospitalization when it is clearly indicated, but he urges that it be taken seriously because it is a significant source of emotional stress, which carries a potential risk to certain vulnerable children and families. The thoughtful physician may be able to prevent unnecessary hospitalization and the resourceful community might help by providing hospitals with a wide range of facilities such as house calls, ambulatory, day-care, night-care, care-by-parent, and home-care services.

The Hospital Environment

A hospital is not a home. It cannot be and does not need to be a home, despite the fact that for some children it serves of necessity in this capacity. Hospital facilities vary, depending on the hospital's size, location, architecture, and orientation towards research, service, or teaching.

From the child's point of view, however, the emotional climate or atmosphere is crucial. Children's furniture, decorations, and play-materials can reflect thoughtfulness and relieve the child's apprehension, but a wholesome emotional climate extends beyond the provision of material things into the creation of optimal staff-patient relationships. These relationships must reflect understanding of the child's reactions to his illness and the child's needs for continuing psychosocial development even while he is in the care of the hospital. Although medical intervention is the primary reason for the hospital's existence, the care of children in the hospital should not be confused with, or limited to, the treatment of their diseases. Treatment, for example, may require prolonged immobilization, but care demands an active social and education program for that child to counter boredom, depression, and school failure. Treatment may require that a two-year-old be hospitalized far away from home, but care may demand that the child's mother live in the hospital for a short time as well. Treatment may be minor surgery to be performed under local anaesthetic, but care requires considerable psychological preparation because of the major impact that needles, masks, lights, sounds, and blood may have on the child who is conscious during the operation. If the procedure involves the child's head, abdominal, or genital area, he will feel particularly threatened.

Hospital staff need to be aware of their own possible contributions to the disturbances in the hospital climate. Staff tensions and arguments are perceived and responded to by patients, just as children at home respond with anxiety to their parents' marital tensions and discord. Physicians and nurses should be aware that in the fantasies of their child patients they may be seen as having unnatural power. This fantasied power can be destructive if, because of it, the child is unable to express his reasonable anger with certain aspects of the treatment, fearing retaliation by the doctor or nurse on whose continued affection he feels his health and life depend. There is also a tendency for staff to be unaware of the impact of their own frustration, annoyance, anxiety, or feelings of professional impotence, which may unwittingly affect patient care. The reflection and self-examination engaged in during conferences or ward rounds sometimes reveal previously unrecognized attitudes such as hostility towards patients with messy illnesses, competitiveness with parents, avoidance manouvres to escape difficult parents or patients, and subtle desertion of the dying child, which, if not recognized and properly controlled, will inevitably affect patient care adversely.

The University Hospital

There is a potential conflict between the medical student's objective of gaining clinical experience for his own professional development and the patient's expectation of the physician's devotion to healing his disease and relieving his misery. We need to understand what can make clinical teaching a reassuring, even delightful experience for some patients, and what can make it hazardous to the emotional health of others.

Patients usually tolerate a degree of embarrassment, discomfort, and even pain inflicted for the sake of teaching, provided the teaching physician maintains through the session a wholesome doctor-patient relationship, which could serve as a model to the students.

Patient variables, such as personality, age, illness, length of stay in hospital, quickly identify those patients who are at risk because of their vulnerability. For example, shy, overly anxious, deprived, or homesick children are more vulnerable than those who are happy and well adjusted. Age variables may be illustrated in the reactions of four children to the same small group of medical students: a baby may enjoy the handling; a ten-month-old child may be frightened and overwhelmed by all the strangers; an inquisitive school-age child may relish the challenge and try to learn as much as possible; a self-conscious teenager may speak of her embarrassment and show awkwardness during the physical examination.

Obviously, some children are too ill to be exposed to the stress of teaching. External manifestations of diseases are easier to demonstrate than the internal findings, which require physical examination of the patient. Teaching of rectal examinations and genital inspection require special consideration. Painful examinations need to be restricted in teaching hospitals.

Certain illnesses tend to make certain patients "interesting cases" or "good teaching material", which creates the emotional hazards implied in the label. Teaching usually calls for a certain amount of repetition, which may lead to recurrent exposure of the patient's personal, confidential information or of his emotionally painful experiences related to sexual problems, body-image anxiety, hereditary illnesses, neglect, grief, etc.

Patients with long-term or recurrent admissions bear the brunt of teaching related problems, which adds to the already massive burden of chronic illness. In teaching hospitals, these patients face an extraordinary amount of undergraduate and postgraduate student turnover, resulting in discontinuity of care, in staff confusion, and in unwarranted repetition of history-taking and physical examinations. The transient nature of the contacts between patients and students may erode the human quality of patient care. The problems of clinical teaching can be reduced, however, by recognition of patients' vulnerability, by adequate psychological preparation of patient and students prior to the teaching session, by awareness of the patient's emotional needs, and by good judgment when discussing the patient or illness in his presence.

The Family

The parents whose child is in hospital are frequently under considerable stress. They have to cope with their uncertainty and anxiety about the sick child, their feelings about the hospital and its staff, the additional expenses, and the inconvenience involved in frequent trips to the hospital. The hospitalization of the child, and the attendant problems, may constitute a crisis that may lead to family growth, but often leads instead to family disruption. Feelings of love and concern for the sick child are in conflict with anger and frustration about the trouble he has created, and the conflict may be difficult for the parents to resolve. Siblings often perceive parental preoccupation with the hospitalized child as favouritism and respond by feeling relatively deprived and resentful, at times showing signs of neurotic, regressive, or acting-out behaviour.

Not infrequently, parents reduce in number, or stop altogether, the visits to their hospitalized children. This is rarely because of wilful rejection or abandonment, but usually because of an unfortunate combination of errors. The following story is typical:

> As the parents enter the room to visit their child, the child starts to cry. When they leave, the child cries again, clinging to them and making a scene. This is quite appropriate under the circumstances, but the parents may interpret this as an embarrassing sign of weakness in their child. It may, to them, be an indication of their failure to raise a well-behaved child. A well-meaning nurse or doctor tells them not to worry, because their child is really quite good and does not cry when they are not around. The parents interpret this as a suggestion that the child only cries because their visit must in some way upset him. So they stay home, increasing their own and their child's emotional pain, resulting in an even greater turmoil at the time of their next visit, confirming their belief that visits indeed upset the child too much.

Any failure of the parents to visit on a regular basis may indicate that they are immobilized by their reactions to their child's illness and hospitalization. Failure of the attending medical and nursing staff to recognize and assist in relieving such a situation is poor practice in that it represents a clear and unnecessary hazard to the mental health of vulnerable children.

The Child

The hospitalized child has many fears: fears of symptoms, pain, damage, exposure, and loss of control; fear of strangers, separation, abandonment, and death; fears of the unknown and of his own terrible fantasies. The child's response will depend on age, previous adjustment, illness, and hospital climate. Sadness, anxiety, refusal to accept unpleasant things, and attempts to secure mothering are normal reactions. It is hoped that the hospital environment can accept these; otherwise there is the danger of labelling the patient childish, silly, stubborn, or spoiled. If hospital staff react with anger and rejection, they may further increase the child's distress and symptomatic behaviour, eliciting further rejection. If the staff's natural tendency to please a sad child becomes overly solicitous and feeds into the child's wish to be completely taken care of, unnecessarily regressive behaviour may emerge such as spoon feeding, wheelchair rides, and other types of babying that prevent the child from functioning at optimal developmental levels. Hospitalization of children who are in developmental transition carries an increased risk of the child losing newly gained ground such as self-care, bowel control, or social skills, so that his pride in his achievements turns into a sense of loss or failure.

With so many reasons for children to be upset in hospital, it is sometimes difficult to know the difference between normally expected behaviour and the behavioural signs indicative of pathological reactions to hospitalization. There are no rules, but we ought to be alarmed when staff or parents recognize new behaviour as incongruent with the child's previous behaviour pattern. Such new behaviour might include sucking, rocking, self-injury, food refusal, incontinence, refusal to sleep, extreme fears, inability to play, withdrawal, or absence of crying.

When children's tears and protests are not effective in getting them out of hospital, some may become resigned to the fact and allow the staff to do with them as they please. This makes for an "easy" patient, but unfortunately many "easy" patients are actually depressed, and because they are withdrawn and undemonstrative they receive less attention, which only aggravates the situation.

Hospitalization is a Separation Experience

How stressful a particular child will find hospitalization depends upon a number of factors. These include how vulnerable that child is to being separated from his family, the response of the child and his family to the disease itself, and the quality of hospital care provided. While all these factors are important, the experience of being separated from mother and family is of particular significance for the infant and younger child.

Infants under five months have not yet developed the type of attachment to the mother that creates the "separation anxiety" so typical of toddlers. Nevertheless, infants do show a "global" reaction to hospitalization that consists of changes in feeding, sleeping, and elimination patterns. These disturbances continue for a few days to several weeks after the infant's return home.

Around six months of age, the child begins to be upset when strangers approach or when mother leaves him in unfamiliar surroundings (separation anxiety); we can expect similar anxiety upon hospitalization. Separation anxiety peaks probably in the second year. A sick child of two, finding himself in hospital without familiar toys and clothes, left to the care of strangers, separated from his mother for an extended period of time, would probably show the characteristic sequence of protest, despair, and detachment described by Robertson and Bowlby.[5, 22, 23] Fortunately, parents or relatives can usually maintain daily contact, and their presence quickly transforms the strange hospital into a familiar environment. The child can usually bring his own clothes, pictures, and toys, and sensitive staff can offer good substitute parenting. As a result, the child may show only a minimal degree of upset. Robertson found that separation from mother *per se* does not have to result in emotional deprivation or even produce protest, despair, and denial, provided the environment is optimal and offers adequate substitute parenting. Hospitals will never be perfect in this respect, however, and the additional stress of illness and treatment will accentuate the separation experience.

Separation from home is more tolerable for the older child, particularly when adequate communication is maintained. Some school-age children, however, become intensely homesick, and their suffering is often aggravated by a tendency for adults to be intolerant of such behaviour.

Long-Term Hospitalization

A universal problem with long-term hospitalization is that it carries a risk of serious emotional deprivation, which can result in chronic depression, failure to thrive, delay in development, poor impulse control, or erosion of relationships.

In contrast to the sudden, sharp, traumatic, but time-limited experiences of acute hospitalization, the long-term patient is expected to make an adaptation to the very peculiar social milieu of a hospital. His life-style will reflect the relationships, attitudes, and priorities he observes among the doctors, nurses, technicians, physiotherapists, students, cleaners, etc. Unless the total staff is organized to present a goal-directed, child-centred treatment plan, the hospital will be perceived by the child as disease-oriented, undemocratic, disorganized, manipulative, and superficial as compared with his own home environment. These perceptions will be reflected in the child's adaptation in hospital, which will include similare undesirable methods of handling people, feelings, and situations.

In addition to the behaviours he acquires from the hospital atmosphere, the long-term patient loses many experiences for normal development by reason of being in hospital. He is deprived of his own committed environment, his freedom, and his social and educational opportunities. Autonomy and responsibility are diminished by all the things he has done to him or done for him.

There is a distinct possibility that the kind of case presentations and staff conferences that physicians are so familiar with during medical training make them well organized but rather intellectual and disease-oriented. They can tend to lapse into medical jargon and, without noticing it, lose sight of the person who is going through the intensely threatening experience of illness. For example, a physician might describe the illness of a fifteen-year-old boy with Wilson's disease in the following terms:

> Wilson's disease is a familial, recessively inherited disorder, which is due to the defective management of copper. As a result copper is deposited in the liver, cornea, kidneys, and brain. This disease runs a progressive course with periodic exacerbations and leads to cirrhosis, Kayser-Fleisher rings in the cornea, renal failure, and brain damage. If started early, copper-removing agents such as penicillamine are usually effective. This fifteen-year-old boy unfortunately started treatment one year after the onset of his symptoms, hence has permanent brain damage with rigidity, spasms, tremors, and a Parkinsonian appearance.

The boy, however, might describe his experiences from a different perspective and in a different language:

> I am here in hospital hundreds of miles from home without my parents. I have lost my friends and failed my year in school. I am scared. I can't even move any more and talking is impossible. People get so frustrated in caring for me because I'm helpless.

> Why me? I guess my parents should not have married: our whole family seems doomed. I might die just like my two sisters. What have I done wrong? All these lab tests—it is blood, sweat, and tears. Even what they call "therapy" means an awful diet and painful needles. I hate it all. The fear of the unknown I find terrible. I look kind of stupid; that is why they sometimes treat me as if I am stupid.

This boy obviously needs more than penicillamine; he needs help to become a person who can function despite his handicaps.

There is an increasing recognition of the need for comprehensive treatment planning for groups of children who require long-term and intermittent hospitalization, in addition to ambulatory care for conditions such as haemophilia, diabetes, burns, cerebral palsy, heart disease, fibrocystic disease, leukemia, or renal disease requiring dialysis-transplantation. These programs should carry a mental-health component that ensures psychological preparation, ongoing counselling of children and their parents, multidisciplinary planning meetings, and adequate provisions for social and educational experiences.

Summary

Care of the hospitalized child might be summarized in the following prescription, which is applicable to any hospital situation. The hospital must reduce social disruption to a minimum by providing adequate space, activities, visiting, parent participation, privacy, self-care, day-care, and educational programs. Children under three, those in developmental transition, those with previous disturbances or current family crisis, and those suffering from chronic illness should be identified as vulnerable children and receive special attention. Developmental specialists, psychologists, social workers, and psychiatrists should be consulted with a view to prevention rather than treatment of developmental and emotional disorder. Hospital staff should learn to recognize their own reactions to illness and learn to anticipate and accept the patient's normal responses such as dependency, fear, anger, denial, and depression. To function as a person, the child needs continuity, understanding, preparation for traumatic events, and people he can trust. To establish such an environment, the health team must have regular periods of reflection, above all, and contact through in-service education, interdisciplinary discussions, and regular ward meetings.

Finally, the institution should, by continued critical evaluation of the hospital milieu, maintain the child at an optimal level of activity, autonomy, initiative, learning, and socialization.

Appendix:
Literature Review

Bakwin,[1] Jackson,[11] Levy,[14] Senn,[25] Jensen and Comly,[10] and Langford[13] are some of the first clinicians who reported their observations and concerns about short-term hospitalization in children.

At the same time, in the forties, Spitz[26, 27] reported his research on what be called "hospitalism", in which he described the shocking effects an emotionally sterile foundling home has on the development of the infants placed there at four months of age. The condition of physical and psychological disturbance and retardation, increased susceptibility to illness, apathy, and profound sadness as a consequence of institutional deprivation is called hospitalism (not to be confused with hospitalization). The work of Spitz led to increased awareness of the occurrence of hospitalism in paediatric hospitals and the need for its prevention.

In the fifties, we find the stimulating work of Robertson, who produced his film *A Two-Year-Old Goes to Hospital*[21] in 1952 and his book *Young Children in Hospital*[22] in 1958. Others should be mentioned, such as Schaffer and Callender[24] on infants, Prugh et al.[20] on pre-school and school-age children, Vaughan and Lord[29] on eye operations, Jessner et al.[12] and Faust et al.[8] on tonsillectomies.

Another important development took place in 1952, when Bowlby[5] prepared his report *Maternal Care and Mental Health* on behalf of the World Health Organization. Although somewhat controversial, it offered a tremendous stimulus for improved child care in general and research into the specific factors that constitute deprivation of care. An excellent review, prepared in 1962, is offered by the World Health Organization.[30]

In the sixties, we find some interesting material. Provence and Lipton[19] published their research study *Infants in Institutions*, which gives "a comparison of their development with family reared infants during the first year of life". More directly related to hospitalization is Bergmann's *Children in Hospital*[4] which describes twenty years of experience as child therapist in a long-stay hospital. *Planning for Children in the Hospital*[18] is a monograph based on the proceedings of a workshop organized by the American Orthopsychiatric Association in 1965. The participants address themselves to the role of the family, staff relationships in hospital, and strategies for the initiating of change in hospitalizations, for children.

Engel's textbook, *Psychological Development in Health and Disease*[7], provides a clear and thorough analysis of child development, with special reference to illness, hospitalization, stress, and deprivation.

Of the recent literature we might mention "Child Psychiatry and Pediatric Practice",[17] which describes three models of psychiatric consultation that aim at improving patient care in hospitalized children. Belmont[3] offers a transcript of a lecture on hospitalization given to resident psychiatrists. McKim[15] in "Child Health related to a Children's Hospital" puts the role of the hospital in perspective to the total community health-care plan involving care-by-parent units, child-health nurse, home visits, prevention, etc. Bakwin and Bakwin[2] offer a valuable review based on their own extensive experience in paediatrics.

RECOMMENDED FOR FURTHER READING

1. BAKWIN, H. "Loneliness in Infants". *Amer. J. Dis. Child.* 63: 30–40, 1942.
2. BAKWIN, H., and BAKWIN R. M. *Behavior Disorders in Children.* Philadelphia, W. B. Saunders, 1972.
3. BELMONT, H. S. "Hospitalization and Its Effects upon the Total Child". *Clin. Pediat.* 9: 472–83, 1970.
4. BERGMANN, T., and FREUD, A. *Children in Hospital.* New York, International Univ. Press, 1966
5. BOWLBY, J. *Maternal Care and Mental Health*. 2nd ed. Switzerland, World Health Organization Monograph no. 2, 1952.
6. DEBUSKY, M. *The Chronically Ill Child and His Family.* Springfield, Ill., C. C. Thomas, 1970.
   —this 200-page book deals well with the "orchestration of care" for the chronically ill children in general and with the special needs arising from eight different illnesses in particular. The contributors are mainly associated with Johns Hopkins Hospital, Baltimore, Maryland.
7. ENGEL, G. L. *Psychological Development in Health and Disease.* Philadelphia, W. B. Saunders, 1962.

8. FAUST, O. A., JACKSON, K.; CERMAK, E. G.; and WINKLEY, R. "Problems of Emotional Trauma in Hospital Treatment of Children". *J. Amer. Med. Assoc.* 149: 1536–38, 1952.

9. HARDGROVE, C. B. and DAWSON, R. B. *Parents and Children in the Hospital: The Family's Role in Pediatrics.* Boston, Little, Brown and Co., 1972.
—describes the day-to-day activities in a sampling of United States hospitals currently carrying out new and innovative programs for the needs of both the hospitalized child and his family.

10. JENSEN, R. A., and COMLY, H. H. "Child-Parent Problems and the Hospital". *Nerv. Child.* 7: 200–203, 1948.

11. JACKSON, E. B. "Treatment of the Young Child in the Hospital". *Amer. J. Orthopsychiat.* 12: 56–67, 1942.

12. JESSNER, L.; BLOM, G. E.; and WALDFOGEL, S. "Emotional Implications of Tonsillectomy and Adenoidectomy on Children". *Psychoanalyt. Stud. Child.* 7: 126–69, 1952.

13. LANGFORD, W. S. "Physical Illness and Convalescence: Their Meaning to the Child". *J. Pediat.* 33: 242–50, 1948.

14. LEVY, D. M. "Psychic Trauma of Operations in Children and a Note on Combat Neurosis". *Amer. J. Dis. Child.* 69: 7–25, 1945.

15. Mc KIM, J. S. "Child Health Related to a Children's Hospital". *Canad. Med. Assoc. J.* 105: 726–30, 1971.

16. MONNELLY, E. P.; IANZITO, B. M.; and STEWART, M. A. "Psychiatric Consultation in a Children's Hospital". *Amer. J. Psychiat.* 130: 789–90, 1973.
—analyses the psychiatric consultations done in a children's hospital during an eleven month period. Common psychiatric disorders which were found were hysteria, hyperactive child syndrome, depression, and organic brain syndrome. Brief.

17. PAKES, E. H.; VANLEEUWEN, J. J.; and GOLDBERG, B. "Child Psychiatry and Pediatric Practice". *Ont. Med. Rev.* 41: 69–75, 1974.

18. *Planning for Children in the Hospital: "Red Is the Color of Hurting".* Based on proceedings of the workshop on Mental Health Planning for Pediatric Hospitals held in New York, 1965. Bethesda, Maryland, National Institute of Mental Health, National Institutes of Health, 1965.

19. PROVENCE, S., and LIPTON, R. C. *Infants in Institutions.* New York, International Univ. Press, 1967.

20. PRUGH, D. G.; STAUB, E, M.; SANDS. H. H.; KIRSCHBAUM, R. M.; and LENITHAN, E. A "A Study of the Emotional Reactions of Children and Families to Hospitalization and Illness". *Amer. J. Orthopsychiat.* 23: 70–106, 1953.

21. ROBERTSON, J. *A Two-Year-Old Goes to Hospital.* Film. 16mm. 45 mins. Sound. Tavistock Child Development Research Unit, London. New York University Film Library, United Nations, Geneva, 1952.

22. ROBERTSON, J. *Young Children in Hospital.* New York, Basic Books, 1958.

23. ROBERTSON, JAMES, and ROBERTSON, JOYCE. "Young Children in Brief Separation—A Fresh Look". *Psychoanalyt. Stud. Child.* 26: 264–315, 1971.

24. SCHAFFER, H. R., and CALLENDER, W. M. "Psychologic Effects of Hospitalization in Infancy". *Pediat.* 24: 528–39, 1959.

25. SENN, M. J. E. "Emotional Aspects of Convalescence". *The Child.* 10: 24–28, 1945.

26. SPITZ, R. A. "Hospitalism: An Inquiry into the Genesis of Psychiatric Conditions in Early Childhood". *Psychoanalyt. Stud. Child.* 1: 53–74, 1945.

27. SPITZ, R. A. "Hospitalism: A Follow-Up Report". *Psychoanalyt. Stud. Child.* 2: 113–17, 1946.

28. VANLEEUWEN, J. J., and MATTHEWS, D. E. "Comprehensive Mental Health Care in a Pediatric Dialysis-Transplantation Program". *Canad. Med. Assoc. J.* 113: 959–62, 1975.

29. VAUGHAN, G. F., and LOND, M. B. "Children in Hospital". *Lancet.* 1: 1117–20, 1957.

30. World Health Organization. *Deprivation of Maternal Care: A Reassessment of Its Effects,* WHO Public Health Papers, no. 14, Geneva, 1962.

ED PAKES

18. The Dying Child and His Family

The physician treating the child who is suffering from a potentially lethal illness must deal not only with the disease itself but also with the emotional reactions of the child and his family to the illness. Research indicates that families with a dying child constitute a high-risk group. The severe stress precipitated by a fatal illness may generate a broad variety of problems, ranging from jealousies and unresolved grief reactions in siblings to separation, divorce, or mental illness in parents.[4, 5, 9, 17]

As the acute infectious diseases come under better control, physicians and nurses will increasingly be required to provide care for patients suffering other life-threatening and ultimately fatal illnesses, such as cancer, renal diseases, and certain congenital disorders. But doctors and nurses, too, experience considerable strain in dealing with the dying child and his family. Studies have shown that physicians generally have an excessive fear of death,[7] and that their choice of medicine as a career may be one way of dealing with these fears.[8] Physicians are torn between the duty to become professionally involved with a dying child and his family and the wish to remain emotionally detached to protect themselves from painful feelings generated in the course of involvement. While the specific reactions of the child and his family to the illness may vary with the age of the child and with factors unique to the particular family, many physicians find the process of helping the child and his family deal with their feelings about the illness exhausting and frustrating. Others recognize that the possibility of doing something active and useful for the family, even if the child dies, can prove helpful not only to the family but also to the physician's own need to maintain his professional vitality.

An understanding of some of the basic psychological aspects of death is essential in preparing to deal with such situations. Many of the issues involved in the management of the chronically ill child overlap with those faced in treating the dying child and his family. As treatment improves yearly, even patients who are destined to die can be kept alive and, in some cases, in remission for increasing periods of time. The uncertainty of the future can in itself produce a chronic stress reaction.

Factors Affecting the Psychology of Death

1. THE AGE OF THE CHILD

Up to the age of three, the child's main concern is his fear of being separated from those he loves and depends upon for his security.

> Three-year-old Danny, who was dying, cried out, "I'm falling, I'm falling!" His nurse, sensitive to his fear of being separated, held him and replied, "I'm catching you, I'm catching you." The nurse's awareness of Danny's separation anxiety allowed her to relieve his distress in the face of death.

In middle childhood, the child cannot conceive the finality of death. He is, however, fearful of mutilation. He may have seen a beloved pet run over by a car or a bird torn up by a cat. He is concerned about the integrity of his body and frightened of anything that can destroy it. At this age, children typically consider the immobility of the dead as a response to external circumstances rather than as a consequence of death itself. A four-year-old may say, "He cannot move because he's in the coffin," while another remarks, "The dead close their eyes because sand gets in them". Death is thus identified with sleep and viewed as a response to the outside world rather than as a change in the self. At times, especially around the ages of five and six, degrees of death are described, as evidenced by the child who said, "He could get out of the coffin if he wasn't stabbed too badly."

Since death at this stage is attributed to outside intervention and often thought of as a bogey or death man who comes to take people away, the child may believe magically in some action that he feels can miraculously reverse the process. This is why a simple object like a Band-Aid can have such significance at this age.

> Brian, age seven, was a very bright boy with leukemia who understood that he would soon die from his disease. He had many procedures during his hospitalization, and prior to his death began to accuse the doctors and nurses of being murderers and killers because they stuck needles into him that hurt. To him, they became outsiders who were invading his body and causing his pain. When the staff could recognize and deal successfully with their own feelings of guilt, they were better able to administer his medications.

We often do not realize that children of this age are more aware of their impending death than seems evident. This is an age at which children frequently avoid discussing their thoughts and feelings about their illness with their parents who, they recognize, are trying to hide the truth from them.

By the age of nine or ten the child, for the first time, is able to view death realistically. Death begins to be seen as a permanent biological process. Typical of this stage would be the ten-year-old girl who likened death to the withering of flowers.

To the adolescent, the prospect of dying is extremely traumatic. He can appreciate the meaning of death, but often has trouble accepting the reality that he, personally, is about to die. Bursting with a lust for life and on the verge of self-sufficiency, the teenager often sees death as an unfair punishment. The adolescent, more so than younger children, asks, "What have I done to deserve *this*?" The normal age-specific emotional reaction of the newly mature to the prospect of personal death is rage. Feeling that life was just within his grasp, he sees death as a ravisher and destroyer that washes away his dreams. Whereas both young children and mature adults can turn to others for support, the newly emancipated adolescent may have too much pride in his newfound independence to allow himself to accept support and understanding as he moves towards death.

A group of medical students was surveyed about whether or not adolescents should be told they are dying. There was general agreement that they should, because adolescence is a time when long-range plans are made. These may be unrealistic if the patient's prognosis is poor. They agreed that the adolescent had the right to some choice in how he would spend the remainder of his life. While one would need to avoid taking away any hope that was helping him face his limited but uncertain future, too rigid a commitment to unrealistic long-term goals (e.g. preparing for university) might stand in the way of his getting the most out of the time he had left.

2. THE LENGTH OF ILLNESS

A sudden death, for example death by accident, may result in an unresolved grief reaction, especially if the parents hold themselves responsible for the accident. The sudden-infant-death syndrome frequently leaves parents weighed down by guilt and wondering if they were neglectful. In such cases, it is essential that they receive a proper explanation of the current knowledge in this field, but merely hearing the facts on one occasion may not be enough to dispel their guilt. In situations involving sudden death, the primary physician should make it a practice to see the parents at intervals following the death in order to assess how they are coping with their reactions to the loss. A prolonged illness, on the other hand, may result in the family wishing the child dead. This, also, may be a source of persistent guilt, which will interfere with the completion of mourning. In either case, should the family reaction appear extreme or excessively prolonged or should the nuclear family's relationships with each other, with members of the extended family, or with long-standing friends show evidence of severe or persistent strain, psychiatric referral should be considered.

3. THE SPECIFIC ILLNESS

a) Some families may react to certain illnesses differently than to others. This is particularly true with diseases that are genetically transmitted, as the partner carrying the gene may feel considerable guilt, which may be aggravated by the reactions of the relatives of the non-affected partner.
b) There is chronic stress associated with diseases requiring extensive, continuing care, such as cases of renal failure or fibrocystic disease.
c) Behavioural problems and a self-destructive failure to observe the treatment regime associated with illnesses such as diabetes or cystic fibrosis may represent depressive or suicide equivalents, particularly in adolescents (see Chapter 7).

4. THE FAMILY

The psychological stress of having a dying child can have a profound effect on the adaptation of a family. They may fall apart or, rallying to each other's support, may come out of it a stronger unit than ever. Although there are common reactions, which will be elaborated upon later, each family is and should be treated as a unique group, which handles feelings in its own characteristic way. Whereas some families are plunged into lasting despair by the diagnosis of fatal illness, others, in response to the diagnosis, wake up to the realization that they are not getting the most out of life. Some such families have begun to "live" more since learning the diagnosis than they ever did before. Some families may turn to religion for solace; others may turn away from it. Some parents turn to each other for support; others turn against each other, each blaming the other. Parents may gain great support from friends and extended family; alternately, they may turn away from them in bitter alienation. Any widespread or persistent tendency towards withdrawal from previous family or social involvements probably indicates that the family is having serious difficulty handling the stress resulting from the illness and is in need of supportive intervention.

The family's previous experience with death is an area that needs to be explored. Generally, their pattern of mourning may be similar and predictable, although feelings specific to the dying child will influence their response to a particular illness. It is important not to deprive the child and the family of hope. The hope that is given by treatment, by caring, and by procedures is a constant factor underlying their reaction to the illness at various stages.

Siblings

The physician should discuss with the parents how they might best present the child's illness to siblings. Practical issues such as the ages of the siblings, their relationships with the sick child, or the likelihood that they might feel that the patient is favoured because of the amount of parental time and attention focused on him in view of his illness must all be considered in arriving at the appropriate decision for a particular family. Younger children frequently believe that their wishes may come true. Such children may feel intense guilt and remorse in response to the death of a sibling because at some time they were angry enough to wish him dead. One of the greatest dangers is the possibility that, because of their guilt or through a lack of parental understanding and support for their hostile feelings, they trap their own grief inside. Should this occur, it might well form the basis for later emotional disturbances (see Chapter 16).

5. PREVIOUS OR OTHER CURRENT STRESSES

Because of the family's preoccupation with the illness, other sources of stress affecting the family may be neglected. Financial stress, marital difficulties, problems in child-rearing, and neurotic difficulties of the parents which might otherwise be dealt with more successfully may become exaggerated and much less accessible to intervention when compounded by a co-existing fatal illness in a family member.

6. THE DYING PATIENT HIMSELF

All too often the patient with a potentially lethal illness is psychologically treated as if he were dead while he is still very much alive. He may be left alone because he is depressed and won't talk, or shunned because he frequently makes "unreasonable" demands. In each such instance, active intervention with this "alive" person can result in gratifying work.

> A nineteen-year-old young man was dying of Ewings sarcoma which had metastasized throughout his body. Everyone knew he knew his prognosis except his divorced mother who looked closer to death than he. This young man had been the "acting father" in the family since the father had left. He felt part of his job was to care for his mother, including protecting her from the knowledge that he knew his prognosis. The rest of the family colluded with this scheme. A group discussion with the family members resulted in their agreeing that the mother and boy should share their feelings about his impending death as had other family members. This resulted in the boy dying secure in the knowledge that his mother would survive in spite of his death, and the mother was more able to mourn the loss of her son and carry on with her own life.

7. CULTURAL ATTITUDES

In our Western world, the anger that mourning relatives at times feel towards the dying person is not culturally acceptable. Therefore, grieving relatives tend to turn this anger—which is part of the normal reaction to the threat of being separated from those we love—on each other or on those who care for the patient. While this may add considerably to the difficulties of those contributing to the medical and nursing care of the patient, it must not be allowed to disrupt treatment. If the origin of this anger is understood, staff may respond to it less personally. This may free them to help the family channel this anger into more constructive outlets, such as volunteer work through cancer societies.

8. THE CARING STAFF AND THEIR RESPONSES

Each staff member will react to the impending death of terminally ill patients in his own way. Since most of us in the healing professions get our greatest gratification from patients who get better, the treatment of dying patients frequently becomes a source of anxiety, frustration, and guilt rather than satisfaction. Our unconscious feelings might be verbalized, "I've done all I can, yet in spite of it this child is still dying. How can I continue to remain involved and allow myself to care about him when it makes me feel so helpless, inadequate, and guilty?" Each professional, if he is to help the child with a fatal illness, must first come to peace with his own feelings about the child's impending death and the limitations of his own therapeutic effectiveness. Many physicians deal with their feelings of helplessness and passivity by excessive intellectualization and by flights into activity. While the younger or middle-age physician may intellectualize his denial of impending death, the older physician may be unaware of how fiercely—and, at times, how inappropriately—his young resident is struggling to keep the patient alive. He may repeatedly examine and submit the dying patient to a multitude of diagnostic procedures in an attempt to reduce this insoluble, emotionally unbearable problem to the level of an intellectual exercise, thus creating for himself the feeling that he is indeed doing something worth while.

> An eight-year-old child was admitted to hospital with a lump in the neck. Great lengths of time were spent trying to decide the diagnosis, but it was only casually mentioned that the father was threatening to take the patient home. He did not want his child traumatized any more. Meanwhile suggestion after suggestion was made about what lab procedures should be performed on this patient who was figuratively halfway out of the door already.

Many physicians choose to share the responsibility of treating the terminally ill child with their colleagues in nursing, social work, or other allied professions. Should the family be the ones to request a consultation, however, this should be seen not as an expression of dissatisfaction with the attending physician but rather as an expression of the parents' need to be certain they have done everything possible for the child in order that guilt at the time of death is reduced to a minimum.

Stages of Emotional Reactions to Impending Death

PATIENT AND FAMILY

Kubler-Ross[14] has described stages of typical emotional reactions through which individuals progress in their adjustment to death. Each person and family goes through each of the stages in their own characteristic way. The physician and his team can do much to facilitate movement from one stage to the next and to assist in the process of mourning both before and after death. An individual can get stuck at any stage if stressed beyond his limit of tolerance, either because of additional factors that increase the burden or because of a pre-existing vulnerability. A return visit, several months to a year following the death, is a useful monitoring device, giving the family the needed support as well as allowing the physician an opportunity to detect unresolved grief that may become a psychiatric problem.

The stages in the emotional reaction to impending death as defined by Kubler-Ross are:

1. *Shock and denial.* The typical reaction, which may be explicitly stated or merely subjectively experienced is, "No, it's not true!" This stage allows the patient and his family to collect themselves, giving them time to mobilize other less radical defences against the painful feelings stirred up by the diagnosis.

2. *Anger and protest.* Here the typical reaction is expressed by the repeated and bitter demand, "Why me?" or "What have I done to deserve this?" This occurs as the denial gradually yields to anger or protest. There is increasing use of projection as, at an unconscious level, the patient and his family experience their affliction and other sources of discontent, real or imagined, as inflicted on them by the environment or God. Their reaction is to fight off whoever and whatever is around. This is a most difficult stage because it may disrupt their relationships with family, friends, medical personnel, and the community at large, all so

necessary to sustain life and avoid increasing isolation and alienation. At this stage, parents are typically complaintive and critical of the care their child receives. If doctors and other hospital staff take these attacks personally and respond to them with hostility and rejection, they merely increase the parents' suffering.

3. *Bargaining.* The typical reaction is contained in the statement, "I'll make a deal with you." The angry, difficult child may remember that in the past if he was good he was rewarded. In a magical way, he may attempt to bargain with medical staff, his parents, or even God to obtain relief from his disease. He may announce, or merely decide within himself, that if he is a good boy for a day his mother will take him home from hospital, he will be spared further paintful treatments, he will get better, etc. When the bargain does not work, the child may respond with intensified anger and protest, or alternatively with despair. The family, like the child, may be reduced to bargaining, responding much as he does to their inability to alter the progress of the disease.

4. *Depression.* In time, inevitably, child and family can no longer avoid the recognition that the bargaining has failed and a profound depression takes over. There are two types of depression:

a) The attempt to accept one's losses, including all that has been missed out on either prior to or because of the illness.
b) The attempt to prepare for possible loss or death in the future, including an anticipatory mourning for the life that might have been.

5. *Acceptance (or adaptation).* Acceptance, the final stage of preparation for death, is reached only when the other stages have been traversed. When the illness is a lethal one, this stage may sometimes be seen as the acceptance of defeat.

MEDICAL TEAM

Not only the child and his family, but all members of the medical team must proceed through these same stages if they are to reach the point where they are emotionally prepared to accept the ultimate loss. Like patient and family, medical staff may get stuck at any stage. The result of such an arrest will be not just a prolongation of that particular stage, but signs of increasing distress and, frequently, pathological and disruptive behaviour by members of the medical team. One might summarize the various reactions of those involved to each of the stages as follows:

1. *Shock and denial.* Members of the medical team may feel overwhelmed by the diagnosis and its implications. In their shock, they may

continue to question the diagnosis even when the evidence is unequivocal, or they may seek to shield themselves from the psychological impact of the diagnosis by prolonged laboratory investigation which no longer has either practical meaning or relevance. Dreading to share the diagnosis with the family and fearing their ability to handle the resulting upset, they may put off dealing directly with the parents or, alternately, may overwhelm them with more facts than they can assimilate. Much of what parents perceive as insensitivity and lack of concern on the part of physicians results, in fact, from behaviour arising out of their doctor's attempts to deal with his initial shock.

2. *Anger and protest.* Physicians frequently rebound from their initial shock and respond to the families of their dying patients with resentment and even rage. This may be directed against the family of the patient who, not without reason, may be seen as difficult, demanding, or unappreciative. It may be displaced to other members of the medical team—family practitioner, surgeon or other specialist, nurses—who are blamed for supposed mishandling of the case. Rage may be vented periodically, through angry explosions in the operating room or on the ward; when these occur, they are related to feelings of helplessness and frustration. Resentment may be displaced onto the child, who is attacked for being uncooperative and acting "like a baby" or turned on the parents, who are seen as overprotective and uncooperative. At times, the physician's anger may be trapped within himself, leading to draining and unproductive self-pity around the fact that so many difficult cases land on his doorstep.

3. *Bargaining.* Physicians and nurses, like the family, may attempt to bargain for the life of their dying patient. They may pledge to be more conscientious in the future, to read journals regularly, even (in the case of nurses) to go on night duty if only a particular child of whom they are fond can recover to go home one more time before she dies.

4. *Depression.* Physicians frequently experience short-lived frustration and discouragement, which can at times grow into unrealistic feelings of inadequacy or self-blame. The physician may become unduly critical of his own work, blaming himself because, for a defined period of time, his statistics are worse than those reported by other centres while ignoring the fact that for some months previously they were better. The self-criticism may develop into full-blown episodes of clinical depression, which may greatly decrease the efficiency of functioning not only as a physician, but as a husband, wife, or parent. This is reflected in the

high incidence of marriage breakdown and emotional problems in physicians' families. Alternately, various forms of escape which serve as defences against the threat of emerging depression (compulsive overwork, abuse of alcohol or drugs, etc.) may be prominent.

5. *Acceptance.* When this stage is reached, the physician is able to live comfortably with the fact that he did all that he could do to prolong the life and decrease the suffering of child and family. He may be aided by the thought that through death the child has been spared further suffering or that from what he has learned from this case he may be more effective in dealing with other similar problems in the future.

Conclusion

While there is a common pattern of reactions to the fatally ill child as outlined above, each situation and each patient or potential patient (which includes all significant family members) must be considered individually. If the physician and his team consider fully and deal appropriately with the stresses that a lethal illness produces, they can have an active role in preventing emotional problems in the patient, in that patient's family, and in the medical and hospital staff treating them.

RECOMMENDED FOR FURTHER READING

1. ANTHONY, E. J., and KOUPERNIK, C., eds. *The Child in His Family.* Vol. 2: *The Impact of Death and Disease.* New York, Wiley and Sons, 1973.
—a highly recommended collection of papers dealing with problems and reactions of children and parents to disease, death, and mourning.

2. BARTON, D. "Teaching Psychiatry in the Context of Death and Dying". *Amer. J. Psychiat.* 130: 1290–91, 1973.
—discusses the interpersonal and socio-cultural dimensions of death as well as ethical considerations and individual responses.

3. BERNSTEIN, D. M. "After Transplantation—The Child's Emotional Reactions". *Amer. J. Psychiat.* 127: 1189–93, 1970–71.
—in this study it was found that anxiety about fear of death was often aroused whether or not there were signs of kidney rejection. Urges the psychiatrist, surgeon, and nephrologist to be alert and compassionate in dealing with the emotional problems which often arise in child transplant patients.

4. BINGER, C. M.; ALBIN, A. R.; FEVERSTEIN, R. C.; KUSHNER, J. H.; ZOGER, S.; and MIKKELSEN, C. "Childhood Leukemia—Emotional Impact on Patient and Family". *New Eng. J. Med.* 280: 414–18, 1969.
—good for the medical reader.

5. BOZEMAN, M. F.; ORBACH, C. E.; and SUTHERLAND, A. M. "Psychological Impact of Cancer and Its Treatment (III); The Adaption of Mothers to the Threatened Loss of their Children through Leukemia (II)". *Cancer.* 8: 1–33, 1955.
—describes parental reactions to diagnosis of acute leukemia in their young children, including shock, denial, anxiety, guilt, depression. Hostility to doctors and inability to comprehend information given are common reactions to the crisis precipitated by the illness and the ability of the physician to establish and maintain a supportive relationship with the parents may be crucial. An excellent discussion of the difficulties faced by hospital staff.

6. EASSON, W. M. "Care of the Young Patient Who Is Dying". *J. Amer. Med. Assoc.* 205: 203–7, 1968.
—reactions vary with age; clinical management must reflect this.

7. FEIFEL, M., and HANSON, S. "Physicians Consider Death". *Proceedings of Seventh Annual Convention, American Psychological Association,* 201, 1967.
—physicians frequently have particular problems with death.

8. FEIFEL, M. "Death", in Farberow, M. L., ed., *Taboo Topics*, pp. 8–21. New York, Atherton Press, 1963.
—it's time death was no longer taboo!

9. FRIEDMAN, S. B. "Care of the Family of the Child with Cancer". *Pediat.* 40: 498–507, 1967.

10. HOROWITZ, L. "Treatment of the Family with a Dying Member". *Fam. Proc.* 14: 95–106, 1975.
—focuses on the uses of transference and counter-transference in the treatment of families with a dying member.

11. KAPLAN, D. M.; SMITH, A.; GROBSTEIN, R.; and FISCHMAN, S. E. "Family Mediation of Stress". *Soc. Work.* 18:60–69, July 1973.
—deals with the impact of stress on the whole family.

12. KLIMAN, G. *Psychological Emergencies of Childhood.* New York, Grune and Stratton, 1968.
—excellent little book emphasizing the need to move towards an approach that can prevent the development of psychological emergencies.

13. KOOCHER, G. P. "Talking with Children about Death". *Amer. J. Orthopsychiat.* 44: 404–11, 1974.
—after describing responses of seventy-five children, ages six to fifteen, to questions about death, offers suggestions for discussing death with a child who has suffered a loss.

14. KUBLER-ROSS, E. *On Death and Dying.* Toronto, Collier-Macmillan, 1967.
—classic book—should be read by all medical and nursing students, and all who deal with seriously ill children and their families.

15. LANSKY, S. B. "Childhood Leukemia: The Child Psychiatrist as a Member of the Oncology Team". *J. Amer. Acad. Child Psychiat.* 13: 499–508, 1974.
—preliminary report of an ongoing study of the leukemic child and his family. Discusses the impact of prolonged anticipation of death on child and family recommending that a child psychiatrist be part of the treatment plan.

16. LURIE, M. J., and GALLAGHER, J. M. "Innovative Techniques for Teaching Psychiatric Principles to General Practitioners". *J. Amer. Med. Assoc.* 221: 696–99, 1972.
—illustrates the need to remain "involved" to learn, although learning may be painful.

17. MARSTEIN, B. "The Effects of Long-Term Illness of Children on the Emotional Adjustment of Parents". *Child Devel.* 31: 151–71, 1960.
—emphasizes that disease produces "other" diseases.

18. PAKES, E. H. "Child Psychiatry and Pediatric Practice; How Disciplines Work Together". *Ont. Med. Rev.* 41: 69–71, Feb. 1974.
—deals with the important bridge between child psychiatry and paediatrics. The new physician should bridge that gap!

22. SCHOWALTER, J. E.; FERHOLT, J. B.; and MANN, N. M. "The Adolescent Patient's Decision to Die". *Pediat.* 51: 97–103, 1973.
—compassionate definitive discussion of the problems faced by the medical team caring for an adolescent patient who chooses to die.

23. SOLNIT, A. J., and GREEN, M. "Psychologic Considerations in the Management of Deaths on Pediatric Hospital Services: The Doctor and the Child's Family". *Pediat.* 24: 106–12, 1959.
—sound advice regarding the management of the family of the child who dies.

24. TOOLEY, K. "The Choice of a Surviving Sibling as 'Scapegoat' in Some

Cases of Maternal Bereavement—A Case Report". *J. Child Psychol. Psychiat.* 16: 331–39, 1975.
—describes a pathological variation of the mourning process in mothers who suffer the psychologically damaging loss of a child whereby a surviving sibling is chosen as a scapegoat for their guilt and self-hatred. Suggests that counselling at the time of bereavement would help prevent this scapegoating. Interesting case report and analysis.

ADDITIONAL READING

19. RICHMOND, J. B., and WAISMAN, H. A. "Psychologic Aspects of Management of Children with Malignant Diseases". *Amer. J. Dis. Child.* 89: 42–47, 1955.

20. ROTHENBERG, M. B. "Reactions of Those Who Treat Children with Cancer". *Pediat.* 40: 507–10, 1967.

21. SCHOWALTER, J. E. "Death and the Pediatric House Officer". *J. Pediat.* 76, 5: 706–10, 1970.

25. WEINER, J. M. "Attitudes of Pediatricians Toward the Care of Fatally Ill Children". *J. Pediat.* 76: 700–705, 1970.

SIMON KREINDLER

19. The Battered Child and His Family

The battered-child syndrome, first described in 1962, refers to a constellation of signs and symptoms seen in children who have received non-accidental physical injury as a result of acts of commission or omission on the part of their parents or guardians.

Incidence

Estimates place the incidence between 250 and 350 cases per million population per year in urban areas. One extensive study suggests that the actual incidence of abuse substantially exceeds officially reported figures.[4] The sex distribution is about equally divided between boys and girls, although boys outnumber girls in every age group below age twelve, whereas girls significantly outnumber boys among teenagers. Child abuse is not confined to very young children, as is frequently thought to be the case. One recent survey in the United States found that over 75 per cent of battered children were over two years of age and nearly 50 per cent were over six years.[2, 10] The most serious injuries, however, occur in the under-three age group, and in this group 65 per cent of those forty children who were fatally injured in Canada from 1965 through 1970 were girls.

Prematurely born infants as a group are well recognized to be at high risk for subsequent physical abuse. Problems in mother-infant bonding are accentuated and complicated by prematurity and probably play a significant role. A major study now in progress suggests a number of factors that may contribute to the failure to develop an adequate bond between infant and mother. These include the very large number of nurses caring for each premature infant in comparison with that experienced by the average newborn in regular contact with his mother.

Child abuse occurs within all ethnic groups and within all socio-economic levels of society. The larger number of cases reported among ethnic minority groups is a reflection partly of discriminatory reporting attitudes and partly of a higher incidence among these families of socio-economic deprivation, fatherless homes, and large families, all of which have been found to be strongly associated with child abuse.

Diagnosis

A diagnosis of child abuse should be considered when some of the following findings are present:[6]

When the parent:

1. presents a history that cannot or does not adequately explain the child's injury or that is otherwise contradictory;
2. is hostile and uncooperative in providing a history;
3. has delayed unduly in bringing the child for medical examination or hospital care;
4. seems detached and inappropriately unconcerned by the seriousness of the child's injury;
5. expresses concern about the possibility of losing control and hurting the child or gives other indications of previous loss of control;
6. refuses hospitalization of the child or further diagnostic studies;
7. has a tendency to "shop around" from hospital to hospital;
8. does not visit the child in hospital, visits only infrequently, or visits only for the sake of appearance;
9. does not relate to the child during visits;
10. lacks usual concern regarding the child's prognosis;
11. is disliked by the hospital staff;
12. is often difficult to locate and frequently moves the family to new locations;
13. gives a history that indicates that he has suffered serious emotional deprivation and physical abuse himself;
14. has an unstable marital relationship;
15. has few friends and no reliable sources of outside help to turn to when under stress;
16. has unrealistic expectations of the child;

17. gives a history of misuse of alcohol and/or drugs.

When the child:

1. has an unexplained injury;
2. shows over-all evidence of poor care;
3. shows evidence of dehydration and/or malnutrition without obvious cause;
4. has been given inappropriate food, drink, or drugs;
5. is unusually fearful;
6. cries very little in general but does so hopelessly when examined in hospital;
7. does not look to the parents for reassurance;
8. is wary of physical contact or, in the case of the older child, seeks the attention of adults indiscriminately;
9. is apprehensive when other children cry;
10. seems hyperalert to the environment;
11. shows injuries that are not mentioned in the history provided by the parents;
12. shows evidence of previous injury or repeated recent injury;
13. shows evidence of multiple and/or old fractures;
14. shows a pseudomature ability to respond to parental expectations;
15. is viewed as "different" or "bad" by parents regardless of the reality;
16. in the older child: seems afraid of parent(s); gives a contradictory history of how the injury occurred; parrots the parental explanation of the injury; denies the existence of parental conflict or family problems; denies previous abuse where this is known to have occurred.

Psychodynamic Factors

Parents who abuse their children may manifest just about any type of psychopathology. With the exception of a small number who are clearly sociopathic or psychotic, the majority do not fall into any one diagnostic category although they have a good many features in common. Parents who abuse children frequently manifest a pattern of behaviours that can exist either in combination with, or independently of, other psychological disorders. Characteristic findings are that:

1. abusive parents expect and demand a great deal from their infants and children;
2. their demands for performance are not only great, but premature and

clearly beyond the ability of the infant to comprehend what is wanted and to be able to respond appropriately;

3. these parents feel uncertain of how lovable they themselves are and look to their children for reassurance, comfort, and love. They relate to their children as if they were adults capable of providing them with comfort and love—a phenomenon described as "role reversal".

If these characteristics are present *the parent will likely have a high potential for being abusive*. In order for battering to occur, however, it is necessary that there be the simultaneous interaction of at least two other variables. These include *factors in the child* him/herself. These involve the child who is somehow special, for example, because of prematurity, specific physical defect, or because he/she is psychologically different from other normal children or is viewed by the parent(s) as different. Finally, *there must be a crisis*, which may be major, such as abandonment by a spouse, loss of a parent, an unwanted pregnancy, or loss of a job, or, which may be minor, such as a hairstyle that did not come out just right or an imagined rejection when a parent feels that a spouse prefers one of the children to him/her.

Many abusive parents give a history of having been raised in much the same way that they are raising their own children. Many of these parents when they were young were denied an opportunity to have the kind of mothering necessary for the development of a sense of confidence or basic trust. This deprivation, which results in a lack of the deep sense of being cared for and cared about from the beginning of one's life can, and often does, occur in the presence of considerable maternal attention and material abundance.

The distinction has been made between the practical or mechanical aspects of mothering (the feeding, holding, clothing, and cleaning of the infant) and the more subtle ingredients of tenderness, awareness, and emotional interaction with it. *Breakdown and failure in the more mechanical aspects of mothering* seems to result in the *neglected* child or the infant with *failure to thrive*. On the other hand, *physical abuse* is associated with *a failure in the development of an empathic relationship between parent and child.*[5]

Treatment

Once the diagnosis of physical abuse has been made and even in cases where it is only possible to have a high degree of suspicion, a multifaceted treatment approach must be instituted. In the first place, the abused child may require medical and/or surgical treatment for which hospitalization may be necessary. If hospitalization is not necessary, one then has to decide whether it is safe to return the child to his home or whether a temporary alternative placement is indicated. At a somewhat later date we can assess the child's development and psychological status to better decide whether any form of psychological intervention seems necessary. Simultaneous with the immediate paediatric and environmental management of the child is the very important task of approaching the parents (or parent) in a sympathetic, non-punitive way. If the child has been hospitalized, the initial approach may have already been made by a paediatrician who should share with the parents the physical findings and any further investigations that are planned. There is a great temptation in all of us to respond to an abusing parent in one of two ways. Either we become very angry or we identify with the parent and deny the possibility that he/she could, in fact, have been responsible for the abuse. Neither of these approaches is of any value. The physician or worker who attempts to help the abusing parents must remain empathic even in the face of sometimes considerable anger directed at him and must attempt to convey to the parents the wish to understand the kinds of internal and external stresses which they have, unsuccessfully, been attempting to cope with.

The immediate management of the parents most frequently involves the intervention of a caseworker from a social agency that has the authority under law to protect and, if necessary, provide care for children who, in their own families, are neglected or abused. These agencies, which are called either children's aid societies or child welfare associations can, in addition to providing a therapeutic relationship, help to arrange for a number of environmental supports such as homemakers; day-care or nursery placement for the abused child and/or siblings; assistance with finding and/or paying for a babysitter; help with finding employment; assistance with arranging educational upgrading, etc. Later one may want to consider referral to self-help groups such as Parents Anonymous. In some cases, referral for marital counselling or individual psychotherapy may be indicated.

In the vast majority of cases a fairly prolonged period of therapeutic involvement on the part of the children's aid society worker is necessary in order to bring about any change in this type of parent. If a psychiatrist is not directly treating the parent or child he may be called upon to act as a consultant to the worker responsible for the case or, at other times, to make recommendations regarding the need for treatment of the abused child, and possibly also his/her siblings. It is important that all physicians and workers be aware that many children raised in an abusive environment demonstrate developmental delays of one sort or another to the point where they may be diagnosed as "retarded." If the situation is recognized early enough, functional retardation of this type can be reversed by providing the child with a loving environment where he receives the previously missing stimulation. The longer the condition goes unrecognized, the harder it is to reverse this problem. Even where the situation has been recognized early, it is important to remember that it sometimes takes several months before improvement may be seen. For instance, it has been noted that over a three to six month period a previously abused child, with what appears to be a normal intellectual potential, will start to demonstrate increased attention span; increased imitativeness; increased interest in problem solving; a more positive response to praise; more creative play; and a greater interest in the people and things around him. Once these new behaviours start to appear the child seems capable of an accelerated development. However, a further six months may be needed to demonstrate changes on test scores.

One of our major tasks in helping the abused child in his subsequent development involves the superficial quality of his/her relationships with others. On the surface, these children often seem fairly normal although when observed over a longer period of time it becomes clear that they have only casual associations with peers and much difficulty in having a relationship of genuine trust with someone special. These children often rely on cues from other people in helping them decide what would be an appropriate response at a particular time. Only if this problem is adequately dealt with will it be possible for these children to develop a healthy self-esteem and, as adults, to be capable of intimacy.

Once an adequate plan of treatment has been instituted, it may be necessary to face the question of the child's placement once again. In general, it is not safe to return the abused child home until there is strong evidence that the parents have found ways of getting satisfaction and pleasure in life so that they no longer have to turn to the child to satisfy their own emotional needs. The parents' abilities to help each other and to reach out for professional help in times of crisis are good indications of the safety of the home. If the parents continue to misperceive the child and to have unrealistic expectations of him, return home is contra-indicated. Parents who pressure the child welfare association or court to return the child because of fears of public or family disapproval should alert us to the likelihood that little has changed where the safety of the child is concerned.

The following list of guidelines can be used to assess the safety of the home when return of the child is being contemplated.[6] The home is more likely to be safe if:

1. the parents have demonstrated a willingness and ability to use others in time of need or crisis;
2. the parents are developing some outside-the-home interests;
3. the parents are developing an improved self-image;
4. help is available to the parents on an on-call basis twenty-four hours a day;
5. the spouse is able to recognize when his/her partner needs help and is willing to do something about it;
6. obvious, previous crises, for example, housing, food, job, illness, etc. have been resolved;
7. obstacles to getting help are minimal; for example, is a telephone available?
8. the parents no longer perceive the child as bad or different;
9. the parents' expectations of the child are realistic;
10. the child is pleasing to the parents, who see the child as an individual with needs of his own;
11. the parents are willing to accept help for the child to meet his special needs (medical, social, psychological, etc.);
12. the parents have been conscientious in keeping follow-up appointments for the child with special needs.

Finally, it must be remembered that the child under three is statistically at a much higher risk of being reinjured than is the case with the child over three.

After the child has been returned home, however, it is essential that treatment continue, as Kempe and Helfer advise:

> When all has gone well and the parents have improved and the child has returned home, there is often a tendency for either parent(s) or worker to consider that everything is now all right and that treatment should be discontinued. This should never be done. The continuation of treatment is crucially important at

this time, since not only is there a need to consolidate gains which have already been made, but it is necessary to see that the inevitable shifts in emotion and changes in living patterns caused by the return of the child can be managed without regression to previous unhealthy patterns. The purpose of treatment is, after all, not just to return the child home, but to improve the total living pattern of the family and to significantly alter the parent-child interaction.[6]

Prognosis

It should be evident that the prognosis in cases of child abuse depends on many variables. Probably more than 50 per cent of battered children have been physically abused prior to the incident that brought them to the hospital for medical attention. In fact, it has been suggested that physical abuse of children is more often than not an indication of a prevailing pattern of caretaker-child interaction in a given home than an isolated incident. It is also estimated that there is a 25 to 50 per cent risk of permanent injury or death if an abused child is returned home without there being any intervention. Where intervention takes place, the prognosis for the child depends not only on the prognosis for rehabilitating the parents but also on the type and severity of the injury sustained by the child. Obviously the effects of severe head trauma or long-standing physical neglect and emotional deprivation are going to be much more devastating than a broken leg or bruised buttocks.

As for the abusive parents, they are generally not "good patients" in the traditional sense. Those who actively resist all manner of therapeutic involvement have the poorest prognosis. These parents generally compose the least stable families in terms of frequently changing marital partnerships, abuse of drugs and alcohol, unemployment, frequent moves from one community to another, etc. The prognosis becomes more and more guarded as the number of these adverse variables increases and is probably poorest where the situation is compounded by a parent who is either sociopathic or frankly psychotic. For parents who can be involved in a therapeutic relationship, however, and can learn to reach out to helping individuals in times of crisis, the prognosis is probably good. It is even better if the parents can come to have a more realistic view of the child and be able to accept him/her as an individual with certain capabilities and needs of his own. If the parents can, in addition, develop a more worthwhile sense of themselves, the prognosis is probably excellent.

Prevention

Preventive measures to be undertaken to combat child abuse would include the following:

1. cultural and legal sanctions against the use of violence or physical force in child-rearing or education;
2. the elimination of poverty and assurance of an equal opportunity to enjoy life for all members of society. This measure would involve adequate income, health care, social services, housing, educational, cultural, and recreational facilities for all members of the community without discrimination;
3. comprehensive family-planning programs, including abortions, in order to reduce the number of unwanted and rejected children, who are the major victims of child abuse;
4. family life education and counselling programs for adolescents and young adults preparing for marriage and parenthood;
5. high-quality, locally available social and medical child-welfare and protection services, which can decrease the environmental and internal stress on family life;
6. improved co-operation and communication between family physicians, hospitals (particularly emergency services and family-practice units), children's aid societies or child-welfare associations, police, courts, and other community agencies.

RECOMMENDED FOR FURTHER READING

1. GELLES, R. J. "Child Abuse as Psychopathology: A Sociological Critique and Reformulation". *Amer. J. Orthopsychiat.* 43: 611–21, 1973.
   —highly technical but useful and relevant critical evaluation of a psychopathological theory of child abuse, suggesting greater emphasis on sociological and contextual variables for a more balanced approach to cases involving abuse.

2. GIL, D. G. *Violence Against Children: Physical Abuse in the United States*. Boston, Mass., Harvard University Press, 1973.
   —reviews the literature and documents of a scientifically conducted nationwide survey regarding the incidence, contributing causes, age distribution, etc., of all cases of abuse reported in the U.S. in 1967 and 1968.

3. GREEN, A. H.; GAINES, R. W.; and SANDGRUND, A. "Child Abuse: Pathological Syndrome of Family Interaction". *Amer. J. Psychiat.* 131,2: 882–86, 1974.
—child abuse is described as the end result of: the abuse-prone personality of the parent(s); characteristics of the child that invite scapegoating; current environmental stress.

4. GREENLAND, C. *Child Abuse in Ontario.* Research Report 3, Toronto, Ontario Ministry of Community and Social Services, Research and Planning Branch, 1973.

5. HELFER, R. E.; and KEMPE, C. H. *The Battered Child.* Chicago, University of Chicago Press, 1974.
—a classic text with excellent chapter on the psychiatric aspects of abuse.

6. KEMPE, C. H., and HELFER, R. E. *Helping the Battered Child and His Family.* Philadelphia, J. B. Lippincott, 1972.
—a very practical text for those who must deal directly with the battered child and the abusing parent.

7. MINDE, K.; FORD, L.; CELHOFFER, L.; and BOUKYDIS, C. "Interactions of Mothers and Nurses with Premature Infants". *Canad. Med. Assoc. J.* 113: 741–45, 1975.
—studies the interaction between mothers and their premature infants in a premature nursery, defining criteria that can be used to predict a possible failure of bonding and an increased incidence of parenting disorders.

8. NEUBERGER, E. H. "The Myth of the Battered Child Syndrome: A Compassionate Medical View of the Protection of Children". *Current Medical Dialogue.* 40: 327–34, 1973.
—this excellent, concise article seeks a coherent and humane approach to child abuse, which is viewed as a symptom of distress in a complex family system.

9. OLIVER, J. E., and COX, J. "A Family Kindred with Ill-Used Children: The Burden on the Community". *Brit. J. Psychiat.* 123: 81–90, 1973.
—discusses the problems of ill-used children in the family, mental and personality disorders in family members, and community support for the family.

10. VAN STOLK, M. *The Battered Child in Canada.* Toronto, McClelland and Stewart, 1972.

GRAHAM BERMAN

20. Family Disruption and Its Effects

Under ideal circumstances, a child is born and grows to maturity within an intact and stable family. Such a family does more than merely meet the child's physical needs. It helps children develop a sense of security and supports them as they mature and develop. In such a family, the needs of the children are reliably met, and their actions and communications bring predictable responses from familiar people in familiar surroundings.

Not all children are so fortunate. The incidence of nuclear-family breakdown is showing a striking increase. Any break in family continuity may cause great distress. It faces the child with all the contradictory feelings stirred up by the absence of the missing parent. He may also find that his needs are neglected or now met in a different way, and that his ways of communicating no longer bring the expected responses.

Factors That Affect the Child's Reaction to Family Disruption

Not all children respond in the same way to the disruption of their family. A given child's reaction to family disruption and to prolonged separation from those on whom he has relied for care and security will depend on:

1. *The characteristics of the individual child.* Some children react with relative tolerance, others with great distress to the same disruptive event in their lives. Some in time will be able to accept a substitute caretaker.

Others will continue to reject and to invite rejection as a reaction to the disruption.

2. *The phase of development.* A child under six months does not usually show prolonged ill-effects. Older children tend not only to experience distress at the time, but may regress in their development, often continuing to show long-term emotional after-effects.

3. *Previous experiences.* A child who feels secure with the present parents can be expected to show much distress on prolonged separation. On the other hand, children who have had repeated disappointments in relationships are more likely to protect themselves from a further hurt by remaining superficial or apathetic both within their relationships and at times of separation.

4. *The preparation for separation.* Stories and free discussion about an expected change in their living situation can help children understand and to some extent prepare themselves emotionally for the experience. If they are to be in the care of a stranger or living in an unfamiliar place, it is valuable to spend some time familiarizing them with the new situation in advance. A new caretaker should become familiar with the habits, routines, and communication patterns that were typical of the previous adult-child relationship.

5. *The nature of the separation.* It is easier for children to cope with an expected separation in controlled circumstances with a familiar person available to offer support. However, separations are often initiated in frightening circumstances, for instance, during a violent argument or a drunken brawl. Not infrequently a social agency, having judged the parents incompetent and having obtained an appropriate court order, apprehends the child on the street and takes him to an unknown foster home.

6. *The experience during separation.* It is an exceptional parent or foster parent who has both the sensitivity and the patience to support a child through the fear and rage that follow loss of the primary caretaker. Ideally the adult should be available to help the child express his feelings of loss, to accept his feelings of abandonment and rage, and to learn the child's modes of communication and special needs. More often the child is left to withdraw into apathy. Sometimes his protest is punished, and an interminable war is launched between adult and child. It is helpful for the child to continue contact with the missing parent when this is possible. The more familiar the new living situation, the less difficult it will be for the child to adapt.

7. *Care after reunion.* If a child is reunited with parents after a period of separation, there may be periods of apathy, of great anger, and of regressive behaviour as he copes with feelings of uncertainty, suspicion, and rage at what he sees as their initial desertion. To some degree such reactions may follow even such trivial (to adults) absences as the parents going away on a holiday or the mother entering hospital to give birth to a new baby. Should the reaction persist, parents may need counselling to help them understand and support the child until he again feels secure enough to give up his disturbing behaviour.

Examples of Disruption of Family Continuity

1. *Simple separation.* The above principles apply, for example, to the care of children when their parents go on vacation. The birth of a sibling introduces additional problems, in that the mother may have less time or a changed routine on her return. Because of this, the older child then experiences, and is expected to adjust to, a permanent loss of some parental attention.
2. *Hospitalization.* This is discussed in more detail in Chapter 17, "Hospitalization and Its Meaning to the Child and His Family". The child is separated from family, familiar environment, and activities, and is looked after by a series of caretakers who have no time to get to know him. Often he is subjected to procedures that may be both frightening and painful. The presence of parents in the hospital can reduce the difficulties, but the parents, too, are often frightened and confused. They may also have other children at home, who may experience and present difficulties as they react to the parents' anxiety and preoccupation with the sick child (see Chapter 16).
3. *Marriage breakdown (separation and divorce).* Children are frightened by parental fighting and are very sensitive to unacknowledged parental disagreement. It is possible that parental separation will be better for the children than being raised in an atmosphere of chronic marital tension and discord. Continuity of care is provided by the custody of one parent and by visits with the other. Often, however, the children suffer from the separation. They may feel guilty, blaming themselves unrealistically for the marriage problems. Frequently they are, indeed, drawn into the problem as the parents compete for the child's affection or use custody, visiting rights, or the withholding of child-support money to needle the estranged partner. The single parent, still struggling with his or her own reactions to the marriage breakdown,

often has difficulty getting relief from the children's demands. The introduction of a new sexual or marital partner may create crises as step-parent, partner, and children work out their relationship.

> Brian, age twelve, remarked to his step-mother, "You may be a very nice person, and my dad chose you because he wanted you to be his wife. But I had no choice about whether I wanted you to be my mother." The step-mother had earlier stated that she felt like an outsider in her new family, excluded from the intimacy that she felt her husband shared with his two sons by a previous marriage. She felt resented and unappreciated when her initial overtures to her step-sons were rejected, and she responded by resenting and scapegoating the boys, whom she saw as rivals for her husband's affection. She was afraid to express this resentment for fear it would antagonize her husband and undermine her marriage. She felt, and not without reason, that Brian unfavourably compared her with his natural mother, whom, since he rarely saw her, he perceived in idealized terms, and whom he played off against her. Her husband, upset by her increasing rejection of Brian and her increasing withdrawal from him, unsuccessfully attempted to mediate between the two of them only to blame each in turn for not trying hard enough and jeopardizing his remarriage.

4. *Custody disputes.* The legal process has yet to develop an effective method for giving due consideration to the child's interests in a custody dispute. Disputes are usually between adults competing for custody. Evidence concerning the needs of the child may or may not be introduced, depending on the lawyers' estimates of the probability of advantage to their clients. While the law presumes that parents will act in the best interests of their child, two parents locked in bitter conflict following the breakdown of their marriage are frequently so preoccupied with their struggle with each other that the interests of the child are frequently ignored. At times, there may be attempts to induce psychiatrists or other mental-health personnel to take sides in this struggle. This has, on occasion, led to courtroom battles of the experts, in which his psychiatrists battle hers in a further escalation of the marital conflict. An increasing number of psychiatrists and other mental-health personnel are refusing to be drawn into the struggle on these terms. They make clear

their readiness to provide an assessment of the situation and any recommendations regarding custody, access, or related matters arising from this assessment, but only if both parties and their lawyers agree to their involvement on these terms. When the dispute is between a biological parent and, for example, an adoptive parent who has not yet had the child long enough to complete the legal adoption process, then the wishes of the biological parent tend to be considered ahead of the interests of the child. The parents' tensions during periods of waiting for litigation and during litigation itself frequently are upsetting, and if the court orders a change of caretaker, the child usually will be affected adversely by the disruption of his relationships. It is for these reasons that proponents of child advocacy argue that the child should be separately represented in court by someone able to determine and to speak for his best interests during any litigation where custody is in dispute.

5. *Death of a parent.* The effects depend on the child's developmental status and the relationship with the dead and surviving parent. The child may show varying degrees of searching for the missing parent or a replacment. He may express rage and grief, withdrawal or simple denial of loss, acting as if nothing has happened. The child may feel guilty, as if responsible for the death. Childhood bereavement may result in certain lasting difficulties in interpersonal relationships, as when the subject repeatedly and compulsively demands that others fulfil his excessive craving for gratification and affection derived from earlier developmental needs left unsatisfied as the result of the parental loss.

6. *Adoption.* Ideally, adoption should occur soon after birth, so that the child can immediately form a relationship with the parents who will continue in his life. When this occurs, the adoptive parents, as those who on a day-to-day basis meet all the child's needs, will naturally over a period of time become his psychological parents. This means that they will be the ones to whom the child will turn and on whom he will rely to meet both his physical demands and his need for security. Most infant adoptions are successful. If problems occur in later years, the fact of adoption may be seized upon by parents as the only or the sufficient cause for the difficulties. Should the parents insist that the child is congenitally tainted ("bad seed") and that obvious tensions between him and the family do not exist or are unrelated to the child's difficulties, this will usually reflect a serious degree of parental rejection, which may be a major contributor to the total problem.

It is advisable that parents be willing to discuss the child's adoption as soon as he is able to understand and ask questions, so that it becomes accepted as a normal fact of the family life. These discussions will probably have to be repeated on occasions as the child grows and matures. Explanations that would be appropriate at one age are totally inadequate at another. Parents of a teenager who are being pressed to explain why their child's biological parents gave him up for adoption cannot dodge the issue by a rhapsody on how they chose him as an infant and how much they valued him. It would be equally inappropriate for the parents of a three-year-old to go into an extended discussion of the reasons why his unmarried mother decided against raising him herself. While there is no set formula as to exactly what to say to the child at a given age, the general principle of telling the child what he wants to know as he asks it in a way that can be understood by someone of his age remains a good one. The child usually integrates the biological parents into his fantasy life, imagining reasons why they might have abandoned him (because he was no good, they wanted him but were too poor, etc.), imagining meeting them or escaping to them.

The child who moves to new parents after establishing a relationship with earlier caretakers faces considerable difficulty. Consider, for example, the child raised in a foster home and later placed for adoption. After a brief "honeymoon period", new parents should expect to be faced with the child's distress, rage, and grief at being separated from those he saw as his psychological parents. The child may lose some acquired skills, withdraw, fight, reject, and oppose new parents, or wander off seeking the lost parents. This adjustment process can last for years, and may fail despite the best intentions and efforts of all involved.

7. *Foster homes.* In most cases foster-home placement is originally undertaken in response to the temporary or permanent breakdown of the nuclear family's ability to care for the child. Children placed in foster homes are frequently already quite disturbed as a result of their years of living in a family that, for a variety of reasons, has been chronically unable to meet their need for acceptance, consistency, and security. The disturbance frequently may be aggravated by the separation that led to the foster-home placement. Foster parents must face the fear, anger, despair, and withdrawal that represents the child's reaction to his unhappy life situation. Foster parents often have a caseworker assigned to them by the children's aid society or child welfare association that assumed responsibility for the welfare and care of the child when he was

removed from his parents. These caseworkers, whose job is to help foster parents deal with problems arising as the foster child attempts to adjust to life within their home, have caseloads often too great to allow them to give foster parents the available consultation and support they need. A further difficulty is that since the child is the "property" of the agency, the foster parents are often not free to form a permanent commitment to the child. This sense of impermance may impair the child's efforts to find security and the foster parents' efforts to provide it. As a result, foster-home placements are inherently unstable. They frequently break down. Multiple changes of foster homes are not uncommon. The more frequent the changes, the greater the degree and permanence of the resulting disturbance. These realities should be born in mind before recommending that a child be removed even from a family situation that is far from ideal.

Despite these difficulties, many able foster parents succeed in giving excellent care to their foster children, forming bonds of affection that survive many years. Ideally, foster-home placement should be preceded by skilled work with the child and if possible with the child's family, with the aim of helping them understand, cope with, and hopefully help prepare the child for the change. The foster parents may need much help in understanding the child's reactions, if they are to respond to them appropriately. Finally, great care should be taken to help the child feel some sense of continuity in his life rather than, as is often the case, experiencing it as divided into discontinous and isolated segments. Feelings and memories of natural parents and previous foster parents, both positive and negative, may persist long after the child has been moved away. If recognized, these may prove vital in helping the child obtain the sense of historical continuity and identity he so badly needs.

8. *Group foster homes.* The group-home development results from attempts to provide the close personal interactions of a foster home in a more professional and organized way while avoiding the impersonal character of a larger institution. Frequently group homes are used for those who have failed to stabilize in alternative settings. They allow skilled foster parents or social workers to care for the child as an individual while at the same time helping him in his social relationships. The child's difficulties in adjusting to a group home are similar to those he may experience in other settings following separation from his family. Group homes of seriously disturbed children place enormous

demands on staff. Foster parents or staff can provide warmth and help only as long as they can withstand the continuous strain and frustration. Their discouragement and frustration are exacerbated when no encouraging signs of change and maturity in the children are evident.

In selecting a group-home placement for a given child, one would want to understand the nature of the difficulties of children already in the home, the personal and professional qualifications of the staff, and the professional back-up from social workers or psychiatrists available to help the staff understand the needs of the children and sustain the pressures without having either to retaliate or to withdraw emotionally from the children.

RECOMMENDED FOR FURTHER READING

1. ADAMS, P. L. "Functions of the Lower-Class Partial Family". *Amer. J. Psychiat.* 130: 200–203, 1973.
—compares functions regarding sexuality, economic life changes, authority, and honour between complete and partial (fatherless) lower-class families. Describes the partial family as functioning defectively in biologic maintenance, social control, enculturation of children, status placement, and emotional maintenance.

2. BENEDEK, E. P., and BENEDEK, R. S. "New Child Custody Laws: Making Them Do What They Say". *Amer. J. Orthopsychiat.* 42: 825–34, 1972.
—presents ten guidelines relevant to child custody laws in Michigan and discusses their application.

3. BOHMAN, M. "A Study of Adopted Children, Their Background, Environment, and Adjustment". *Acta. Paediat. Scand.* 61: 90–97, 1972.
—summarizes results of a three-year study of adopted children and their families. Investigates reasons for behaviour disturbances in adopted children. Clear and concise.

4. BRODY, E. M. "Aging and Family Personality: A Developmental View". *Fam. Process* 13,1: 23–37, 1974.
—discusses some issues of death, loss, separation, and aging, as they relate to individual and family development and to shifting roles and responsibilities of family members.

5. CALDWELL, B. M. "What Does Research Teach Us About Day Care for Children Under Three?" *Children Today*. Vol. 1: 6–12, Jan.-Feb. 1972.

—discusses such issues as intellectual, social, emotional development, and health of children under three who are separated from their parents for all or part of the day. Also discusses effect of separation on parents.

6. CLARK, M. B. "A Therapeutic Approach to Treating a Grieving Two-and-a-Half-Year-Old". *J. Amer. Acad. Child Psychiat.* 11: 705–11, 1972.

—demonstrates how timely, brief therapeutic intervention can help a young child and mother suffering from unresolved grief and mourning following the death of the father and husband.

7. CRUMLEY, F. E., and BLUMENTHAL, R. S. "Children's Reactions to Temporary Loss of the Father". *Amer. J. Psychiat.* 130: 778–82, 1973.

—discusses the child's long-term loss of his/her father as a developmental interference which results in a disturbance in the typical unfolding of the child's personality. Interesting case reports.

8. DESPERT, J. L. *Children of Divorce*. Garden City, New York, Dolphin Books, Doubleday, 1962.

—one of the earlier books in this field. Provides a good general discussion of related issues based on the author's extensive clinical experience.

9. EPSTEIN, J. *Divorced in America: Marriage in an Age of Possibility*. New York, E. P. Dutton, 1974.

—a moving, personalized account by a journalist which views the historical and social aspects of divorce.

10. FREUD, A. "Painter v. Bannister: Postscript by a Psychoanalyst", in *The Writings of Anna Freud*. Vol. 7: 247–55. New York, International Univ. Press, 1968.

—a comment on a legal decision, discussing the needs of the child.

11. FURMAN, E. *A Child's Parent Dies*. New Haven and London, Yale University Press, 1974.

—theoretical and clinical detail of children's reactions to and the consequences and management of the loss of a parent.

12. GARDNER, R. A. *The Boys and Girls Book about Divorce*. New York, Science House, 1970.

—intended for children or laymen, this book is somewhat oversimplified. It is suitable for parents wanting to provide a book for their children to read on the subject.

13. GOLDSTEIN, J.; FREUD, A.; and SOLNIT, A. *Beyond the Best Interests of the Child.* New York, The Free Press, 1973.
—excellent discussion of interacting psychological and legal problems related to child-custody decisions.

14. GRAUER, H. "Psychodynamics of the Survivor Syndrome". *Canad. Psychiat. Assoc. J.* 14: 617–22, 1969.
—explores some of the psychodynamics of concentration-camp survivors and the effects of this traumatic experience on the family.

15. KITTRIE, N. N. *The Right to Be Different.* 102–68. Baltimore, Johns Hopkins Press, 1972.
—a highly technical work. One would probably need some experience with courts and the law to find it useful. The therapeutic approach is somewhat oversold.

16. KOGELSCHATZ, J. L.; ADAMS, P. L.; and TUCKER, D. McK. "Family Styles of Fatherless Households". *J. Amer. Acad. Child Psychiat.* 11: 365–83, 1972.
—through the study of 105 children from fatherless families, explores characteristics, symptoms, and diagnoses of the families, the mother's emotional worlds, and the children's perspectives. Good illustrative cases.

17. KRANTZLER, M. *Creative Divorce.* New York, Signet Books, 1975.
—a highly personal but relatively effective book discussing the problems in adjusting to divorce from the viewpoint of the divorced person.

18. KRONBY, M. C. *The Guide to Family Law.* Toronto, New Press, 1972.
—another book dealing strictly with the legal aspects of divorce and family law in Canada.

19. LEWIS, M. "The Latency Child in a Custody Conflict". *J. Amer. Acad. Child Psychiat.* 13: 635–47, 1974.
—examines the legal practices allowing changes in custody from the psychological viewpoint, stressing the importance of the social context and the desirability of work with child and parents both prior and subsequent to custody proceedings.

20. Mc CONVILLE, B. J.; BOAG, L. C.; and PUROHIT, A. P. "Mourning Processes in Children of Varying Ages". *Canad. Psychiat. Assoc. J.* 15,3: 253–55,1970.
—reports qualitative aspects of mourning processes occurring in children after the loss of parents or other loved persons. Supports the idea that the patterns of children's mourning are determined by age and developmental stage.

21. MC DERMOTT, J. F.; BOLMAN, W. M.; ARENSDORF, A. M.; and MARKOFF, R. A. "The Concept of Child Advocacy". *Amer. J. Psychiat.* 130: 1203–06, 1973.
—discusses the development of the concept of child advocacy.

22. MC DERMOTT, J. F. "Divorce and Its Psychiatric Sequelae in Children". *Arch. Gen. Psychiat.* 23: 421–27, 1970.
—a study of children from divorced families, identifying characteristic reactions to divorce. Less impressionistic than reference # 21.

23. MILLER, J. B. M. "Children's Reactions to the Death of a Parent: A Review of the Psychoanalytic Literature". *J. Amer. Psychoanalyt. Assoc.* 19: 697–719, 1971.
—reviews and capsulizes much of the psychoanalytic literature dealing with the nature of children's reactions to object loss by death of a parent.

24. PAVENSTEDT, E., and BERNARD, V. W. *Crises of Family Disorganization.* New York, Behavioral Publications, 1971.
—clinical examples of family breakdown and appropriate management of the problems.

25. ROBERTSON, J., and ROBERTSON, J. "John, 17 Months: 9 Days in a Residential Nursery". Film. England, Tavistock Child Development Research Unit, 1969.
—a moving and convincing record of a child's reaction to separation from home and parents, and to unsatisfactory temporary care.

26. RUTTER, M. "Parent-Child Separation: Psychological Effects on the Children". *J. Child Psychol. Psychiat.* 12: 233–60, 1971.
—reviews literature on parent-child separation and reports findings from an intensive longitudinal study of patients' families. Concludes that a child's separation from his family is a potential cause of short-term distress but separation is of little direct importance as a cause of long-term disorder.

27. RUTTER, M. "Maternal Deprivation Reconsidered". *J. Psychosomat. Research.* 16: 241–50, 1972.
—suggests that the syndrome of acute distress is due in part to a disruption of the bonding process (to either parent); and that affectionless psychopathy may result from failure to develop family bonds by three years of age.

28. SHERESKY, N., and MANNES, M. *Uncoupling: The Art of Coming Apart.* New York, Dell Publishing Co., 1973.
—a highly technical book dealing with the legal aspects of divorce in the United States.

29. TAYLOR, D. A., and STARR, P. "The Use of Clinical Services by Adoptive Parents: A Review of Some Practice Assumptions". *J. Amer. Acad. Child Psychiat.* 11: 384–99, 1972.
—discusses the findings of this study and of other clinical and research reports related to the issues of the disproportionate incidence of adoptive families in clinic caseloads. Also discusses the aetiology of family problems leading to the use of clinical resources.

30. TIZARD, B., and REES, J. "The Effect of Early Institutional Rearing on the Behaviour Problems and Affectional Relationships of Four-Year-Old Children". *J. Child Psychol. Psychiat.* 16: 61–73, 1975.
—compares the behavioural problems and affectional relationships of four-and-a-half-year-old children reared in institutions since early infancy with similarly aged children living at home. Also studies same-aged children who had been living in an institution but who were later adopted or restored to their natural mother.

31. WALLERSTEIN, J. S., and KELLY, J. B. "The Effects of Parental Divorce: Experiences of the Preschool Child". *J. Amer. Acad. Child Psychiat.* 14: 600–616, 1975.
—reports upon part of a larger, ongoing inquiry into the effects of parental divorce on children and adolescents. Describes sixty families shortly after the initial separation of the parents and a year later. Very good.

32. WALLSTON, B. "The Effects of Maternal Employment on Children". *J. Child Psychol. Psychiat.* 14: 91–95, 1973.
—attempts to integrate research dealing with the effects of maternal employment on infants, pre-school children, school-age children, and adolescents.

33. WESTMAN, J. C.; CLINE, D. W.; SWIFT, W. J.; and KRAMER, D. A. "Role of Child Psychiatry in Divorce". *Arch. Gen. Psychiat.* 23: 416–20, 1970.
—short paper, based on personal experience of the authors, reviewing the contribution the child psychiatrist can play.

SOL GOLDSTEIN

21. The Child's Reactions to Dental Care

Visiting the dentist has always been at best an anxiety-producing experience, evoking in some patients visions of outright panic and trauma. There may have been some realistic reasons for this in the past, when certain procedures were quite painful. Although modern dental techniques afford far less pain and a shorter period in the chair, dental visits remain, for most, a dreaded and troublesome experience. Usually adults can control their anxiety and discomfort without interfering with the dentist. Children, however, typically translate anxiety into action, in this case non-cooperation with the dentist. This may seriously interfere with the treatment being attempted. How then does one obtain the co-operation of the child?

To answer this question globally would be impossible. This chapter cannot provide a comprehensive guide to the dentist's dealings with all children, nor can it supply a way of avoiding all traumatic experiences. Instead it will outline some of the factors involved in the interaction, in the hope that an understanding of them will allow a greater opportunity for working in an empathic way with the child dental patient.

Anxiety, fear, panic—all of these, at times, may appear irrational to the observer unless he can understand what is going on in the mind of the person experiencing them. What is being demanded of the child dental patient? He is told, "Sit down quietly in the chair, open your mouth wide, do not close it until you are permitted. Do not move, fuss, kick, bite, or pinch. Do not touch any of the equipment. Do not talk. Please sit and co-operate." In short he's being told, "Sit quietly and passively. Open your mouth and allow strange hands bearing strange equipment to enter and to work on your teeth. Do not try to protect yourself, no matter how it hurts or how frightened you feel".

That the mouth has great emotional significance is evidenced by the importance that eating, smoking, drinking, and sucking the thumb and other objects play in our lives. We use all of these to reward, punish, comfort, and console ourselves. Thus the mouth is an area central to conflict, symbolically important to all "taking-in" activities and a vehicle for expulsion activities, including speech. We are all aware of how our moods affect our appetities, how emotional turmoil can lead us to vomit, or at other times, to overindulge ourselves with food and with alcohol. It is into this very important area that the dentist intrudes. Here is where he works, manipulates, and at times removes parts of our body.

In the first, most important, formative year of our lives, the mouth is the area around which most pleasure revolves. This is an age when the child is most helpless and yet, as he is doted upon, at his most omnipotent. Mother can comfort him, and through the mouth he can make her come at his demand by crying. This is the most *active* function of the first year. It is his call that makes things happen. Either the infant is picked up and changed, or the breast or its substitute are thrust into the open mouth to relieve his hunger. It is through the mouth that he regurgitates if too much food is taken, or expels air if too much is swallowed. It is through the mouth that the sucking reflex works, relieving tension and bringing pleasure. Thus the period of time when the child feels most omnipotent corresponds with the period when pleasures are brought to him through the mouth.

But the world must change, and there comes a time when the infant realizes that he is not omnipotent. He becomes aware that he is neither the whole world nor the ruler of it, but rather a small and helpless part of it, very dependent on others to help sustain him. This realization occurs when the infant begins to notice other people, to recognize parents, to differentiate between their smiles and their frowns. It also coincides with the normally developing child's first experience with unrelenting, unrelievable pain. This pain, caused by the eruption of the first teeth, also occurs in the mouth. At this time the child can obtain some relief through biting down. The breast-fed child finds that when he does so, his mother withdraws. At the same time, the mother is affected by the biting, irritating personality of the child during his teething period, since she finds herself unable to relieve his distress. The resultant frustration produces a pulling away, a beginning separation between mother and child.

After that first year, during which the mouth plays such a key role in the child's development, comes a period during which the child begins to establish himself as a more separate individual. Now comes the time when his mother begins to demand that he control his excreta. Toilet-training has begun. The child learns that he has the power to please or displease those around him by controlling or by not controlling his bowel and bladder evacuation. At this stage, the child is more mobile and is told, "Don't touch", "Stop", etc. Demands are made for behaviour control, for the delay of immediate pleasure in exchange for later approval from the important adults in his world. For the first time, the child is expected to co-operate. How this is handled and the experiences gained at this stage set the tone for situations demanding co-operation in the future. The co-operation the dentist requires closely resembles this process. The child is asked to give up his personal comfort in order to gain the dentist's and his parents' approval. He is expected to be able to trust and conform to another adult, another authority figure.

If training has gone well, the relationship concerning most matters of control likely has gone equally well. If training has involved struggles, however, then the child may see any request for co-operation as a demand for submission which elicits feelings of being intruded upon, with lowered self-esteem resulting if he complies. Any of these may stir up rage in the child in similar situations. In cases where the withholding of faeces has been met with the repeated use of enemas, the child might experience them as an actual physical attack, an intrusion on his body. Similarly, such a child in the dental chair may experience the dentist probing inside his mouth as a frontal attack on his body which threatens his physical well-being and psychological survival.

Not only does the dentist have to deal with the result of early child-parent relationships, but as an authority figure he may encounter resistance due to the child's mistrust of other such people as a result of previous meetings with doctors, barbers, teachers, etc. Parental attitudes and behaviour may compound the problem. How do the parents speak of the dentist? Do both parents agree on the child's need for dental care, or does one believe that since the first set of teeth fall out anyway there is no point in spending time, energy, and money to maintain their well-being? Has the child overheard either parent talking of his or her fear of the dentist? Has the dentist been used as a threat if the child does not behave, does not eat the right food, or does not brush his teeth regularly? What has the child heard from his siblings about the awful things that go on in the dentist's office, about how large the "needle" or "pliers" are? What about the child's trust in the dentist who reports the presence of two or three cavities in spite of brushing with "Brand X", which the television commercial has promised will prevent cavities? The list can go on and on.

Let us now continue our look at the child's conception of the actual dental procedure. After the age of control and co-operation comes an age in which children begin to compete with their peers and with the adults around them. Although this occurs through the medium of rather harmless games, the fantasies of the growing child are anything but innocent. In fantasy, children at this stage deal with their adversaries in very violent, destructive ways, just as they deal with their loved ones in very romantic ways. In their dreams and in their play, they become the spouse of the loved one, the parent of his or her children, the murderer and destroyer of those who get in their way. Any game of "house" or "school" or "cops and robbers" or "cowboys and Indians" will show how stringently they would punish and how severely they would be punished, how intensely they would love and how ardently they would be loved. Theirs becomes the world of "an eye for an eye and a *tooth* for a *tooth*". This leads to a great preoccupation with hurting or being hurt.

The child at this stage becomes very sensitive to bodily injury, to concerns about the wholeness of his body. It is one of life's coincidences that during this stage the child normally begins to lose his primary teeth. Whether the child experiences this loss as traumatic, or whether his fantasies of a benevolent and rewarding "tooth fairy" predominate will help determine how the dentist, whose work with the teeth actually threatens the child's feeling of body intactness, will be seen and reacted to. Again, the question of trust arises. Now, however, the patient has to trust not only that the dentist will not assault his self-esteem, but also that the dentist will not destroy him physically, in retaliation for hostile fantasies and wishes the patient may have had or may still have.

Later in a child's life (ages seven to eleven) there comes a period when fair play is of the utmost concern. As this time, the dentist may be faced with the child's anger and disappointment, because, in spite of his complying with good rules of dental hygiene, cavities still occur or teeth do not grow in properly. Children may attempt to make deals with the dentist, deals which are unrealistic. Still, in the process of learning that the world is not run according to strict rules of cause and effect, children are at times angry that they are none the less expected to adhere to rules and to co-operate. In his relationship with the dentist, the child finds a concrete example of the disillusioning world. Therefore, why co-operate?

Then comes adolescence, when, among all else that goes on, the developing teenager begins to keep secrets from adults. His most closely guarded secrets are about his sexual life—the fantasies entertained, the activities performed. Can the dentist determine what these secrets are by looking inside the mouth? Some adolescents believe that their teeth show changes in colour and an increased number of cavities as a result of masturbation. Their reluctance to co-operate with the dentist has nothing more to do with him than the fact that they attribute to him the power of perceiving their sexual impulses and their methods of handling them.

Having reviewed some of the psychological significance of the mouth, the teeth, and the co-operation expected at various levels of development, let us look at some typical emotional responses to the dental situation, and at ways in which these may affect a child's response to the dentist.

In the dental chair the child can see himself as a victim, the dentist as an aggressor. In such a situation the victim has several forms of action open to him. As one is blocked, he can fall back on another. As each of his attempts to neutralize the situation is blocked, his anxiety level increases, at times assuming panic proportions. This must be borne in mind to avoid this panic.

Confronted by an aggressor, a victim experiences fear. The first line of defence is that of "fight or flight". Either of these in the dentist's office is generally considered inappropriate behaviour. Nevertheless, such behaviour is the major complaint of dentists who deal with young patients or, for that matter, older ones with minimal control over their impulses. When the patient accepts that he cannot run, his next line of defence is to yell for help. This is difficult to do when the aggressor's hand is filling one's mouth. Finally, unable either to run away or to scream, all he can do is plead for mercy from the source of the threat. Again this is not possible for the same reason. Unable either to escape from or to neutralize the threat, the child experiences mounting feelings of danger arising from the procedure itself, from the psychological meaning of the procedure, and from the loss of self-esteem which may result from the shame he feels in response to his fear. No one is proud of having fled the scene, or screamed, or pleaded for mercy. Often the patient's belligerent behaviour is as much a cover-up for the shame he feels because of his fear and the ways he has exposed his cowardice through his behaviour as it is a reaction to the dental experience itself.

What can be done, then, to reduce the anxiety and resultant behaviour in the dentist's office? The dentist cannot alter the child's basic development or the fact that the area he works in is so loaded with psychological fantasies and significance. It is not his job to be the child's psychiatrist; to interpret to the child the unconscious reasons for his anxiety would merely heighten it and accentuate his behaviour. It is hoped, however, that the dentist will understand and respect the anxiety of his patient rather than put it down to childishness, cowardice, or any other esteem-reducing cause. The dentist must somehow manage to engage his patient as an ally so that together they can work to overcome this anxiety. As an ally, he can talk with the patient about the latter's "feeling nervous" in a matter-of-fact, empathic way, presenting this as a universal response, not one to be ashamed of but something to be worked on. Then, to reduce the fantasies of aggressor and victim, the dentist can further the partnership by explaining in a language and at a level that the patient can understand what needs to be done and in what stages.

The unknown is very frightening, but anxiety is reduced when what lies ahead is made more concrete and definite. Informing the patient what he may experience and at what point will allow some predictability. If the child knows that there may be some bleeding, that it is not cause for alarm, and that it will soon stop, he will not be so upset when the bleeding does occur. Similarly with pain. If the type of pain and how long it will last are predicted it will become more tolerable. The element of surprise is removed and trust is established. The patient should know that he is not being made uncomfortable on purpose or for an unnecessarily long time, and that the work is necessary and will be done. If a patient detects that a dentist is unsure of what he is doing or feels overly apologetic about performing a certain procedure, anxiety increases. This should not, however, prevent the dentist from apologizing for an unexpected or quite severe pain.

Time is very important. Procedures should be kept as short as possible, since time passes much less quickly for the patient than for the dentist. Whenever possible there should be periodic breaks that allow the patient to exercise his mouth, to rinse, and especially to talk for a minute, informing the dentist how things are going. When the patient is talking he is active, temporarily relieved of the role of being the passive recipient. This shift from passivity to activity facilitates the relief of tension. For quite long procedures it would even be helpful to allow the patient to get up for a moment, or at least to stretch and flex his taut muscles. When one is tense, muscles tighten up, leading to further tension and discomfort. Anything that interferes with the dentist's relationship with his patient should best be avoided, such as unnecessary phone calls, conversations not concerning the patient, or excessive moving from room to room and patient to patient. Periods of being left alone while waiting for a procedure to be done allow anxiety to rise rapidly. When the dentist is talking to his assistant about matters other than the patient, the child is also virtually alone, isolated, and vulnerable to anxiety. Instead, the child will be helped if the dentist is available to tell him what is being done and how much longer it will take, sparing details which may disturb him but allowing the child to feel part of the team.

The relationship between a child and his dentist, and the establishment of successful communication between them, are of the utmost importance. A rapport will already be partially accomplished if the dentist has responded with warmth and understanding despite any initial discomfort or anxiety on the part of the child, and if he has explained what is being done, as outlined above. In view of the fear that arises when the child cannot run, yell, or plead, communication is possible, even though one's hands are in the patient's mouth, by giving the patient a signal, for example, raising the left index finger, to indicate excessive discomfort or the need for a break. Having such a signal does much to alleviate the anxiety and feeling of total helplessness, usually making it possible for the "alarm system" to be used infrequently while at the same time avoiding a major blow up.

When the procedure has been completed, it would be important to allow the child to express how he felt about the experience, including offering him a chance to express any negative feelings he had towards the dentist. When it seems to be the case, a statement such as "You must have felt pretty angry with me!" may prove much more helpful than one such as "That wasn't so bad, was it?" It is good practice to show the child that the relationship is a continuing one by arranging for his next appointment before he leaves. If the procedure resulted from something the patient neglected to do or should not have done, this should be explained showing the child how he can avoid further discomfort.

The question whether or not dentists should give rewards is a rather personal one which depends a great deal on the personality and preference of the dentist. Should one choose to give rewards, they should somehow be related to dental hygiene—a book about dental care, a toothbrush, tooth paste, etc.

What has been presented could all too easily be dismissed as requiring too much time and concentration on each patient. Generally, however, dentists are very much involved in prophylactic work, requiring time and energy not directly involved in treatment. The concepts and procedures outlined above would, it is hoped, be seen as a form of prophylaxis against undue and unnecessary anxiety during the present and future dental procedures.

RECOMMENDED FOR FURTHER READING

2. AYER, W. A. "Use of Visual Imagery in Needle Phobic Children." *J. Dent. Child.* 60: 125–27, 1973.
—discusses the extreme fear of injection and of extractions in some children visiting the dentist. Describes some successful approaches to the elimination of this kind of phobia, which are based largely on Wolpe's behaviour therapy technique (which attempts to condition various stimuli that are incompatible with anxiety).

3. CLARK, C. A. "An Effective Program for National Children's Dental Health Week". *J. Dent. Child.* 61: 30–32, 1974.
—reports on a program in Cleveland that teaches children about dental diseases, methods of prevention, and sources where further information may be obtained which leads to positive behavioural changes.

5. FRAIBERG, S. *The Magic Years*. New York, Scribner's, 1959.
—delightful, easy-reading, enlightening book dealing with the early years of childhood.

9. GORDON, D. A.; TERDAL, L.; and STERLING, E. "The Use of Modeling and Desensitization in the Treatment of a Phobic Child Patient". *J. Dent. Child.* 61: 102–5, 1974.
—describes a technique for modifying and eliminating maladaptive behaviour for a phobic child who must undergo dental treatment. Demonstrates a practical management plan for a very fearful parent and child.

10. MURPHY, L. *Personality in Young Children*. Vol. 2. 1st ed. New York, Basic Books, 1956.
—techniques used in assessment of personality in young children. Excellent case illustrations.

11. ROSENBERG, H. M. "Behaviour Modification for the Child Dental Patient". *J. Dent. Child.* 61: 111–14, 1974.
—stresses the need for dentists to be aware of the role that behaviour plays in determining his success in treating young patients. Suggests that dentists become proficient in using techniques of behaviour modification.

12. SAWTELL, R. O.; SIMON, J. F. Jr.; and SIMEONESSON, R. J. "The Effects of Five Preparatory Methods upon Child Behaviour During the First Dental Visit". *J. Dent. Child.* 61: 367–75, 1974.
—compares the effects of different experimental manipulations of the child's first dental visit. Discusses such procedures as desensitization, behaviour modification, and vicarious symbolic modeling.

13. SERMET, O. "Emotional and Medical Factors in Child Dental Anxiety". *J. Child Psychol. Psychiat.* 15: 313–21, 1974.
—reports the investigation of aetiological factors of child dental anxiety, and considers the role of emotional and medical factors in this regard. Technical presentation.

ADDITIONAL READING

1. ABRAHAM, K. "The First Pregenital Stage of the Libido (1916)". *Selected Papers,* I.P.L. no. 13, London, L. & V. Woolf, 248–79, 1949.

4. ERIKSON, E. H. *The Theory of Infantile Sexuality. Childhood and Society.* 2nd ed. New York, W. W. Norton, 1963.

6. FREUD, ANNA. *The Ego and the Mechanisms of Defense*. New York, International Univ. Press, 1967.

7. FREUD, ANNA. *The Psychoanalytical Treatment of Children*. New York. I.U.P., 1965.

8. FREUD, S. "Three Essays on the Theory of Sexuality" in Freud, S., ed., *The Standard Edition of the Complete Psychological Works of Sigmund Freud (1901—1905). Vol VII: 125*–45. London, The Hogarth Press, 1953.

9. FREUD, S. "Sexual Enlightenment of Children" in Freud, S., ed., *The Standard Edition of the Complete Psychological Works of Sigmund Freud (1906-1908).* Vol. IX: 129–39. London, The Hogarth Press, 1959.

UNIT FIVE: Principles of Intervention

DAVID N. MUSHIN

22. General Principles of Treatment in Child Psychiatry

From the preceding chapters it should be clear that emotional and behavioural problems in children arise from an interplay of biological, psychological, and social factors. Treatment, to be effective, must be directed towards one or more of these three areas. Thus for a child whose presenting symptom is hyperkinesis, the child psychiatrist might choose to intervene at the biological level (e.g. through medication), at the psychological level (e.g. helping the child find more acceptable ways of dealing with his anxiety), or at the social level (e.g. helping the parents develop more adequate techniques of managing the child's behaviour, helping them to cope more appropriately with their frustration, consulting the child's teacher about problems in learning and classroom behaviour). This multilevel approach, of course, is not unique to psychiatry. The treatment of tuberculosis, for example, extends beyond a chemotherapeutic attack on the tubercle bacillus to include such preventive measures as eliminating malnutrition, treating alcoholism, and upgrading substandard living conditions, as all these social problems increase susceptibility to tuberculosis.

In considering the general issue of treatment in child psychiatry there are three basic principles to be kept in mind.

1. The child is a developing individual. Emotional and behavioural problems my interfere with development. Correction of interferences may be at least as important as dealing with the identified problem.

2. The child is dependent on his environment, either immediate (family) or more distant (school). Treatment will therefore usually require dealing with environmental factors as well as intervening directly with the child.

3. A third important general principle involves the conceptualization of three basic levels of treatment. In *primary prevention* the psychiatrist seeks to modify factors likely to produce an illness. Just as improving living standards will decrease the incidence of tuberculosis, so may the development of community cohesion, the improvement of a school system, and the provision of adequate recreational facilities diminish the incidence of psychiatric problems in a community. In primary prevention, we try to identify groups of vulnerable individuals, then intervene to abort the development of the disease. For example, Tay-Sachs disease is a hereditary condition resulting in mental retardation with rapid deterioration and death by age five. This disease is transmitted by a recessive gene most commonly found in Jews of Eastern European origin. A simple blood test can identify the carrier from the population at risk (i.e. the Jewish community). Where both spouses carry the recessive gene, genetic counselling and termination of affected pregnancies can prevent the condition.

Other conditions, for example, schizophrenia and alcoholism, are thought to develop out of an inherited predisposition (i.e. genetic loading) activated by environmental influences. Attempts are being made to identify genetically vulnerable children in order to pinpoint the types of familial and social conditions that cause some children but not others to develop psychotic features.

Secondary prevention involves the management of conditions once they occur. Intervention at this level seeks to reverse an existing pathological process and its effects, thus allowing a return to normality. Examples would include the treatment of pneumonia with antibiotics or of phobias with psychotherapy. This chapter will deal primarily with psychiatric treatment aimed at the level of secondary prevention.

Tertiary prevention involves the management of irreversible problems, usually requiring prolonged and continuous care. This is the basis of a large part of medical and, in particular, hospital treatment. The stroke patient with residual disabilities has a poor prognosis if one thinks of complete recovery. But many such patients can learn to compensate for their disabilities. They can be helped to walk and possibly to talk again, to become self-sufficient rather than to remain unnecessarily dependent on nursing staff or relatives, and to approach as closely as possible their earlier level of function. They cannot be cured, but they can be helped. Similarly, the autistic child has a poor prognosis if we think of his fitting into our concepts of normality. But we may be able to do much to help him develop speech, to promote more acceptable behaviour, and to teach whatever skills are within his capacity.

In treating a given patient, we may choose to intervene at various levels at the same or different times. For example, one might treat a child with a behaviour disorder in psychotherapy, hoping to promote a return to normal feelings and behaviour (i.e. secondary prevention). Concurrently one would counsel the parents, both to identify and minimize their feeding into the particular child's disturbance (secondary prevention) and to decrease the risk of disturbance developing in the siblings (primary prevention). At the same time, the child might need help in adjusting to educational deficits whose results could not entirely be undone (i.e. tertiary prevention).

Psychiatric treatment of a child occurs within the context of his ongoing development. His capacities will change as his development proceeds. What one expects of a child—and whether a particular form of behaviour will be considered normal or abnormal—will depend on his stage of development. Thus we would not be concerned if a five-year-old has not learned to read. If a seven- or eight-year-old, however, had not learned to read, investigation and probably some form of remediation would be indicated. Similarly, on an emotional level, it is normal for a two-year-old to be anxious if left with a babysitter, whereas an eight-year-old should be able to tolerate this without significant distress. Many of the symptoms of emotional disturbance in children can be seen as resulting from a block in the normal process of development that has caused a child to remain fixated at an earlier level of development. The six-year-old who has frequent temper tantrums and stubbornly resists any parental suggestions is behaving in a manner normal for a two-year-old but inappropriate for a child of his age. Treatment for such a child would consist of freeing the child to proceed once more with the previously arrested process of development.

The child's developmental level will also affect the form of treatment needed. Thus a three-year-old with a poorly developed ability to express abstract feelings verbally might be helped to resolve troublesome thoughts and feelings through play (i.e. play therapy) whereas a ten-year-old should be more able to discuss such issues more directly.

Remember, too, how dependent the young child is on his environment. His parents do much more than merely meet his physical needs. They provide him with a sense of security—or a lack of it. Through their expectations, their example, the limits they set, and the decisions they make, they will shape his attitudes and his behaviour. As the child gets older and enters school, a whole new series of demands and expectations are presented. Treatment of a child, therefore, is difficult if not impossible outside the context of his environment. At least parents, and often siblings, teachers, and guardians, will need to be involved in the treatment process in view of the extent of their influence on the day-to-day functioning of the child.

These, then, are general principles to be considered in deriving a plan of management for a particular child. What forms of treatment are available in child psychiatry?

1. Biological Therapies

Biological therapies in psychiatry include medication, electroconvulsive therapy, and psychosurgery. The latter two are rarely used with children as, unlike ECT with adults, there is little evidence of their effectiveness. Drugs are used with children to deal with certain symptoms, particularly problems of behaviour (e.g. hyperactivity, poor control of aggression, bizarre psychotic behaviour). Generally part of an over-all treatment plan, the drugs and other medications used will be discussed in detail in the following chapter.

2. Psychological Therapies

Psychological therapies are interventions to change an individual or group (e.g. a family) identified as having problems. The change is usually brought about through the relationship between a therapist and a patient. The patient may be either an individual, a group, or a family seeking help. In order to succeed, the patient must recognize that there is a situation requiring help, and he, or at least the parents, in the case of a child, must have some desire and commitment towards effecting change. The therapist tries to form an alliance with the patient so that together they can search for more successful ways of dealing with the problem. Clearer identification of the nature and source of the difficulties may point to alternative ways of dealing with them. Initial successes, the relief which accompanies the ventilation of long-pent-up feelings and the supportive relationship with the therapist may provide encouragement and relief. These in turn will further strengthen the relationship with the therapist, leading to increased expectations and, it is hoped, an even greater willingness to work together in the direction of recovery.

These general comments apply to all forms of psychological treatment. But there are many distinct forms of psychotherapy, differing from one another both in their theoretical base and in the techniques they use to bring about change. The various forms of psychotherapy can be divided broadly into two main groups: (a) therapies aimed at modifying behaviour without directly attempting to resolve the conflicts that lead to that behaviour; (b) therapies aimed at dealing with conflicts and modifying defence patterns to allow for more adaptive (i.e. successful) behaviour.

a) THERAPIES AIMED AT MODIFYING BEHAVIOUR WITHOUT DIRECTLY ATTEMPTING TO RESOLVE THE CONFLICTS THAT LEAD TO THAT BEHAVIOUR.

The behaviour therapist believes that all behaviour—including symptoms—represents a response to stimuli which can be clearly identified and then manipulated. Unlike the dynamically oriented psychotherapist, he does not see the need to view behavioural symptoms as an outward expression of inner conflicts that must be resolved through treatment. He is less interested in learning about past conflict situations than he is in identifying and measuring the behaviour he seeks to change.[8]

The basic model of the behaviour therapist is that *a stimulus provokes a response*. An example is the classical experiment in which Watson had a young child play with a white rat in his laboratory. Initially the child responded to the rat with interest and curiosity. Watson then repeatedly presented the rat to the child along with a loud noise. The noise immediately frightened the child (i.e. the noise was an unconditioned stimulus producing a fear response). As the child learned to associate the appearance of the rat with the feared noise, the fear generalized and became associated not just with the noise but also with the rat. By this stage, the presence of the rat, even without the noise, was enough to frighten the child. Thus the child had learned (i.e. had been *conditioned*) to fear the rat so that the rat's presence was a *conditioned (learned) stimulus* evoking a fear response. Another way of conditioning the child to fear the rat would have been to punish him each time the rat was presented (i.e. negative reinforcement). Similarly if the child's mother screamed and jumped on a chair every time the rat was presented, the child might *model* himself on her and develop a fear of white rats. The fear might extend to include other white furry animals, which would be an example of *stimulus generalization*. If the rat was then presented repeatedly in the absence of any other fearful stimuli he might, in time, lose his fear through the process of *extinction*. If the rat was presented in association with a pleasant stimulus or if playing with the rat was associated with a reward, the child might lose his fear through *counterconditioning*. The child's mother might also help overcome the fear by playing calmly with the rat in his presence, again providing a *model*, this time for a non-fearful response.

These concepts are basic to the theory of behaviour therapy.[25] A good description of its use as a treatment technique is provided by Werry and Brown.[9,2] Initially, the problem is defined. Certain symptoms, which are most distressing to the patient, his parents or those around him are identified. Examples might include a fear of dogs or disturbing classroom behaviour. These may be his only problems (e.g. an isolated phobia) or part of a more generalized pathological process (e.g. stealing as a symptom of severe and long-standing rejection and emotional deprivation). The problem is then analysed to define stimuli which elicit the behaviour and responses which either sustain or alter it. For example, temper tantrums may occur when a child is ignored by his mother, and they may intensify when she becomes frustrated and throws up her hands in despair or yells and spanks him. On the other hand, they may diminish when she firmly sends the child to remain in his room until he is ready to deal reasonably with what is upsetting him.

In initiating therapy, one first tries to establish a therapeutic alliance with child and family whose co-operation is essential if the therapy is to succeed. Then, therapist and family agree on the behaviour that is to be changed (i.e. the *target behaviour*) and seek to define factors which evoke and maintain it. The therapist draws on his understanding of the family and his knowledge of behaviour theory to propose ways in which the target behaviour can be eliminated. These might include: (i) identifying and eliminating stimuli that regularly produce the target behaviour; (ii) identifying and avoiding responses that positively reinforce the target behaviour; (iii) prescribing a regime which negatively reinforces unwanted behaviour (thus encouraging its extinction) while positively reinforcing (rewarding) more desired forms of behaviour. This approach is called *operant conditioning*:

Melody, age twelve, resisted doing her chores around the group home in which she was living, and was antagonistic and quarrelsome in her dealings with both children and staff. Any attempt on the part of staff to hold her to her responsibilities or to explore the reasons for her oppositional behaviour met with endless arguments, accusations, and blaming of others followed by her storming out of the house. She had recently resumed shop-lifting, and staff had been totally unsuccessful in their attempts to encourage her to deal with her feelings in a less antisocial manner. The situation had deteriorated to the point where she was on the verge of being discharged from the group home, although neither she nor the staff really wanted this. Staff were feeling helpless, angry, and out of control. Melody was frightened but angry and, at that point, incapable of modifying her behaviour. Since the usual treatment approaches of the group home did not seem to be helping, it was decided to try a behaviour modification program.

Accordingly, Melody was approached by the staff who pointed out that unless she managed somehow to bring her behaviour under control there was danger of her placement breaking down. Melody agreed. The staff suggested a behaviour modification program and Melody accepted. Together they drew up a list of target behaviours which were to be eliminated (e.g. messy room, disobedience, fighting, swearing, stealing). For each of these, Melody would spend a designated time sitting alone in her bedroom. Failure to serve her time, arguing, or leaving the group home when there was time to be served would automatically lead to additional time spent in the bedroom. All the unacceptable behaviours and the time allotted to each were listed on a chart posted on the kitchen wall. On a second chart was a list of points that Melody could earn for behaving in certain specified ways, e.g. cleaning up her room, washing the dishes, doing one hour's homework, earning a satisfactory weekly report from her teacher, etc. These points could be used to earn privileges that otherwise would be unavailable to her. The "rate of exchange" had been negotiated between Melody and the staff in setting up the program (e.g. she must earn five points to be allowed to go downtown on her own, two points to wear make-up, etc.) Each week there would be a regular meeting between Melody and staff in which penalties, rewards, and ways in which Melody could spend points she had earned were adjusted to keep the program both fair and therapeutically effective.

The above example illustrates how Melody and the staff clearly identified certain forms of behaviour they wished to extinguish. They attempted to achieve this end both by negative reinforcement of unacceptable behaviour (i.e. time spent in the bedroom) and by positive reinforcement of desirable behaviour (i.e. points which could be exchanged for privileges of her choice). As the disruptive or socially unacceptable behaviour was given up, the general environment—staff, peers, teachers, or, in other cases, parents—spontaneously reinforced the change. Generalization occurred; for example, Melody was negatively reinforced only for aggressive or antisocial behaviour that occurred within the group home, but her new patterns of behaving more acceptably spread so that her relationships with children in the neighbourhood and at school also improved.

Another form of behaviour therapy involves the extinction of unwanted behaviour through the process of desensitization. This has proved useful in the treatment of phobic behaviour and certain somatic conditions. First, the child is trained in a technique of deep relaxation. He is then asked to imagine fear-provoking situations, and these are arranged in hierarchy with those provoking least anxiety at one end and those provoking the most at the other. If a child had a fear of riding in elevators, he might feel little anxiety when imagining himself approaching a tall building with his parents, more anxiety at entering the elevator, and most anxiety when imagining himself alone in a moving elevator. Different situations in order of increasing anxiety are presented to the relaxed child who is told to indicate when he feels anxious. At such a point he is relaxed further until he can tolerate such a situation without anxiety, and then further situations are presented. This process is repeated until he feels comfortable with the idea of riding in an elevator by himself. Thus gradually the systematic presentation of increasing amounts of stress (the phobic stimuli) concurrent with relaxation leads to a gradual desensitization of the stimulus whose capacity to provoke anxiety is hereby extinguished. A further example is that of the treatment of certain asthmatic attacks. It is even possible to detect early wheezing through elaborate electronic equipment attached to the child which then transmits this message to a central radio receiver which automatically retransmits to the child's receiver a stimulus conditioned to evoke bronchial relaxation.

Behaviour therapy may be performed by the therapist in a clinic setting, but the therapy is frequently extended by training parents to continue the program within the home. This part of the program consists of teaching the parents to identify and reinforce appropriately pertinent factors occurring in the home. At the same time, alteration of the parents' attitudes and behaviour may provide positive models for the child. In some cases, intermittent reinforcement of the desired behaviour will be necessary to prevent extinction of the change. Behaviour therapy has proved helpful for modifying unwanted symptoms and behaviour in a wide range of conditions including neurotic disorders (e.g. phobias), psychophysiological disorders (e.g. enuresis and asthma), behaviour disorders and psychoses (e.g. autistic children).

b) THERAPIES AIMED AT DEALING WITH CONFLICTS AND MODIFYING THE DEFENCE PATTERNS TO ALLOW FOR MORE ADAPTIVE (I.E. SUCCESSFUL) BEHAVIOUR.

These therapies work on the assumption that symptoms and behaviour are the result of underlying pathology, that is, conflicts between the basic drives and the defences against those drives, which have not been comfortably and successfully resolved. In a child with a behavioural problem, the presenting symptoms, such as stealing, lying, disobedience, or the inability to get along with other children, are seen as the outward behavioural expression of inner conflicts, such as feelings of deprivation and rage resulting from parental rejection. There may be multiple causes for such pathology: the same symptom (e.g. hyperactivity) may derive from a variety of factors acting either singly or in combination. What may have begun as an organic problem affecting the central nervous system may be complicated by parental anger and rejection secondary to the child's difficult and disruptive behaviour or by guilt at having a damaged child. These additional factors may then stir up further anxiety and increased activity in the child. *In such cases, therapy would be aimed at identifying and reducing conflict in the child and at helping him find more adaptive and appropriate ways of dealing with conflict when it arises.*

One might illustrate this with reference to the above examples. If the child's behavioural problem was seen as a response to conflicts in the child secondary to feelings fo rejection, one might attempt, through therapy, to achieve several goals:

i) That of helping the parents recognize the importance of their attitudes and of helping them become more accepting of the child.
ii) That of helping the child learn, in the meantime, to deal with his feelings of anxiety, deprivation, and rage in ways other than those that invite further rejection. This may involve helping him gain more control over his anxiety or aggression and channelling these into more constructive or adaptive outlets.

Similarly, in the case of the hyperactive child, in addition to treating the neurological component of the hyperactivity with medication, one might also:

i) Counsel the parents (help them develop a program of management that would compensate for the child's tendency to hyperactivity by systematically training him to control his behaviour) and simultaneously help them deal with feelings of frustration and guilt that are contributing to their anger and rejection of the child.
ii) Work with the child, to help him become aware of the part he plays in the vicious circle of hyperactivity and rejection existing between him and his parents, to assist him in gaining control over his impluses and finding other more successful ways of dealing with anxiety, frustration, and rage.

Within this group of therapies there are a number of treatment modalities which may be employed. These include:

Individual Psychotherapy

This involves direct interaction between a therapist and a child, directed towards resolution or more effective handling of the child's intrapsychic problems. The therapist first attempts to form a therapeutic alliance with the child. The use of this alliance would depend on whether the therapist was performing *intensive* or *supportive* psychotherapy.

In *intensive* psychotherapy, the therapist's emphasis is on helping the child *recognize* and *understand* the nature of his conflicts and the ways that the anxiety and the defences they generate distort his perceptions and interfere with his functioning. The child is seen one to three times per week over a period of months or years. He is encouraged to talk and play freely, and his fantasy productions are used as a guide to understanding his intrapsychic conflict. In intensive psychotherapy, the relationship between child and therapist becomes exaggerated and distorted. A times, the child may feel rejected, while at others he may see the therapist as overprotective. In response to these feelings, he may behave in a manner that would seem incomprehensible to someone with no understanding of the process of therapy: alternately or simultaneously vengeful, timid, stubborn, affectionate, disobedient, or seductive. The goal of intensive psychotherapy is to have the child realize that many of these perceptions and responses arise not from the attitude or actions of the therapist but from his own private distortions and maladaptive responses. They are *transferred* (displaced) onto the therapist by the child as a result of his experience with other key adults, especially his parents. It is the recognition and understanding of these *transference reactions* that makes intensive psychotherapy much more than purely an intellectual exercise. Intensive psychotherapy should only be considered for the child with a long history of neurotic and relationship difficulties who has failed to respond to parental and other efforts at change.

Supportive psychotherapy is directed less towards the uncovering of conflict and the development of insight than towards using the therapeutic alliance to direct the child away from conflict situations and to more appropriate patterns of behaviour. Therapy is used to drain off anxiety and to help him deal with day-to-day problems in a realistic and effective manner. Here, the therapist is more likely to answer the child's questions than to help the child find his own answers. Fantasy material is de-emphasized by the focus on the child's handling of day-to-day problems. Supportive rather than intensive psychotherapy is indicated if a child is in danger of being overwhelmed by the turmoil of daily living —for the child whose intellectual limitations stand in the way of his working out the questions posed in intensive psychotherapy; or for families and children unprepared to explore conflict situations in depth.

Intensive and supportive psychotherapy as defined above represent the two ends of a spectrum. The psychotherapy of most children contains both exploratory and supportive elements. In addition, some children are seen in *planned short-term psychotherapy*. Here a decision is made in advance to treat a child for a predetermined number of weeks (usually six to ten). The therapist actively and directly engages the child in a therapeutic alliance, which he then uses in a highly structured way to help the child identify and learn to deal more effectively with a selected and limited number of key conflict areas.[1]

Combined (Collaborative) Therapy

Children greatly depend on their environment and in particular their parents to provide for their changing needs during the course of their development. Generally, the younger the child, the greater the influence of parental attitudes and behaviour on his feelings and development. Even concerned parents may, inadvertently, have an adverse effect on a child's development. Unresolved personal conflicts that each parent brings to the marriage or difficulties in the marital relationship may result in major distortions in their ability to perceive accurately and respond effectively to the needs of one or more children. The reverse also holds true. Disturbed children are frequently disturbing, and parental anxiety and distress will often interfere with their most conscientious attempts to understand and minister to the needs of their children. The younger the child, the more important it is to include the parents in some way in the treatment process. The aim is to help the parents recognize and modify feelings, attitudes, and behaviour that are supporting continued disturbance in the child and undermining the child's development and response to psychotherapy. Occasionally, one or other parent may be disturbed enough to require personal psychotherapy. More frequently, either the child's therapist or a second therapist, social worker, or counsellor will work with the parents. If a second therapist is involved, the two will collaborate regularly to exchange information and co-ordinate the two streams of therapy.

Another approach to dealing with a patient is to see his family as a group in *family therapy*. The theoretical basis for family therapy is discussed in detail in Chapter 3. Each family member is seen not as an isolated person with his individual assortment of conflicts and defensive manoeuvres but as an integral part of a system in equilibrium. Within this system, family members are continually interacting with each other. The development of symptoms in a problem child is seen as evidence that the system's function is disturbed or distorted. This process is recognized in part in combined therapy, but much of the information about interaction between parents and child is gained at second hand and the contribution of the other siblings to the disturbance in the family system is often largely ignored. When the family is seen together in family therapy, the therapist deals primarily with the disturbances in the relationships between family members (i.e. with the interpersonal level of the family's equilibrium). The therapist can observe and reflect back gaps and distortions in family communication, helping to clarify ambiguities and breakdowns that evoke frustration and misunderstanding while interfering with problem identification and resolution. The therapist, as a trained and objective outsider, can often listen and help others hear accurately what members are trying to say, thus providing an antidote for some of the confusion and discouragement. While the therapist cannot, of course, solve the problem for the family, he may help them accurately define the issues and work productively towards solutions.[15] (For additional references on the topic of family therapy, see bibliography at end of Chapter 3.)

Group Therapy

Group therapy has particular value in treating the child with difficulty in his peer relationships. The format varies with the age and needs of the children in the group. Whereas younger children may play together in the presence of the therapist (activity group therapy), adolescents are more likely to discuss their difficulties more directly. The group is usually balanced to include some children who are overcontrolled and others who are frequently overwhelmed by explosive outbursts of intense feeling. The more inhibited members may benefit from the stimulation obtained from their more rambunctious peers, while at the same time they put the damper on the impulsiveness of members whose controls are precarious. Group members help each other both by serving as a model and by confronting others with conflict areas and directing them towards new ways of managing. The exposure to other group members promotes emotional expression, and the bonds formed between the children in a group may be important in enhancing self-esteem and in helping a child develop the confidence and social skills he needs to risk himself in less protected social situations.[10, 13]

The various forms of psychotherapy described up to this point are not mutually exclusive. The choice of type of therapy for a particular case is a complicated issue involving many factors. In any one family the form of therapy may change depending on that family's needs at a given time. The decision to employ any one of the psychotherapeutic techniques described above does not necessarily preclude the selective use of environmental manipulation, educational techniques, or behaviour modification under appropriate circumstances.[5,6]

Environmental Manipulation

As the child is more dependent on his environment than the adult, he may be more vulnerable to a pathogenic environmental situation and less able to deal successfully with the resulting stresses without outside help. Substandard housing and poverty may play an important role in family disintegration. Some families may benefit greatly if directed towards community resources which can support them and improve their living conditions. Help is needed particularly in times of crisis and transition. Immigrant families, who move into a community in which even the language is strange, find the life-style the teenagers rush to assimilate clashes with their own old-world and religious traditions. Social and ethnic agencies may help such parents make contact with a group within their new world with whom they can identify, a group who may be able to interpret the mores of the alien community and provide the security they need to avoid alienating their adolescents permanently. Schools and teachers may do much either to alleviate or to aggravate a learning or behavioural problem. Even if organic or psychological components of such a problem exist, a modified approach or special placement on the part of the school may be necessary if the child's potential for learning and adjusting is to be salvaged.

Finally, there are some children who are rejected, neglected, or abused emotionally and even physically by their parents. Such situations may urgently demand some form of community intervention, though the exact nature of this may vary from counselling the family or providing a specially trained homemaker to, in the last resort, removing the child and making him the ward of a children's aid society or child welfare association.

In-Patient Treatment of Children

Wherever possible, the child in need of treatment should receive this without being removed from his own family. Sometimes, however, it may be necessary to remove the child at least temporarily. Some parents may be so depriving and abusive—which usually means that they were similarly deprived and abused as children—that the child needs placement for his own protection. Some children are so upsetting to family and community because of a severe behaviour disorder or the symptoms of psychosis that, despite attempts to support and guide the family, the child provokes severe family and even community disorganization, rejection, and attack. In other cases, the problem may have proved refractory to even an adequate trial of out-patient therapy. In any of the above circumstances, it may be appropriate to place the child in a setting more suited to his physical, emotional, and therapeutic needs. Such a move is not to be taken lightly, as the very act of removing a child from his family may prove more damaging than the situation from which one is seeking to rescue him. A variety of resources exist, ranging from foster homes and group homes which provide an alternative living situation with some degree of supervision, guidance, and support for the child, through more structured staff-operated group homes and treatment centres. Treatment centres provide more external controls over the child's total living situation. Many such settings have cottage or group home arrangements with eight to ten children of the same age in each unit. Trained child-care workers are assigned to each group, both to act as surrogate parents and to deal with the emotional and behavioural difficulties of the child as they occur in the course of daily living. This form of treatment is know as *milieu therapy*. It may be supplemented by direct treatment of the child individually or in a group or by some form of therapeutic involvement of the family. These latter functions may be performed by other members or an interdisciplinary team consisting of psychiatrists, psychologists, social workers, and child-care workers. The team will evaluate the child's status and progress at various times, reformulate the treatment goals, and work out techniques of intervention whereby these can best be achieved. Intervention aimed at identifying and resolving the child's conflicts or at modifying his behaviour through the application of learning theory may be used on a round-the-clock basis. In-patient settings can sometimes push the autistic child towards socialization, more appropriate behaviour, and the development of speech. For the severely retarded child, a protective environment with constant nursing care may be required.

The majority of even seriously disturbed children can be treated without separating them from their families. If residential treatment is required, one must realize that the act of removing the disturbed child from his family may produce a sense of relief that this thorn has been removed from the family flesh. Ideally, this period of relief will be used to help the family work towards a more stable situation to which the child will eventually return. Not uncommonly, the family may see the placement of the child as proof that he and he alone has a problem. This may cause them to resist attempts to become involved in ongoing counselling or therapy as they close ranks to permanently exclude the "bad" or "sick" child. Thus, removal of a child from his family must be viewed as a point of crisis in his relationship with the family, so that every effort to keep them involved with the child and the therapeutic program should be exerted.[16, 19]

These, then, represent the major therapeutic approaches used in the treatment of the emotionally disturbed child and his family. The principles of chemotherapy and a practical guide to the use of drugs with children are to be found in the following chapter.

RECOMMENDED FOR FURTHER READING

1. ALDRICH, C. K. "Office Psychotherapy for the Primary Care Physician", in Arieti, S., and Caplan, G., eds., *American Handbook of Psychiatry*. 2nd ed. rev., Vol 5: 739–56, New York, Basic Books, 1975.
—after discussing the role of the primary care physician, provides an excellent review of major issues involved in the process of diagnosis and psychotherapy. Clinical examples and bibliography.

2. ANTHONY, E. J. "Psychotherapy of Adolescence" in Caplan, G., ed., *American Handbook of Psychiatry,* 2nd ed. Vol. 2: 234–50, New York, Basic Books, 1974.
—a clear, readable discussion of the preconditions for psychotherapy and the problems and techniques of individual psychotherapy with adolescents.

3. BALSER, B. H. *Psychotherapy of the Adolescent.* New York, International Univ. Press, 1957.
—a comprehensive description of different levels of psychiatric practice, with special emphasis on the role of the school.

4. BARTEN, H. H., and BARTEN, S. S. *Children and Their Parents in Brief Therapy*. New York, Behavioral Publications, 1973.
—the papers included illustrate a range of short-term approachers to psychotherapy with children and their families.

5. BERMAN, S. "The Relationship of the Private Practitioner of Child Psychiatry to Prevention." *J. Amer. Acad. Child Psychiat.* 13: 593–603, 1974.
—discusses the contribution of the child psychiatrist in private practice to child mental-health services and the importance of coordinating his/her participation with programs related to prevention, mental-health legislation, and mental-health training.

6. BIJOU, S.W., and REDD, W.H. "Behavior Therapy for Children", in Freedman, D.X. and Dyrud, J.E., eds., *American Handbook of*

Psychiatry. 2nd ed. rev., Vol 5: 319-44, New York, Basic Books, 1975.
—presents a number of theoretical models and discusses a variety of therapeutic procedures. Extensive bibliography.

7. BLOS, P., and FINCH., S.M. "Psychotherapy with Children and Adolescents", in Freedman, D.X., and Dyrud, J.E., eds., *American Handbook of Psychiatry*. 2nd ed. rev. Vol 5: 133-62, New York, Basic Books, 1975.
—a clear, well-organized description providing the theoretical framework and discussing many issues and technical problems involved in psychotherapy with children and adolescents. An excellent introduction to the area with an extensive bibliography.

8. BROWN, D. G. "Behaviour Modification with Children". *Mental Hygiene*. 56,1: 22–30, 1972.
—a clear statement of applications of behaviour modification to treatment of children.

9. CAREY, W. B. and SIBINGA, M. S. "Avoiding Pediatric Pathogenesis in the Management of Acute Minor Illness". *Pediats*. 49: 553-62, 1972.
—outlines mistakes psysicians commonly make in managing acute minor illnesses which leave the child's and parents' emotional adjustment at risk. Contains suggestions for primary prevention and research.

10. CHURCHILL, S.R. "Social Group Work: A Diagnostic Tool in Child Guidance". *Amer. J. Orthopsychiat*. 35: 581-88, 1965.
—the use of a diagnostic group by a social group worker may assist greatly in evaluating a child's social skills and liabilities. The description and clinical examples give an understanding of how this form of group work with children can be used in treatment as well.

11. EASSON, W.M. *The Severely Disturbed Adolescent*. New York, International Univ. Press, 1969.
—description of in-patient residential and hospital treatment of seriously disturbed adolescents.

12. FREUD, A. *The Psychonalytical Treatment of Children*. New York, International Univ. Press, 1965.
—an authoritative description of the psychoanalytic treatment of children from one of the pioneers of the field.

13. GINOTT, H.G. *Group Psychotherapy with Children*. New York, McGraw-Hill, 1961.
—a comprehensive introduction to the area.

14. GRAZIANO, A.M. *Behavior Therapy with Children.* Chicago, Aldine/Atherton, 1971.
—a highly technical survey of the area; a useful reference for the serious student of behaviour therapy.

15. Group for the Advancement of Psychiatry. *The Field of Family Therapy.* Vol. 7, GAP Report no. 78, 1970.
—a competent, fairly recent review of the area.

16. LAUFFER, M. W.; LAFFREY, J.J.; and DAVIDSON, R.E. "Residential Treatment for Children and its Derivatives", in Caplan, G., ed., *American Handbook of Psychiatry.* 2nd ed. rev. Vol. 2: 193–210, New York, Basic Books, 1974.
—surveys the types of settings, criteria for placement, techniques and problems of treatment in a variety of residential and day-care treatment settings.

17. LESTER, E. P. "Brief Psychotherapies in Child Psychiatry". *Canad. Psychiat. Assoc. J.* 13: 301–9, 1968.
—describes issues related to time-limited intervention.

19. NOSHPITZ, J.D. "Residential Treatment of Emotionally Disturbed Children", in Arieti, S., and Caplan, G., eds., *American Handbook of Psychiatry,* 2nd ed. Vol. 5: 634–51. New York, Basic Books, 1975.
—a good introduction to issues of administrative structure, selection, and fit of patients; good discussion of milieu therapy and life space interviewing; some discussion of role of psychotherapy, problems in role clarity, collaboration, and accountability; issues around schooling and discharge.

21. ROSENTHAL, A.J., and LEVINE, S.V. "Brief Psychotherapy with Children: Process of Therapy". *Amer. J. Psychiat.* 128: 141–46, 1971–72.
—examines techniques and content of brief psychotherapy with children.

22. SATIR, V. *Conjoint Family Therapy.* Rev. ed. Palo Alto, Science and Behaviour Books, 1967.
—written mainly in point form, this small but useful book is a good introduction to understanding the family as a social system in equilibrium. The chapter on the inclusion of children is particularly helpful. (136–59).

23. SCHOPLER, E., and REICHLER, R.J. "Parents as Co-Therapists in the Treatment of Psychotic Children". *J. Autism and Child Schiz.* 1: 87–102, 1971.

—describes and evaluates a treatment program for psychotic and autistic children in which parents are taught to function as effective co-therapists.

26. WERRY, J.S., and WOLLERSHEIM, J.P. "Behaviour Therapy with Children: A Broad Overview". *J. Amer. Acad. Child Psychiat.* 6: 346–70, 1967.
—a competent review of the area.

ADDITIONAL READING

18. MANN, JAMES. *Time-Limited Psychotherapy.* Cambridge, Mass.: Harvard Univ. Press, 1973.

20. REIDY, J. J. "An Approach to Family-Centered Treatment in a State Institution". *Amer. J. Orthopsychiat.* 32: 133–42, 1962.

25. WATSON, J.B. and RAYNER, R. "Conditioned Emotional Reactions". *J. Exper. Psych.* 3: 1–14, 1920.

24. SIFNEOS, P.E. "Two Different Kinds of Psychotherapy of Short Duration". *Amer. J. Psychiat.* 123: 1069–74, 1967.

KLAUS MINDE

23. The Role of Drugs in the Treatment of Disturbed Children

Few topics have created as much controversy among psychiatrists as the role of drugs in the treatment of disturbed children. Some physicians have claimed that psychopharmacological agents, if they function as more than placebos, do so as chemical straightjackets for troublesome children and in fact only retard the recognition of true psychopathology within the individual child or his family. Others have claimed that drugs are the only causal remedies for psychological disturbances as they act upon the brain, which is seen as the ultimate site of behavioural pathology.

This chapter will attempt to deal with some of these issues by examining the value of particular groups of drugs in specific child psychiatric disorders and will give a general outline of the relationship between pharmacological and psychological treatment. It will also discuss some of the factors which may make it difficult to evaluate behavioural changes induced by psychiatric drugs in children and recommend guidelines for the practising physician.

Specific Issues in Drug Research with Children

Assessment of drug effects in children meets with particular problems. Rarely does a child complain about his own behaviour. It is usually the school or the family that does so. Hence any evaluation of behavioural change should include observations from these two sources, as they encompass the biggest portion of the child's natural environment. It has been well established that parents and teachers in general agree highly with each other about a child's behaviour and that their opinions are much more valid than clinical observations made during an interview with a psychiatrist or psychologist. This is of course due to the ability in all children to contain particular symptoms, such as hyperactivity, for short periods of time. An interview with a doctor is also usually much less stressful than an hour in school, where other children may tease or compete for a teacher's attention. Hence it will show less of the typical conduct of the child.

Another important factor in the evaluation of drug effects in children is their sensitivity to variations in their immediate environment. A new teacher or a father who has begun to understand some of his child's present needs can produce dramatic shifts in behaviour. Hence any behavioural changes attributed to drug effects must be carefully evaluated against unexpected new circumstances in the child's milieu, the possible benefit of the accompanying advice to parents, or the different expectations of the teacher who now knows that "something is happening".

A further complicating factor in evaluating drug effects is the child's normal growth and development. A number of objective tests which have been shown to be sensitive to short-term drug treatment of particular types of children, such as the Porteus Maze Test, have very little value for the prediction of long-range behavioural outcome. On the other hand, tests such as measures of intelligence or specific learning patterns that are only responsive to long-term drug therapy are confounded by biological changes associated with normal development.

Finally we must constantly be aware that we still have no completely acceptable system for classifying children's psychiatric disorders. A child who is hyperactive may have brain damage with or without mental retardation, may be very anxious, may show a personality disorder, or may have a combination of all three. Clearly a particular medication will vary in its effect upon the hyperactivity in accordance with the aetiology of the symptom.

In summary, the following factors must be considered when evaluating drugs and behaviour:

1. Evaluations of behaviour must be standardized and should consist of reliable and valid measures of behavioural changes. Such measures in children should always include evaluations by parents and teachers in addition to clinical reassessment.

2. Careful notice must be taken of expectations aroused in both the child and his environment by our intervention, as children respond easily to environmental manipulation.
3. Long-term changes in behaviour may possibly be related not to medication but to ongoing development.
4. Diagnostic classifications in child psychiatry at this time lack general acceptability. Therefore, medication should be evaluated against specific target symptoms such as stealing or bed-wetting rather than broad concepts such as neurotic behaviour.

Specific Drugs and Their Effect on Disturbed Behaviour

GENERAL CONSIDERATIONS

No drug is specific for any one diagnostic category. Drugs never "cure" but they can ameliorate and sometimes remove distressing symptoms such as excessive, aimless activity or hallucinations. They are helpful, therefore, only as adjuncts to psychotherapy or any other efforts that assist the child in his general development. This may mean that in practice a particular drug calms a child sufficiently to return to school and to continue to learn, or that he can now sit down with his mother and they can both enjoy a meal together. The school experience will, it is hoped, lead the youngster to feel more competent and hence in charge of his life. The meal with mother possibly permits him to see his mother again as a person to have fun with rather than as an ever-scolding and admonishing nuisance.

Thus drugs in children must never be used *instead of* other care but always as an addition to care based on human relationships.

When prescribing any kind of psychopharmacological agent to children, the following additional factors should be considered:

1. Children tend to respond with more individual variation to an identical milligram per kilogram dose of medication. In general, they are less sensitive to drugs than are adults and require larger doses per kilogram of weight.
2. A number of investigators have shown that children above the age of ten react qualitatively differently to psychiatric drugs than younger children do. Thus amphetamines and their derivatives may suddenly stimulate rather than calm children, while an identical dose of a phenothiazine may slow down psychomotor activity much more dramatically in an older than in a younger child.

Appendix 23-1 THE PHENOTHIAZINES*
These effects are primarily related to adults but do occur in children as well.

Behavioural Effects	*CNS Effects*	*Autonomic Nervous System Effects*	*Metabolic Effects*	*Allergic or Toxic Effects*
1. Excessive drowsiness (less with piperazine, more with Largactil) 2. Mood: depression 3. Toxic psychosis (rare)	1. Effect on the seizure threshold: some (like Largactil) lower the seizure threshold. Others have no effect (e.g. Mellaril) 2. Extra-pyramidal side-effects (most with piperazines none with Mellaril) a. Parkinsonism b. Akathisia, i.e. uncontrolled restlessness c. Dystonia, e.g. tongue spasms, torticollis, twitching, etc.	1. Lowering of blood pressure 2. Tachycardia 3. Dry mouth 4. Constipation 5. Difficulty in voiding 6. Blurred vision	1. Fluid retention 2. Lactating breasts 3. Amenorrhoea 4. Delayed or absent ejaculation (Mellaril) 5. Impotence (rare)	1. *Agranulocytosis* Very rare. More common in women over 40 years. (Described only for Largactil, Sparine, Pacatal, Vesprin) 2. *Jaundice* Incidence seems to be decreasing. Is fairly rare, about 0.5%. Usually occurs in first few weeks of treatment. Is an obstructive type of jaundice, characterised by biliary stasis (seen by raised alkaline, phosphatase). It begins with grippe-like symptoms followed by jaundice and tender, enlarged liver. It is reversible 3. *Photosensitivity* Similar to bad sunburn of exposed parts. Skin is very itchy. This is common in children especially with Largactil 4. Anemias, purpura, serum sickness have been reported but are very rare.

* Source: Hollister, *New England Journal of Medicine*. Vol. 264, No. 6. Feb. 9, 1961. Vol. 264, No. 7. Feb. 16, 1961.

1. MAJOR TRANQUILLIZERS

These drugs include all the phenothiazine derivatives and on the basis of their chemical structure (see Appendix 23-2) may be divided into three groups.

a) The chlorpromazine model group, which has a three-carbon straight side chain. Examples: Largactil, Sparine.
b) The piperazine group characterized by a piperazine ring in the side chain. Examples: Trilafon, Stelazine, Stemetil.

c) The piperidine group with a piperidine ring in the side chain. Example: Mellaril.

All of these drugs reduce general psychomotor agitation and have an antipsychotic effect. Some members of the piperazine group are also anti-emetics and the groups differ from each other in their specific side-effects (see Appendix 23-1). Consequently phenothiazines work best in conditions associated with psychomotor agitation, brain damage, and general loss of behavioural integration. The more evidence of organic damage the child shows the better will the response to phenothiazines be. In practice, this implies that autistic or young schizophrenic children benefit far more from a phenothiazine if they are also organically impaired, that is, if they have no speech at five or six years of age or show other gross neurological deficits, than if their problem is mainly in relating to other people. This effect on brain-damaged children naturally does not mean that the basic intellectual limitations in mental deficiency or the underlying pathological lesions in a chronic brain syndrome can be modified by phenothiazines. It does mean, however, that some of the disturbing symptoms associated with these conditions, such as the constant rocking or head-banging of very retarded children, which often leads to self-injury, or the hyperkinesis and distractability shown by such children, can be relieved by these compounds.

Behaviour disorders and psychiatric conditions highlighted by fear or general withdrawal such as phobias or extreme shyness normally do not respond to major tranquillizers.

The question of which phenothiazine to give to a particular child is difficult to answer. In general chlorpromazine seems the compound of choice because of its wide margin of safety and the decreased incidence of extra-pyramidal manifestations. Furthermore, chlorpromazine costs less than many other phenothiazines and has stood up against all rival compounds in its general efficacy.

Side-effects. See Appendix 23–1

Recommended dosage

Generic name	Trade name	Daily dose
Chlorpromazine	Largactil	25–300 mg
Perphenazine	Trilafon	2–30 mg
Trifluoperazine	Stelazine	1–20 mg
Thioridazine	Mellaril	25–400 mg

2. ANTI-DEPRESSANTS

Depression in childhood is a somewhat elusive condition as mood swings in children are often reflections of the present environment and hence are easier to change by environmental manipulation than through any medication. Thus anti-depressants should not be prescribed in children for psychiatric reasons.

Tofranil and Elavil are useful anti-enuretics, however, eliminating or at least reducing enuresis in about 60 per cent of all school-age bed-wetters. Enuretic children under the age of six normally do not benefit from these compounds. They are also far less effective in children who have been dry for some years and begun to wet again than in those who have never had total sphincter control. This is possibly related to the cause of intermittent enuresis, which is generally thought to be psychological, whereas continuous wetting is now felt to be related to delayed neuronal maturation. Anti-depressants are also quite ineffectual in children who wet both at night and during the day.

Recommended dosage

Generic name	*Trade name*	*Daily dose*
Imipramine	Tofranil	25 mg at bedtime for children aged 6 to 9. 50 mg at bedtime for children 10 and above.
Amitriptyline	Elavil	as above

Side-effects

These are important because anti-depressants are common adult drugs to which small children may have access, and fatal cases of poisoning have been recorded. Death is thought to be due to profound hypotension or central nervous system depression. Imipramine and Amitriptyline must never be given in combination with mono-amine-oxidase inhibitors, especially Parnate, as deaths in convulsion have been recorded. Overdosage of Parnate (amine-oxidase inhibitor) causes a peculiar reversible picture of decerebrate rigidity.

3. MINOR TRANQUILLIZERS

This group of compounds is frequently advertised as the therapeutic agent of choice for severe anxiety, aggression, and a host of other psychiatric symptoms in adults. The most commonly used minor tranquillizers are diazepam (Valium) and chlorodiazopexide (Librium). There are a variety of others on the market whose chemical structure varies only in details from these two basic compounds. Despite the immense popularity of these agents in adults, none of them has shown any consistent usefulness in a paediatric population. On the contrary, they have led to psychological upheavals in individuals and families. Hence these drugs should not be prescribed routinely in children for any psychiatric indication.

Side-effects

a) drowsiness (requiring reduction of dose)
b) dizziness
c) dysarthria (after excessive amounts)
d) some skin reactions
e) habituation (with withdrawal symptoms resembling those of barbiturate withdrawal reactions)

4. STIMULANTS

Stimulants such as dextroamphetamine (Dexedrine) and methylphenidate (Ritalin) have been hailed as a major breakthrough in the treatment of children with hyperactivity and various types of behaviour disorders. Here, more than in most other areas of child psychiatry, however, the difficulties and ambiguities of our inexact classification have made it difficult to achieve a precise definition of drug efficacy.

Confusion as to the specific meaning of terms such as "hyperkinesis", "minimal brain dysfunction", "hyperactivity", or "learning disorder" make it difficult to evaluate and compare the work of individual investigators and to state principal assumptions which are acceptable to the majority of concerned psychiatrists.

Briefly, hyperactive or hyperkinetic children show an increase in aimless activity, coupled with difficulties in concentration. They are impulsive in their general behaviour and learning, and consequently often develop conflicts with peers. They are not retarded, do not as a rule present specific learning deficits, and may or may not show signs associated with minimal brain damage (e.g. poor balancing or hopping, inferior finger-nose test, poor recognition of numbers traced on the forearm). It is these children who respond best to stimulant medication. The drugs will generally decrease hyperactivity and distractibility and improve attention in these children. Medication will not dramatically alter general learning and the children will continue to be difficult to live with. In fact, one very recent study, which followed hyperactive children who had received no medication for five years and compared them with a group who had received stimulants for the same length of time, found no difference between the groups in the amount of activity or distractibility displayed or in their academic, personal, or social functioning.[12]

Restlessness, a poor school record, and difficulties in relationships are also symptoms often found in children labelled as having a behaviour disorder. Stimulant drugs are usually less effective here, but have nevertheless been increasingly prescribed by psychiatrists and paediatricians alike. This has often led to neglect of the interpersonal aspect of drug treatment such as the counselling of parents or development of a comprehensive remedial program involving teachers and other paramedical personnel for hyperactive children, or the more psychotherapeutic approaches used in children with behaviour disorders. The results of such a "drug only" approach are necessarily less satisfactory and have led to much debate both in and outside the medical profession about the alleged mass-drugging of children.

Of the two main stimulant drugs dextroamphetamine (Dexedrine) and methylphenidate (Ritalin), the latter is less toxic and at present the drug of choice for children presenting with the classical syndrome of hyperactivity.

Guidelines of Administration and Side-Effects

Ritalin is generally useless for the treatment of children younger than five years. Such children often show intensive side-reactions, especially sadness and a zombie-like behaviour, which usually is more disconcerting to parents than the hyperactivity and behaviour disorder.

Ritalin, if at all possible, must always be given in the minimum possible dose and should be discontinued on weekends and during school holidays. These breaks prevent the building up of a drug tolerance in the child and prove to the parents that physicians do not simply want to drug their youngster.

Side-effects of the drug are common (30 per cent) but of varying significance. The most frequent side-effect is loss of appetite. This can often be dealt with by giving the child in question a good breakfast and a heavy snack at bedtime. Generally children on stimulants should eat whenever they want to, and experience has indicated that one is justified in keeping up the Ritalin dosage as long as no real weight loss occurs. Some children also make up for lost calories during the weekend. If actual weight loss occurs, a decrease of the dose will usually take care of it.

Another common problem is the apparent increase in activity after 4.00 p.m. and the loss of sleep or delayed bedtime of children. This is not a side-effect but is related to the short-term effectiveness of the medication and the resurgence of general activity after the immediate effect has worn off. When this pattern develops we have found it best to split the lunch dose and give another dose at 5.00 or 6.00 p.m. This usually calms the child until he is asleep. We thus give 20 mg (or 2 pills) after breakfast and 10 mg (or 1 pill) after lunch and supper.

Rare side-effects are an increase in activity, serious itching, or the belief that small animals crawl under the skin. These conditions require immediate discontinuation of the medication.

Some investigators have recently documented a slowing down of physical growth in children who have been on stimulants for a number of years. These findings have neither been confirmed or refuted at present. It seems nevertheless indicated at present to stop all stimulant drugs in children who approach their adolescent growth-spurt until more detailed data have been collected.

Dosage schedule (each tablet contains 10 mg of methylphenidate)
Day 1. Begin with half a tablet after breakfast
Day 2. 1 tablet after breakfast
Day 3. 1 tablet after breakfast, and half after lunch
Day 4. 1 tablet after breakfast and 1 after lunch
Day 5. 1 and a half tablets after breakfast, and 1 after lunch
Day 6. 2 tablets after breakfast, 1 after lunch
Day 7. 2 tablets after breakfast, 1 and a half after lunch
Day 8. 2 tablets after breakfast, 2 after lunch

It is recommended that the parents be telephoned on days 2, 4, and 7 to see how things are going and that the child be seen again after he has been on the medication for ten days. The drug is not discontinued on weekends during the build-up period, and a report from the child's school four weeks after treatment has been begun is advised.

If the parents report an optimal response after four days of increment, there is naturally no need to increase the dose any further. After each holiday, one should try to keep the child off medication and only if the teacher or other adult complains should one continue for another term.

5. OTHER DRUGS

Haloperidol (Haldol) has been found valuable in the treatment of motor hyperactivity, particularly where biological factors play a large part in the child's hyperkinesis. The drug has also been used for tics, including the Gilles de la Tourette syndrome.* The commonly recommended dosage of haloperidol in children is 0.05 to 0.1 mg per kilogram body-weight in twenty-four hours. The drug is usually given in two divided doses. The build-up of blood level and effect occurs over several days. With doses over about 0.07 mg per kilogram per twenty-four hours, the simultaneous administration of an anti-Parkinsonian drug is advisable. The drug can be given to children from the age of two years on.

Barbiturates are generally considered of little value in the practice of child psychiatry. They do not usually improve restlessness and are not suitable as sedatives.

Meprobamate (Equanil) and diphenhydramine (Benadryl) are still used by some physicians in doses of 400 to 1200 mg (Equanil), and 20 to 150 mg per day (Benadryl), but as their therapeutic value is limited and side-effects can be serious (deaths on Equanil have been recorded) they are not recommended for use in children.

General Principles of Drug Treatment

1. Drugs can be useful agents in managing child psychiatric disorders when chosen appropriately and applied with discrimination.
2. Skill in using drugs requires knowledge of their pharmacological properties and sensitivity to their psychological significance.
3. An old drug is to be preferred to a new drug unless there is good evidence that the new one is superior.
4. Duration of drug use should be as brief as possible.
5. Dosages must be individualized.
6. The use of drugs does not relieve the physician of the responsibility for attempting to identify and eliminate factors which cause the psychological disorder in a particular child.

*The Gilles de la Tourette syndrome is a form of tic, marked by motor incoordination with explosive outbursts of profanity and vulgarity (coprolalia).

Appendix 23-2 Types of Drugs

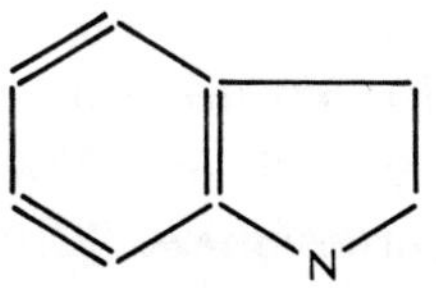

Indol nucleus, present in
Serotin, LSD and Reserpine

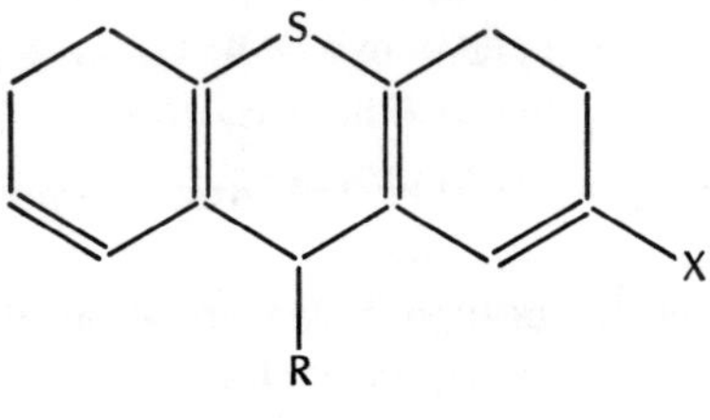

Phenothiazine basic formula
as in Chlorpromazine

Distinguish between

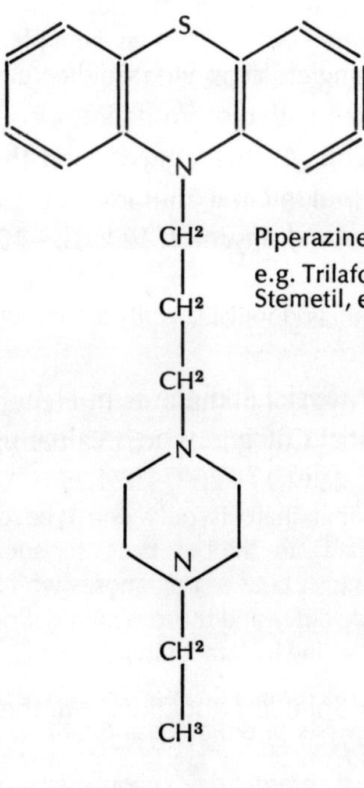

Piperazine group
e.g. Trilafon,
Stemetil, etc.

Piperidine
cl group
e.g.
Thioridazine

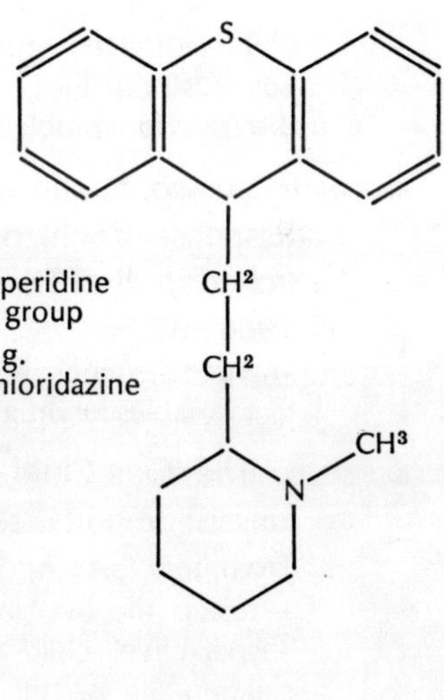

RECOMMENDED FOR FURTHER READING

1. BARKER, P., and FRASER, I.A. "A Controlled Trial of Haloperidol in Children". *Brit. J. Psychiat.* 114: 855–57, 1968.
—a good study demonstrating the efficacy of haloperidol in reducing specific target symptoms.

2. CONNELL, P.H.; CORBETT, J.A.; HORNE, D.J.; and MATTHEWS, A.M. "Drug Treatment of Adolescent Tiqueurs: A Double-Blind Trial of Diazepam and Haloperidol". *Brit. J. Psychiat.* 113: 375–81, 1967.

3. DAVIS, K.V.; SPRAGUE, R.L.; and WERRY, J.S. "Stereotyped Behavior and Activity Level in Severe Retardates: The Effect of Drugs". *Amer. J. Ment. Def.* 73: 721–27, 1968–69.
—discusses ways in which drugs can be used to decrease behaviour that complicates management of the severely retarded.

4. EISENBERG, L. "Principles of Drug Therapy in Child Psychiatry with Special Reference to Stimulant Drugs". *Amer. J. Orthopsychiat.* 41: 371–79, 1971.
—notes that drugs can be useful to the healthy development of children if given appropriately, as a part of the total treatment plan. Suggests principles for the use of stimulant drugs with children and discusses four problem areas.

6. FISH, B.; SHAPIRO, T.; and CAMPBELL, M. "Long-Term Prognosis and the Response of Schizophrenic Children to Drug Therapy: A Controlled Study of Trifluoperazine". *Am. J. Psychiat.* 123: 32–39, 1966–67.
—a good example how dose variation and initial severity are important variables for drug studies.

8. FISH, B. "The 'One Child, One Drug' Myth of Stimulants in Hyperkinesis: Importance of Diagnostic Categories in Evaluating Treatment". *Arch. Gen. Psychiat.* 25: 193–203, 1971.
—rejects the oversimplified myth that there is only one type of "hyperactive" child and that stimulants are the best drugs for such children. Stresses the need to distinguish between diagnoses which define the type of total personality disorder and those which define major developmental symptoms (including hyperactivity).

9. FREEMAN, R.D. "Review of Medicine in Special Education: Another Look at Drugs and Behaviour". *J. Spec. Educ.* 4: 377–84, 1970.
—an excellent short summary of present-day knowledge of psychopharmacological treatment in children.

10. GRINSPOON, L., and SINGER, S.B. "Amphetamines in the Treatment of Hyperkinetic Children". *Harvard Educational Review* 43: 515–55, 1973.
—reviews research and conflicting findings on the effects of amphetamines on hyperactive children. Urges reconsideration of amphetamine administration policy in our schools today because of their unknown long-term risks and possible adverse effects.

11. MINDE, K. *A Parents' Guide to Hyperactivity in Children.* Quebec Association for Children with Learning Disabilities, Montreal, P.Q., 1971
—a booklet which explains the syndrome and the management of such children to parents. Easy reading. Available through the Association at: Suite 8, 4820 Van Horne Ave., Montreal H3W 1J3 ($1.00).

12. MINDE, K.; WEISS, G.; and MANDELSON, N. "A Five-Year Follow-Up Study of Ninety-One Hyperactive School Children". *J. Amer. Acad. Child Psychiat.* 11, 3: 595–610, 1972.
—gives latest results of the outcome of various drugs regimes in hyperactive children.

13. POUSSAINT, A.F., and DITMAN, K.S. "A Controlled Study of Imipramine (Tofranil) in the Treatment of Childhood Enuresis". *J. Pediat.* 67: 283–90, 1965.
—the classical study proving the efficacy of Tofranil in enuresis.

14. SHAPIRO, A.K., and SHAPIRO, E. "Treatment of Gilles de la Tourette Syndrome with Haloperidol". *Brit. J. Psychiat.* 114: 345–50, 1968.
—three cases of the syndrome were treated successfully with haloperidol.

15. SPRAGUE, R. L., and SLEATOR, E. K. "Effects of Psychopharmacological Agents in Learning Disabilities". *Ped. Clin. Nth. Amer.* 20: 719–36, 1973.
—the recent summary of findings in various drug studies.

16. TISCHLER, B.· PATRIASZ, K; BERESFORD, J.; and BUNTING, R. "Experience with Pericyazine in Profoundly and Severely Retarded Children". *Canad. Med. Assoc. J.* 106: 136–41, 1972.
—good article showing the efficacy of high doses of Neuleptil in the behaviour control of retarded children.

17. WEISS, G.; KRUGER, E.; DANIELSON, E.; and ELMAN, M. "Effect of Long-Term Treatment of Hyperactive Children with Methylphenidate". *Canad. Med. Assoc. J.* 112: 159–65, 1975.

—this study presents the behavioural and cognitive outcome of hyperactive children who were treated with medication in comparison with an untreated group.

18. ZRULL, J. P.; WESTMAN, J. C.; ARTHUR, B.; and RICE, D. L. "An Evaluation of Methodology Used in the Study of Psychoactive Drugs for Children". *J. Amer. Acad. Child Psychiat.* 5: 284–91, 1966.
—shows an extremely low agreement between various team partners such as teachers, parents, psychiatrists, and psychologists in noting drug induced changes in children.

ADDITIONAL READING

5. FISH, B., and SHAPIRO, T. "A Typology of Children's Psychiatric Disorders. 1: Its Application to a Controlled Evaluation of Treatment". *J. Amer. Acad. Child Psychiat.* 4: 32–52, 1965.

7. FISH, B. "Drug Use in Psychiatric Disorders of Children". *Amer. J. Psychiat.* 124–1: 31–36, 1967–68.

QUENTIN RAE-GRANT

24. The Primary Care and Referral of Children with Emotional and Behavioural Disorders

Parents and others responsible for children with emotional or behavioural difficulties have available to them a number of channels, formal and informal, through which they may seek help for their children or themselves. Generally they turn first to other family members or to close friends, seeking either confirmation of their worries or reassurance that there is nothing basically wrong and no cause for concern. When convinced that some help is needed, they may then turn to a trusted individual such as their clergyman, family practitioner, or paediatrician. Because these individuals already know the family and have an ongoing rapport with them, they are in many ways more able to establish quickly a working relationship that can be used to help solve the problems. However, because of the social aspect of the relationship the family has with the person to whom they turn for help, they may withhold certain very personal and emotionally charged but rather important information out of a sense of reticence or embarrassment. Thus the personal relationship, while facilitating the early contacts, may impede the investigation and examination of more intimate areas.

The majority of behavioural problems and emotional disorders are, and will continue to be, dealt with by resources other than specific mental-health facilities. If academic or behavioural problems in school have alerted the parents, they may turn to the teacher, the principal, the guidance counsellor, or the school psychologist for help. If the child is behaving antisocially in the community, the police and the courts may be the first to intervene. Should physical symptoms cause concern, the family doctor, a paediatrician, a public-health nurse, or an out-patient clinic may be consulted; a substantial proportion of general and paediatric practice involves problems that are purely emotional and developmental or that occur in conjunction with, or as the consequence of, a physical illness of a family member. If abandonment, neglect, or abuse are or have been suspected, a children's aid society or child welfare association is likely to intervene. Concerns about the development of a younger child may first be discussed with the staff of a day-care centre or nursery school, while an adolescent may refer himself by "rapping" with the staff of a drop-in centre or a free clinic.

Thus a variety of professionals working in a variety of settings may be selected, at times on a random basis, to provide primary, or frontline, care. Since the number of children in need of help is at least ten times the number that can be served by the available mental-health resources, the continuing importance of primary care and the need for primary resources to have available adequate mental-health and psychiatric services for back-up and consultation when required is obvious. This chapter will try to address the questions of general principles of intervention at the primary-care level, when to refer and what to expect on referral.

Evaluation of the Problem

Symptoms of emotional disorder are really only signals of underlying distress. They indicate an imbalance between internal and external forces to which, at times, they may provide a partial solution. Most symptoms occur in a transient form in normal children in the course of development, particularly in times of internal change (e.g. adolescence) or external change (e.g. leaving home to go to school or in response to illness or death of a family member) (See Chapter 5). In fact, if one compares the "symptoms" in a normal population with those in a clinic caseload, the difference lies not in the presence or absence of symptoms but in the number, the degree, the intensity, and the duration of the symptoms in those identified as needing help.

The first question to decide, then, is whether symptoms are normal and age-appropriate and, therefore, likely to disappear in time. Secondly, one must clarify the kind of response that these symptoms are evoking from the environment, as even a "normal" symptom that elicits an overreaction of concern or hostility may become a fixed and more enduring pattern. Thus the longer the duration and the greater the inability of the environment to cope with the child's symptoms, the stronger the indication for intervention. Should one be dealing with more than the normal developmental difficulties, the more immediate the identification of the underlying problem, the more likely intervention will be successful and the more quickly it will prove effective.

Like all interventions and treatments, appropriate help in this area requires a comprehensive history and examination of the situation. (For a more extensive discussion of issues and problems related to assessment, see Chapter 4.) One must have a working understanding of how each family member functions as an individual, a knowledge of how members relate to and influence one another, and some idea of their potential strengths as well as their areas of difficulty. One may begin by tracing developmentally the appearance of the behaviour, who first identified it as a matter of concern, the various opinions expressed about it, those things that have been tried, and the degree of success. Simultaneously, one can explore the interest of the family and of the child in working towards change, given the time and energy that this requires. The family that does not recognize the behaviour as a problem and comes only because someone else had identified it as one, or the parents who do not see that they have had any part in its origin and feel that they can do nothing to effect change, are unlikely to understand at that time the need for their involvement or to be motivated to take part in any remedial program to the extent necessary for its success. At the other end of the scale is the family that assumes some responsibility for the production of the difficulties, is willing to work, and motivated to change.

Primary-Care Interventions

Any request for help represents an opportunity for intervention. The greater the anxiety level of the family—that is, the closer the family appears to be approaching a state of crisis—the more receptive the family may be to a relatively brief intervention (see Chapter 15). It is often to those providing primary care rather than to a mental-health facility that the family will turn at such a time. Generally, the avenues available for intervention include the following:

1. *Review*. Frequently, the taking of a fairly complete individual and family history may in itself have important therapeutic effects. In the process of stock-taking and with the help of the interviewer, certain

issues and actions may become very clear, and the stage is then set for change.

2. *Environmental manipulation* still has a respected place, provided one can clearly demonstrate the relationship between the component in the environment to be altered and the behaviour attributed to it, e.g. supporting a request for public housing. Change for the sake of change is rarely effective, and may be contraindicated if it obscures or complicates the problem. Usually environmental manipulation is effective only when all parties agree to its potential value.

3. *Reassurance.* Many parents seek reassurance because of their concern for their child's future and their doubts about their own competence. If, following adequate exploration of the child's behaviour, his general adjustment, and the over-all family situation, one can be sure that reassurance is justified, supplying it may do much to decrease parental anxiety and to provide a more relaxed and healthy environment in which the child can grow. However, premature or false reassurance is *never* justified, as it may dismiss on an invalid basis behaviour that merits more extensive intervention. Although it is often utilized for the convenience of the counsellor or to save time, it rarely does so in the long run. (For further elaboration and examples, see discussion of Reassurance in Chapter 15.)

4. *Counselling** is a two-way process of helping individuals and families define problems in relationships, recognize what they are doing to one another, elicit alternatives, and develop new skills for coping. The counsellor cannot impose his ideas, as they will be rejected unless they coincide with those of the parents. The counsellor does not have all the answers, nor should he allow himself to be placed in the position of having to provide the solutions. Counselling is a joint endeavour—the counsellor guides, but cannot mandate; he may suggest, he may have to repeat, and he must always be prepared to revise the direction of his advice. The counsellor commits himself to work with people as they struggle, effectively or not so effectively, with their problems. From the beginning, his position contains a number of potential pitfalls.

Although people come expressing a desire for help, they may

*The term "counsellor" will be used generically to describe anyone providing the services defined herein. There is obvious overlap with certain forms of psychotherapy, casework, and much that goes on within the doctor-patient relationship.

also bring an underlying fear of criticism and a sense of failure, since they themselves have not been able to solve the problem. Seeking help confirms this sense of inadequacy, and so may be combined with a covert hope that perhaps the counsellor, too, will fail since in so far as he is helpful, his success can be taken as proof of the client's inadequacy.

The process of counselling is not a popularity contest. The counsellor will not be able to please all people at all times. If counselling is to be effective, it may in fact require pointing out very directly issues that will arouse antagonism and, at times, invite very open hostility. Counselling is a therapeutic alliance. It goes through phases. The counsellor may be placed on a pedestal of knowledge and acumen on one occasion. On another he may be roundly lambasted for not being helpful or for raising unpleasant topics. Both reactions are distortions of the reality. Indeed the examination of how and why the counsellor is being placed in these positions plays an important part in understanding the dynamics of the situation. The counsellor is perceived and dealt with in ways that recapitulate and reflect other key relationships from the present or the past. The process of help involves recognizing these distortions as projections and examining their origins.

> The first day that Dr. S. walked onto the ward he noticed that Michael, age fourteen, was carefully watching him and constantly keeping him at a distance. Later he learned that Michael, who had been through fourteen foster homes, was mistrustful and hostile to all adults. Dr. S. worked intensively with Michael for over a year. He had forgotten the circumstances of their initial meeting until one day Michael, who had become rather friendly, commented that when Dr. S. had first walked onto the ward, "I just took one look at you and your face was so mean, I just knew you were a son of a bitch." When Dr. S. asked how he looked now, Michael laughed and replied, "You look OK. I didn't even know you then. I just figured you'd be mean, because you were a grown-up". Clearly Michael was projecting onto Dr. S. feelings derived from past relationships with adults. From that time on, much of Michael's therapy consisted of demonstrating ways in which his distorted perceptions and hostile behaviour in response to them interfered with his relationships and provoked others to punish and reject him.

Only when the consellor has been able to remain neutral and objective, neither flattered by the plaudits nor devastated by the antagonism, can he make the projective nature of these feelings clear as they occur.

Counselling implies maintaining a position of neutrality, particularly in situations involving conflict between two sides that see the same issue from very different vantage points. Each competes for the counsellor as an ally, inviting him to confirm that its opinions are correct, axiomatically therefore denying the validity of others' views. Once the counsellor loses his objectivity, he loses his credibility and usefulness and becomes co-opted into the ongoing struggle. It is particularly dangerous to reach conclusions and act on them having heard only one side of an issue. In cases involving child custody, for example, the picture given of one parent by the other may be factually correct but emotionally distorted. The same is true where adolescents and parents are in conflict. To become the ally of one side, and therefore the antagonist of the other, is an invitation frequently extended and rarely justified. One should recognize that the child's or adolescent's description of the parents is his perception of them rather than an accurate presentation of the parents as they are or behave.

The counsellor need not work in isolation. There are many helping agencies available for families—the school, social agencies, recreation services—and simultaneous involvement of the family and child with these agencies may facilitate what the counsellor can do individually. Effective collaboration with these agencies with the range of skills and services that they can provide has the advantage of sharing the burden, particularly in dealing with multi-problem families. This ensures that at the appropriate time for termination of counselling, ongoing help of a continuing nature will remain available.

Senn and Solnit[8] have listed a number of common errors in case management. They include: (1) the problems of the hurried interview that does not allow time to deal in depth with family and personal issues; (2) the failure to determine where the problem lies; (3) the temptation towards a too rapid and inaccurate interpretation of data that selects the most obvious and deals with it as if it were the most significant. As most disorders in this area arise from multiple factors, too narrow a view of the origin of the disorder restricts the chance of arriving at a constructive solution. At all times, intervention and exploration should proceed using practical terms that apply to the particular situation under discussion. Theoretical explanations may help the therapist, but given in the course of counselling, they invite intellectualization and rationalization that undermine the family's attempt to derive appropriate solutions acceptable to and likely to be implemented by them.

Referral

When one has been counselling a case over a period of time, it may be difficult to consider referral and natural to view it as a reflection on one's own capacity. Yet the good counsellor is one who has learned to understand and accept the limits of what he personally can do. Not all people are able to deal with all issues with the same equanimity and effectiveness. To recognize that one works better with certain conditions and not as well with others is an indication of maturity and skill as a counsellor. Referral can be both helpful and necessary, but it can also be used in a punitive way. The counsellor's discomfort may lead to its being done in an abrupt, curt, and mechanical fashion that decreases the likelihood of its being followed through. If presented with annoyance, it is likely to be interpreted as a punishment for failure to improve despite the best help that the counsellor could provide. Implicit in the process of successful referral is the preparation of people for disengagement from present attachments and that of helping them get ready to pick up with others who bring different skills. Since often the referral is made as much for the counsellor's purpose as for the client's, it is important to give attention to how the issue is raised and to what it means for those to whom it is suggested. They should have an opportunity to work through their concerns and should terminate feeling free to return when and if this seems appropriate.

Reason for Referral

The patient, client, or family should be referred to more specific mental-health and psychiatric resources in the following situations:

1. When the endeavours of the counsellor or practitioner do not seem to be helping or where a plateau at which no further improvement is occurring seems to have been reached.
2. When a major diagnostic question arises on which the counsellor wishes either a more specialized opinion or further investigation, for example, differentiation of severe neurosis from psychosis, brain damage, or retardation.

3. When the counsellor is faced with certain crisis situations that the family cannot control or tolerate even with his help, such as serious suicidal attempts or threats or massive and continuing misbehaviour. Non-responsive cases of anorexia nervosa and other psychosomatic disorders are also best referred to settings where the physical and emotional components can receive attention simultaneously (see Chapter 9).
4. When the counsellor's own sense of discomfort about what he is dealing with or what he is doing begins to mount, he is wise to seek further advice on the management of the case. Too often these feelings are partially recognized by the practitioner but ignored so that action is delayed. In general, it is better to err on the side of referral than to delay until a crisis forces one's hand.

Referrals can only be recommended; they cannot be forced upon the family or the patient. Without their willing co-operation, the referral is not likely to be helpful. Their co-operation will have to be solicited, and child and family may need to discuss the referral over a period of time before they are able to accept it for what it is, namely, a move in their own interests, suggested and supported by the counsellor. This support may have to continue after the other facility is involved, as the process of transfer is not an easy one, and often the original counsellor has a position of trust, which the new therapist has yet to win. The degree to which a referral may prove helpful is often determined by this process of preparation and the time given to resolving the doubts, answering the questions, and providing the incentive.

The child who is referred should be informed whom he will be seeing, and the reasons for the referral. The more clearly he understands why he is being referred, the more likely he is to benefit from the referral. Often parents are anxious about seeking help from a psychiatrist, and may communicate this anxiety to the child. There is often realistic concern about how the peer group will react if it becomes known. Adolescents in particular may feel apprehension about having to see a psychiatrist, and frequently the resolution of this initial anxiety is the essential first phase of therapeutic work.

The practitioner also has a part to play in paving the way for people getting to a referral source. Usually a mental-health or psychiatric facility appreciates knowing from the referring person the reasons for the referral, something of the background of the family and the problem, what has gone on already, and, in particular, whether or not the practitioner wishes to remain involved in the situation (that is, is this a request for consultation?) or is expecting the psychiatrist or mental-health centre to pick up the treatment. A message via nurse or secretary often leaves many of these questions unanswered, leading to later misunderstanding. Most mental-health facilities like direct contact either by telephone or letter so that they can relate what they do to the specific concerns, being sure to what extent the referring individual is asking for an opinion, advice, collaboration, or the assumption of direct treatment. The most successful referrals generally occur when the two people or agencies involved know each other, have previously worked together on cases, and have developed a sense of trust in each other's competence.

Many mental-health facilities, following such a discussion, will ask that a member of the family phone and set up the initial appointment. This is partly to have the family involved in making the contact right from the beginning, and partly out of the knowledge that the family that lacks the motivation to follow through on a suggested referral is not yet sufficiently prepared to benefit from it.

In referring a case either to a colleague in private practice or to a multidisciplinary setting, what can the referring practitioner or counsellor reasonably expect? At the very least, he can legitimately demand a knowledge of the impressions of each of the disciplines represented in the team and the diagnostic conclusions and treatment recommendations of the team as a whole. He can expect to be kept up to date with the progress of the case and to be invited to participate as a member of the team, at least in the diagnostic and follow-up phases.

Mental-Health Professional Roles

In the heyday of the child-guidance clinics, the roles of the psychiatrist, psychologist, and social worker had an artificial distinction and clarity. The *psychiatrist* was the physician on the team. He physically examined and psychiatrically assessed the child. He also provided the medical component of treatment including psychotherapy and medication, if indicated, for the identified patient. The *psychologist,* though also at times serving as a child therapist, primarily contributed during the assessment, defining the child's intellectual functioning through intelligence tests and assessing emotional development and delineating areas of conflict through projective tests. The *social worker* was responsible mainly for taking a history from the parents, for obtaining information on social functioning, and for providing casework (counselling) for the parents. Together these three constituted a *therapeutic team,* working with each other on a collaborative basis as one person treated the child and another the parents. The psychiatrist, as team leader, assumed responsibility for the team's developing and maintaining an integrated approach to treatment.

The picture has changed considerably as the various professionals involved redefine their aspirations and areas of expertise. Psychologists have moved from a heavy reliance on projective testing to more specific testing in the cognitive areas, particularly useful in delineating difficulties in learning. They have also developed to a greater extent than most psychiatrists and social workers the techniques of behaviour modification. With the increasing range and effectiveness of psychopharmacological agents and an increased emphasis on the art of consultation, many psychiatrists are less involved in ongoing psychotherapy, which they frequently delegate to other members of the enlarged treatment team. In most hospital-associated facilities the contributions of *occupational therapists,* both diagnostically and therapeutically, have been recognized. A major role is often assigned to *speech pathologists;* and *nurses* with specific training in the mental-health area are frequently involved in providing group and milieu therapy. In this their function may overlap with that of the *child-care worker* (milieu therapist), who often supplements generic training preparing him to provide continuing on-the-spot care for children in residential treatment with additional training in group or family therapy. Thus, roles have become blurred. Each discipline brings its own contributions and complements the areas of expertise of the others. No single discipline has all the answers or all the resources. While there remain cases requiring long-term intervention, the pressure of mounting service demands and changing philosophies and techniques of treatment have led to a shift from the traditional fascination with psychopathology and intrapsychic clarification to an increasing emphasis on functioning and coping capacities and short-term and crisis approaches to treatment. Within the same setting, a similar service may be provided—and provided with a varying degree of skill and sophistication—by a number of professionals from a variety of disciplines.

Mental-health facilities for too long operated in isolation, partly of their own choosing and partly because the community was uncomfortable about approaching them. Since the number of children needing help is at least ten times the number that can be served by the available mental-health resources, primary care will continue to be the cornerstone around which mental-health services for the total community must be built. The mental-health facilities themselves can collaborate with and consult those providing primary care, but the primary-care person will remain the one to whom most of those in need will turn first, as well as the community link on which psychiatric or mental-health facilities depend for effective function. Just as effective therapy depends on the therapeutic alliance, so effective delivery of mental-health services depends on fostering and maintaining this set of interlocking relationships between those providing primary care and those staffing mental-health facilities. Only with such a partnership will we be able to deal successfully with the problems that concern and interfere with the lives of a substantial portion of the population.

RECOMMENDED FOR FURTHER READING

1. BALINT, M. *The Doctor, His Patient, and the Illness.* New York, International Univ. Press, 1957.
—somewhat technical, but clear, highly relevant, and practical. Focuses primarily on doctor-patient relationships. A classic.

2. BERMAN, S. "The Relationship of the Private Practitioner of Child Psychiatry to Prevention." *J. Amer. Acad. Child Psychiat.* 13: 593–603, 1974.
—discusses the contribution of the child psychiatrist in private practice to child mental-health services and the importance of coordinating his/her participation with programs to institutions, mental-health legislation, and mental-health training.

3. HODGE, J. R. *Practical Psychiatry for the Primary Physician.* Chicago, Nelson-Hall, 1975.
—useful for the medical practitioner who needs an understanding of basic psychiatry.

4. Mc CONVILLE, B. J "Child Psychiatry—Services for One Million Children?" *Canad. Psychiat. Assoc. J.* 17: 265–72, 1972.
—critically reviews recent surveys on treatment of emotionally disturbed children and proposes a model of child-care services stressing the role of government, local, and regional services.

5. PORTNOY, S. M.; BILLER, H. B.; and DAVIDS, A. "The Influence of the Child-Care Worker in Residential Treatment". *Amer. J. Orthopsychiat.* 42: 719–22, 1972.

—urges residential centres to make more effective use of child-care workers who are seen as major therapeutic agents.

6. RIEGER, N. I., and DEVRIES, A.G. "The Child Mental Health Specialist: A New Profession". *Amer. J. Orthopsychiat.* 44: 150–58, 1974.
—describes a training program for child mental-health specialists which is recommended as essential for nationwide implementation if adequate preventive and treatment services are ever to be produced.

7. RICHMOND, J. B., and SCHERL, D. J. "Research in the Delivery of Health Services". in Hamburg, D. A., and Brodie, H.K.H., eds., *American Handbook of Psychiatry.* 2nd ed. rev. Vol. 6: 731–55. New York, Basic Books, 1975.
—highly technical review of major issues related to research into the delivery of health services, covering such areas as research design, evaluative indices, and studies and consumer participation.

8. SENN, M., and SOLNIT, A. J. *Problems in Child Behavior and Development.* Philadelphia, Lea and Febiger, 1968.
—a most practical and useful text for paediatricians and practitioners that presents diagnosis and intervention within a developmental framework.

9. STEINHAUER, P. D. "The Contribution of the Child Psychiatrist to the Professional Development of Other Mental Health Professionals", in Steinhauer, P.D., ed., *Training in Child Psychiatry in Canada,* pp. 96–101. Available from Laidlaw Foundation, 203 St. Clair Avenue East,, Toronto, Canada, 1974.
—discusses the contribution that the practicing child psychiatrist can make to a child welfare association or children's aid society through ongoing consultation.

10. STEISEL, I. M. and ADAMSON, W. C. "The Use and Training of Allied Mental Health Workers in Child Guidance Clinics". *J. Amer. Acad. Child Psychiat.* 13: 524–35, 1974
—discusses the importance and various roles of allied mental-health workers in enhancing the delivery of care to children in child guidance clinics.

11. TIZARD. J. "The Upbringing of Other People's Children: Implications of Research and For Research". *J. Child Psychol. Psychiat.* 15: 161–73, 1974.
—discusses the association between the behaviour of children in residence and the formal organizational structure and child-care practices of institutional settings, exploring both theoretical and practical issues related to child development.

Glossary

Aetiology The study of the cause of any disease.
Agnosia Lack or loss of the ability to understand the meaning or to recognize the importance of various types of stimuli, especially in the non-language field.
Amenorrhoea Absence or cessation of menstrual flow.
Anorexia Nervosa A psychiatric syndrome usually occurring in young women. The cardinal features are extreme aversion to food, severe weight loss, and amenorrhoea.
Antiemetic A drug that prevents or alleviates nausea and vomiting.
Antisocial Opposed or antagonistic to social values.
Apperception Conscious realization; the awareness of the significance of what is perceived, especially through relating percepts to similar, already existing knowledge.
Asocial Indifferent to social values.
Autoerotism Spontaneous sexual emotion generated by an individual in the absence of an external stimulus preceding directly from another person. Masturbation is a common form of autoerotic activity.
Autonomic Nervous System The autonomic nervous system, at times called the vegetative nervous system, is that part of the nervous system that regulates those bodily activities that are carried out beyond conscious awareness. The beating of the heart and circulation of the blood, breathing, digestion, and temperature regulation are examples of bodily processes under the control of the autonomic nervous system (see BIOFEEDBACK MECHANISM).

Biofeedback Mechanism Biofeedback is the physiological mechanism whereby an individual can control certain bodily functions such as heart rate, basal metabolic rate, blood pressure, etc., which were until recently thought to be totally under the control of the autonomic system. Since people can be trained to develop a greater degree of control over these autonomic functions, they can thereby achieve concomitant changes in mood such as tranquillity, relaxation, the inducement of a dream-like state, etc.

Cachexia Malnourishment resulting in weight loss, usually from a chronic disease process.
Catatonia (Catatonic Schizophrenia) A form of schizophrenia characterized by extreme negativism, phases of stupor or excitement, impulsive posturing, and stereotyped and highly ritualistic behaviour.
Coeliac Disease A disease of infants and young children in which an inability to digest gluten (in wheat flour) results in impaired absorption of ingested foods with resultant diarrhoea and interference with growth.
Cognition The ability to think and reason.
Colic Spasmotic contractions of smooth muscle or duct. *Infant colic,* often occurring in the first four months of life, refers to recurrent episodes of intestinal colic and the associated pain and irritability.
Congenital Receptive Dysphasia An inherited impairment in the ability to understand speech.
Constitution The relatively constant physiological composition and biological make-up of a person, resulting largely from inherited tendencies but to some extent modified by past environmental experiences whose effects have permanently influenced the individual.

Coprolalia Foul speech; often used to refer to the explosive outbursts of profanity in Gilles de la Tourette disease.
Coprophagia The eating or mouthing of faeces.
Counter-Transference One aspect of the professional's emotional reaction to his patient (client). While at times triggered by the patient's behaviour or the ongoing interaction between them, counter-transference results from the often unrecognized influence of the vulnerabilities, attitudes, and conflicts derived from the therapist's past life which are still very much operative in the present. For example, a therapist may believe that a child's refusal to co-operate is the source of

his frustration, not realizing that it is really his discomfort with his own inability to control the situation and to be successful in his attempts to help that child that is accounting for his extreme annoyance.

Decerebrate Remove the brain, either surgically or as a result of an injury which severs the nerve pathways connecting brain and spinal cord. In either case, because of the lack of connection, the organism is deprived of the highly complex and sophisticated functions normally controlled by the cerebral cortex (e.g. speech, hearing, vision, thought, voluntary movements, etc.), and so exists at a brainstem level (i.e. with respiration, circulation of the blood, temperature control, digestion, elimination, and some reflex activities remaining but no more).

Decompensation Failure or breakdown in the normally operative defence system leading to a deterioration of the customary level of adjustment.

Denial A defence mechanism which consists of a refusal to admit the truth or unpleasant reality even to oneself.

Developmental Crisis Symptoms of a brief and transient nature related to and arising from periods of temporarily increased anxiety generated by the process of normal development.

Developmental Deviations Those deviations in personality development which may be considered abnormal in that they occur at a time, in a sequence or to a degree not expected for a given age-level or stage of development.

Displacement A defence mechanism in which strong feelings are shifted or transferred from the original ideas or people to whom they were attached. For example, a child with school phobia may not recognize how angry she is at her mother because she has displaced the anger to her teacher, whom she must then avoid.

Dizygotic Derived from two separate fertilized ova, for example fraternal (as opposed to identical) twins.

Dysarthria Imperfect articulation of speech.

Dysgraphia A disturbance in handwriting, originating from a dysfunction affecting those areas of the brain which govern the act of writing.

Dyslexia Disturbance in learning to read, due to dysfunction or a lesion affecting those areas of the brain governing the act of reading.

Dysphasia Impairment of speech due to a lesion in the dominant hemisphere of the cerebral cortex. This results in a lack of co-ordination and an inability to combine words for effective speech.

Echolalia The meaningless repetition of words or phrases.

Ego In psychoanalytic psychology, the ego is that part of the psyche that mediates between the basic biological drives of the person (the id) and the demands of reality (the socializing forces) in family and community. Its prime function is the perception of reality and the adaptation to it. Its various tasks include: perception, including self-perception and self-awareness; motor control (action); adaption to reality; memory; thinking; feeling; judgment, and the controlled response to anxiety to ensure safety and self-preservation; a general synthetic or organizing function manifested in the assimilation of external and internal experiences; creativity.

Electroencephalogram (EEG) The tracing obtained by recording via electrodes the electrical currents developed in the brain. Commonly used to diagnose and/or localize malfunctioning of the brain.

Enuresis The involuntary discharge of urine. The term "nocturnal enuresis" is synonymous with bed-wetting. "Diurnal enuresis" refers to involuntary wetting during the day.

Epigenetic A theory which holds that development proceeds in an orderly, step-like manner through a series of stages, each of which represents a higher level of function than its predecessors.

Esotropia Deviation of a visual axis towards that of the other eye when fusion is a possibility, as in crossed-eyes or squint.

Extrapyramidal Tract Those nerve tracts whose main action is concerned with automatic movements involved in postural adjustments and with autonomic regulation. Disorders of the extrapyramidal system may occur either from damage to the nervous system (e.g. cerebral palsy) or as a side effect of certain medications (e.g. phenothiazines).

Febrile Having a fever.

Fetish A part of the body or some object associated with a loved person that replaces and substitutes for the loved person. Although sexual activity with the loved person may occur, gratification is possible only in the presence of the fetish or, at least, if it is fantasied during such activity. Typically, the fetishist can obtain sexual gratification from the fetish alone, in the absence of the person for whom it substitutes.

Fugue State A condition in which the patient suddenly leaves his previous activity and begins to wander or goes on a journey which has no apparent relation to what he has been doing and for which he has amnesia afterwards. Fugues may occur in association with epilepsy (twilight state), as a form of catatonic excitement, or as a form of conversion hysteria (dissociative reaction).

Genotype The genetic inheritance; the sum total of the physical and psychological characteristics carried in the chromosomes.

Gestalt The total quality of the image perceived (i.e. the over-all perceptual experience) is more than just the sum of the various stimuli presented. Rather the total response is a pattern (i.e. a gestalt) which differs from the original stimulus in that it is organized and modified by the past experience and integrative mechanisms of the individual exposed to the perception. For example, someone who becomes violently ill whenever he tastes seafood will have a very different response to a broiled lobster than will someone for whom lobster is a favourite food, although what is seen and smelled is the same.

Growth Increase in size and weight, resulting from an increase in the number and size of the cells.

Guilt A feeling of regret or self-recrimination for having done a wrong (or unworthy or evil) thing, experienced by a person who has a basic feeling of self-worth or self-respect (see also SHAME).

Homeostasis The autonomic tendency of an organism to resist changes in the status quo or equilibrium, thus maintaining the constancy and stability of its environment.

Hyperkinesis Excessive muscular activity; exaggerated motility. Hyperactivity.

Hypertonic Condition characterized by abnormally increased muscular tension, spasticity, or rigidity.

Hypoglycaemia An abnormally low level of glucose (sugar) in the blood.

Hypothalamus The principal centre in the forebrain for integrating visceral functions mediated via the autonomic nervous system. Functions of the hypothalamus include regulation of sexual activity, water, fat and carbohydrate metabolism, and body temperature regulation.

Id One of the three psychoanalytic divisions of the psyche, the other two being the ego and the superego. It represents the basic biological drives or instincts present from birth onwards and constantly demanding discharge.

Intrapsychic Originating or taking place within the psyche. The inner mental processes, thoughts, feelings, and conflicts with which an individual is contending.

Identification The process, largely unconscious, of imitation of parental figures and other role models which serves as the basis for much of the child's conscience development, his gender identity, and his concept of the sort of person he would like to be.

Ideation Clear mental presentation of an object, or concept.

Limbic System Sometimes referred to as the "visceral brain", the limbic system is thought to exert an inhibitory effect on brain-stem mechanisms concerned with emotional expression. Lesions within the limbic system may result in restlessness or hyperactivity.

Latency Frequently referred to as *middle childhood*, latency is that period extending from the end of the infantile period (about age six) to the beginning of adolescence during which the child's attention and energies are centred primarily on socialization and his adjustment to the external world (including school). During this period, intrapsychic development is generally considered relatively quiescent, hence the term latency, as psychoanalysts see the stage as offering a biologically determined breathing space between the psychological conflicts of the preceding Oedipal period and the subsequent physiologically increased stresses and conflicts of preadolescence.

Manic (Mania) A form of mental disorder characterized by an expansive emotional state, elation, hyperirritability, overtalkativeness, pressure of speech and behaviour, and loosened mental associations leading to flight of ideas. Specifically refers to the manic phase of manic-depressive psychosis.

Manneristic Behaviour An individual motor pattern that may have had some personal and idiosyncratic meaning but now appears as repetitive and stereotyped behaviour.

Marasmus Emaciation of extreme degree.

Maturation Change in the developing organism resulting from the combined effects of growth and experience.

Megacolon Extreme dilatation and distension of the large bowel. Two forms are recognized:

a) *Aganglionic megacolon* (Hirschsprung's Disease) resulting from a congenital absence of nerve supply to a segment of the large bowel.
b) *Functional megacolon* in which, despite a normal nerve supply to the bowel, there is faecal retention of psychological origin.

Metabolism The sum of all the physical and chemical processes by which living organisms maintain themselves by building up new living matter and supplying the energy necessary for life.

Metastasize The transfer of diseased cells from one organ or part of the body to another not directly connected with it, as in the spread of cancer through the circulatory or lymphatic system. The diseased deposit is called a metastasis.

Monozygotic Derived from one fertilized ovum, as in identical twins.

Multiproblem Family A family which characteristically demonstrates a variety of long-standing and unresolved psychological, interpersonal, social, and economic problems. The extreme instability and tension existing within such families both favours the development of psychopathology in the children and interferes with the likelihood of the family being successfully involved in ongoing psychotherapy. Because of their characteristic patterns of disorganization in response to repeated crises, they may benefit from the well-timed use of crisis intervention techniques.

Neuropathology The abnormal physiological and biochemical mechanisms in diseases of the nervous system.

Neurophysiology Normal physiology of the nervous system.

Oedipal In psychoanalytic theory, the Oedipal period is that phase of development immediately prior to latency, which is characterized by the child developing a sexual interest in the parents, especially the parent of the opposite sex. Determined partly by the strength of innate biological drives and partly by factors within the family environment, the resolution between these feelings and the guilt and anxiety they arouse continues until the latency period, when the Oedipus complex is normally relinquished in favour of extraparental interests and activities. Failure to resolve successfully the complex, which is rekindled by the physiological upsurge initiated by puberty, is seen by psychoanalysts as the nuclear conflict in psychoneurosis, and a decisive influence in adult sexuality.

Ontogeny A biological term referring to the development of the individual organism as compared with the evolutionary or *phylogenetic* development of the species.

Pan-neurotic The simultaneous presence of all symptoms known in neurotic illness in the same patient. Commonly seen in pseudoneurotic schizophrenia, these neurotic mechanisms dominate the clinical picture, constantly shifting but never disappearing.

Parasympathetic One of the divisions of the autonomic (self-controlling) nervous system, the other being the sympathetic nervous system.

Passive-Aggressive The tendency to express aggressive or hostile feeling passively, for example, by withholding satisfaction, failing to meet or complete expectations or assignments, negativistic or oppositional behaviour. May be masked by a veneer of false conformity, as in the child who never openly defies but constantly forgets, agrees to do what he is told "in a minute", etc.

Pathogenesis The way in which a disease or disorder originates or develops.

Pathognomonic Distinctively typical or characteristic so as to be diagnostic of a particular disease.

Pathophysiology The physiology of the disordered function.

Perinatal Occurring in the period shortly before, during, or after birth.

Phenotype The physical and psychological characteristics of the individual. The phenotype reflects the genetic base which has been modified by exposure to the environment.

Phylogeny The genealogical history and evolutionary development of a species or group as distinguished from the ontogenetic development of the individual.

Placebo Any therapeutic procedure or substance that has an effect on a symptom or disease although it has no specific action on the condition being treated. This effect results not from a specific or pharmacological action but from the patient's expectations. (These will depend on the decrease or increase in anxiety produced by the symbolic meaning of the medication, or by the symbolic implications to the patient of the physician's behaviour and attitudes.) More specifically, a placebo is an inactive substance used in controlled studies to determine the efficacy of a particular medication.

Plantar Pertaining to the sole of the foot. The plantar response is the reflex reaction obtained by stroking the sole of the foot, which is altered in some forms of neurological injury or disease.

Potentiate When the combined action of two factors is greater than the sum of the effects of either used alone, then each is said to potentiate the other.

Premorbid Present before the development of disease, as in "premorbid personality".

Primary Caretaker The one individual, usually the mother, who ministers to the infant's needs on a continuing basis and whom the infant learns to associate with survival and security.

Projection A defence mechanism in which the individual throws outward upon another person disowned ideas or impulses, which are then seen as coming from the other person. When the conflict has thus been externalized, the person may then perceive and handle it as if it had always been external. For example, the child who projects his own anger at parents onto neutral figures, such as a teacher or counsellor, whom he then falsely perceives as being angry at him, is using the mechanism of projection. One who relies excessively on this defence mechanism projects painful feelings wherever possible in to the outer, painful world, thus keeping the inner world of self free of pain.

Psychobiological Dealing with both genetic (biological) and psychodynamic factors affecting personality development and adjustment to the environment.

Psychodynamics The study of mental forces in action. Essentially, a theoretical formulation of how the mind develops and of the intrapsychic adjustments to stress and conflict occurring in the process of adaptation.

Psychogenic Originating within the mind or psyche. A psychogenic illness is due to psychic, mental, or emotional rather than to detectable organic or somatic factors.

Psychomotor Relating to movement that is psychically determined as distinct from that which is clearly organically caused, as in psychomotor epilepsy.

Psychoneurosis That group of disorders not dependent on any evident neurological lesion, in which an emotional conflict which remains unconscious is masked and replaced by symptoms resulting from the excessive use of defence mechanisms. The type of defence mechanism (i.e. the choice of neurosis) depends on the nature of the warded-off impulse, the age of the patient when the decisive conflict was experienced, the nature and intensity of the frustrating factors, the availability of substitute gratifications at the time of the frustration, the constitutional make-up and environmental experience, and, particularly, the specific historical situation which predisposes to certain types of reactions.

Psychopathology Disease or disturbance of the mind, behaviour, or psychic processes.

Psychopharmacology The study and use of drugs to influence emotional states and mental illnesses.

Psychosis The psychoses feature a severe and intense disruption affecting all areas of the patient's life; a pervasive withdrawal from affective relationships with other people and from external, objective reality; distorted and exaggerated emotions that may constitute the whole life of the patient; disturbances of judgment, thinking, and reality testing.

Psychotherapy Any form of treatment for mental illness, behavioural problems or other problems presumed to be of an emotional nature in which a trained person deliberately establishes a professional relationship with a patient or client in order to remove, modify, or retard existing symptoms, to alter disturbing patterns of behaviour, and to promote positive personality growth and development.

Psychotropic A drug having an effect on psychic function, behaviour or experience.

Puberty That period of development marked by physical growth spurt and acquisition of secondary sexual characteristics.

Reaction-Formation A form of defence against urges which are unacceptable to the ego, reaction-formulation consists of the development of conscious, socialized attitudes and interests which are the direct opposite of repressed and unsocialized trends which continue to exist in the unconscious. An example is overprotection as a reaction-formation to unconscious hate or rejection.

Reactive Disorder A response to environmental stress that goes beyond the normal. The term implies that the usual coping mechanisms are no longer working, but that the reason for the symptomatic response is more related to the existence and extent of the external stress than to an internalized neurotic process.

Resistance The largely unconscious process by which patients protect themselves from the pain and anxiety associated with the emergence of repressed (i.e. unconscious) conflicts and feelings into consciousness. Analogous to the guarding of the patient with an acute abdomen, it is almost entirely beyond the patient's conscious control. Frustrated mental-health professionals at times use the term "resistance" as if it were synomymous with avoidance, as, for example, "the child is resisting his appointments", or "he resists talking about his difficulties". To the extent that this implies a conscious decision or that the struggle is primarily interpersonal (i.e. between patient and therapist) rather than intrapsychic (i.e. a largely unrecognized struggle against the emergence of repressed conflict) the term is being used incorr.

Reticular Formation The diffuse system of interlacing fibres and nerve cells forming the central core of the brain stem. Considered part of the "reticular activating system" (RAS), which seems to be essential for the initiation and maintenance of alert wakefulness, for focusing of attention, perceptual association and directed introspection.

Sensorium Consciousness and accuracy with regard to time, place, and person. When a person is clearly aware of the nature of his surroundings his sensorium is described as "clear" or "intact". When a person is disorientated and unclear from a sensory (not a delusional) standpoint, his sensorium is described as impaired or "cloudy".

Serotonin A potent inhibitor of the passage of cerebral nerve impulses, serotonin is normally active in the regulation of centres in the brain concerned with wakefulness, temperature, and blood-pressure regulation, and various other autonomic functions.

Sex-Typing The process of learning to behave and see oneself in the manner described by society to be appropriate to one's biological sex.

Shame The pervasive feeling of being a bad, worthless, unacceptable person, in contrast with *guilt* (q.v.).

Situational Crisis A symptomatic reaction, usually of a transient nature, occurring in response to unusual external stresses (e.g. the loss of a parent or severe marital stress) which temporarily upset psychological equilibrium.

Somatic Relating to the organic tissues of the body. At times, the terms *psyche* and *soma* are employed as if they were opposites rather than inseparable constituents of the total person.

Superego One of the three functional divisions of the psyche as described in psychoanalytic psychology. Largely but not entirely unconscious, it represents the internalization of social values within the psyche (i.e. conscience and morality) as well as the aspirations of the individual (i.e. the ego-ideal).

Trait A predisposition to a particular form of response or behaviour. May be inherited, or may have become part of the personality as a result of repeated experiences.

Tiqueur A person who suffers from tics.

Index

*denotes clinical illustration in the text.